A Manner of Living

An Evidence-Based, Realistic, and Sustainable
Approach to the Art of Eating Well, Living Well, and
Being Well for Life.

GENA E. KADAR, DC, CNS

GVPL Publications
Newport Coast, CA 92657
GVPLpublications@gmail.com

ISBN 978-0-692-26426-3
0692264264

First Edition, 2014

Library of Congress Control Number: 2014920544

The information provided in this book is for educational purposes only. This book is not intended as a substitute for the medical advice of your licensed healthcare professional. This book is not meant to be used, nor should it be used, to diagnose or treat any medical condition. The reader should always consult a licensed healthcare professional in matters relating to his/her health and particularly with respect to any symptoms that may require diagnosis or medical attention. The publisher and author are not responsible for any specific health needs that may require medical supervision and claim no responsibility to any person or entity for any liability, loss, damage, or negative consequences caused or alleged to be caused directly or indirectly as a result of the use, application, or interpretation of the material in the book. References and resources are provided for informational purposes only and do not constitute endorsement of any websites or other sources. Readers should be aware that the websites listed in this book may change.

10 9 8 7 6 5 4 3 2 1

Cover images courtesy of Rod Foster Photography.

DEDICATION

To my father and my mother, thank you.

Table of Contents

Acknowledgments

To my father, the most brilliant, fearless trailblazer, and exceptional person I will ever know. You are my inspiration and my motivation. Everything I do, I do to make you proud. Thank you for showing me what is unconditional love. To my mother who is beauty and kindness personified. Your intelligence, generosity, creativity, strength, friendship, and love inspire me. You are my anchor, and you put wind in my sails. Thank you for being the genuine example of goodness and compassion in my life and for always being there to share laughter and *guess what's*. To my brother whose humble greatness sets the bar for me and whose dependable love and confidence in me is an unwavering source of support, the extent of which never ceases to amaze me. I am so lucky to also call you a best friend. To my grandmother, each time I think of you it fills my heart with love, comfort, and joy. To all my true friends, your friendship is priceless and timeless. Together we have explored life, discussed ideas, shared our pasts and pondered our futures; each of you fulfills a part of me. To my mentor, thank you for your heartfelt feedback, guidance, and insight that helped me make my good book into a great one. Your support and inspiration means more than I can express in words and is infused into the essence of this book. To the teachers, writers, academics, researchers, and clinicians that have informed and inspired me, I stand upon the shoulder of giants in the work I do. And last, but most certainly not least, to my patients, readers, and students, your trust in me and your attentiveness to my words continuously drives me to be the best I can be, so I can help you become the best *you* can be.

Preface

Pull up a chair. Take a taste. Come join us.
Life is so endlessly delicious.
— Ruth Reichl

Read the Preface of this Book

Thank you for deciding to read this book. If it was a gift, thank you for not *re-gifting* it! And thank you for reading the preface. I know there is usually a strong urge to skip over the preface and move on to the start of the *actual* book, but in this case, the book begins right here and right now, as does our journey together as reader and author.

Here is the best part, and why I am so glad you chose to read this book; I wrote this book for *you*. I really did! I will elaborate on that sentiment later on, but first allow me to introduce both the concept of this book and myself. I am Dr. Gena E. Kadar, a professor of clinical nutrition, a Certified Nutrition Specialist, a licensed chiropractor and your humble author and tour guide for developing a better you. In the pages of this book, I have gathered the most current evidence from the fields of nutrition, exercise physiology, weight loss, obesity, and stress management, and coupled with my own professional experience, have translated this information into simple ideas and easy-to-do lifestyle change strategies that will not only empower you to transform your life, but also give you the tools to make it happen.

To understand my motivation for writing this book, here is a fun fact about myself: I have read just about every diet book that has ever been written. Why? Part of the reason is that as a professor of clinical nutrition and as an integrative healthcare practitioner specializing in weight/fat loss and in implementing therapeutic lifestyle change programs, I want stay abreast on the latest developments and fads in the field. As a practicing clinician, I also wanted to know what my patients were reading and being sold on as the latest "solutions" to their weight gain woes. In turn, I could offer them informed guidance and clarification regarding the often misleading headlines or unsubstantiated health and diet claims they were being sold on as weight loss gospel. The other main reason why I have read every "diet" book? Well, I hate to admit it, but it was to discover my own panacea for staying thin. Perhaps that explains at least partially, why I ended up specializing in the field of nutrition in the first place.

Weight loss is a fascinating area of healthcare; billions have been spent on it, fortunes have been made off it, but sadly most consumers only seem to be losing the thirty dollars they spent on the latest diet book. How is it that the more we purport to know about weight loss, the fatter we get as a nation? If I had a dime for every time a patient of mine said to me "I know what I should be doing to lose weight but I just can't seem to do it," I would be retired and living in a spectacular chateau somewhere in the south of France - paid for in cash. Ok, I exaggerate, but the point is, there is no shortage of information on what we theoretically *should* be doing to lose weight. After the billions spent on "experts", gadgets, books, DVDs and programs, there is one thing that we do know for certain about weight loss: *diets do not work*.

This is Not a Diet Book

This book is different. It is not a diet book. In fact, it rejects all together the notion of the word "diet" as we currently understand it. Instead, it embraces the true origin of the word "diet" and shatters the current perceptions that this word conjures up. You see, if we look back a few hundred years to the 13th century, we can discover the classical meaning of the word "diet". The word is rooted in the Greek word "diaita" meaning *manner of living."*

The original meaning of the word "diet" therefore refers to how we live our lives; not just what we eat. In fact, the Greek work "diaita" is itself derived from the Greek word "diaitasthai" which means *to lead one's life.* So how is it that we have taken a word that is so universal and so profound in its meaning and significance, and interpreted it to be such a frustrating, limited, and self-sacrificing act?

The concept of the "diet" has become ingrained in our collective modern consciousness as a restrictive, temporary strategy to shed pounds and to torture those of us that may be horizontally challenged. It conjures up thoughts about weight loss, but not optimal body composition (more on this later). We associate diets with what we eat; not how we live our lives. To most people, the word "diet" suggests merely the shedding of pounds as measured on a scale; it does not distinguish between the loss of muscle and the loss of fat. It implies a transient, isolating sacrifice we take on alone. Often hearing the word "diet" resounds of failure for those that have unsuccessfully attempted it in the past, and triggers a feeling of distress among those that wish to embark upon it first thing Monday morning. The word has become such a dreaded term that we use it to punish ourselves when we have over-indulged in delectable delights of the palette: "Now I have to go on a diet." This statement is usually met by our companions with a sigh or something equivocally sympathetic yet disparaging.

Thus, this word no longer reflects its true definition, nor does it reflect a positive notion regarding our intake of food and how we live our life. Sadly, it has now become a word that conjures up feelings of failure, frustration, and folly. This thwarted understanding of the word "diet" is most certainly not the premise I want to build this book upon. Therefore, from here on and throughout the remainder of this book, other than when I refer to manners of eating that are considered "diets" by our conventional understanding or by title, I will intentionally avoid any reference to that four letter word.

Instead, any attempt I make to describe smart eating strategies will be referred to as a manner of eating or a *food plan.* The beauty of this shift in terminology is that while we may not all be on a, *ahem,* diet, we are all in need of a food plan. After all, we all have to eat! So, the objective when I discuss healthful and delicious eating strategies in the pages to come, is not to about going on a "diet" (the last time I use that word gratuitously, I promise!); instead, the idea is simply to refine and improve our current food plan, or our manner of eating, in order to enhance our lives.

This Book is Not about Weight Loss

Not only is this not a "diet" book, but this book is not about helping you lose weight. WAIT! Before you put this book back on the shelf, let me explain. Anyone can lose weight... it's true. In fact, the failure of most diets is in part related to that very fact. Confused? Weight loss alone is most often a combination of water, fat, *and* muscle loss; with muscle and water often being the first to go. The problem is that when we lose muscle we also shed our ability to be efficient fat-burning machines. On the other hand, when we lose fat and preserve muscle, we become more lean, look slender (yet firm), and retain the ability to burn fat at our own individual optimal rate. In other words, we become more efficient at burning energy and less likely to regain the fat. The added benefit is that we also decrease our likelihood of developing many chronic diseases and delay, or in some cases even prevent, age related functional decline. I will explain this in greater detail later on, but for now it is important to know that this book shifts away from discussing "weight-loss" and instead focuses on *fat loss*. While this may appear to be only a small shift in the lingo of this text, its application is a giant leap that will allow you to more effectively and efficiently improve your health and wellbeing.

This Book is Not about Exercise

So far, I have established that this book is not about "diets" (at least not how they are generally understood), nor is it about generalized weight loss. Since I am in process of explaining the vernacular of this book, there is one additional word I need to address: exercise. For many of us the word "exercise" still retains a positive connotation. However (and regretfully), for the rest of us, this term can often conjure thoughts of failure or at the very least a dreaded nuisance. So once again, out of respect to all the disillusioned exercisers out there, I intend to reframe our context in an effort to break away from preconceived notions about exercise. Thus, I shall also refrain from using the word "exercise" in this book. Instead, I will talk about activity and movement. Movement, motion, and activity are all words that I will use to replace the word exercise; so as to conjure up an image of the brilliant functional ability of our body, instead of a treadmill in an unventilated gym. We have all heard someone say "I hate to exercise," but who has ever said "I hate to move?" Movement of the human body in all its wonderful possible combinations is a gift; this book will motivate and inspire you to make the most of that gift so that it becomes the gift that keeps on giving.

This Book is for *You*

With all that said, this book is not only about what we should eat and how to achieve a healthy body composition. This book is about helping you refine your approach to *all* behaviors, activities, and choices that define how you lead your life. This book is not only for those that want to lose fat and get slim. It is also for anyone wanting to be healthier. It is for anyone that feels stressed, tired, and frustrated and wants to be well. It is also for someone that is already healthy and wants to maintain their high quality of life. It is for those looking to live their best life in both mind and body; it is for those who want to prolong the years of their life *and* the life in those years. It is for those that want to learn to live life to the fullest – to achieve their optimal health potential. So whoever you are, this book was written for *you*. Whether you are 4 or 104, this book offers a realistic approach to optimizing your health and well-being, and most importantly, for sustaining these results for life. This book is about refining and re-defining your *manner of living*.

The Process of Developing a Healthier You

The information in this book is designed to reveal itself through a logical progression. I start by establishing a solid foundation, by providing rationale for why making choices that promote a healthy life is a worthy pursuit, and then I provide you with the tools to make that happen.

In order to be successful, it is first important to understand that why, what, and how we eat truly matters. From there, I will answer the million dollar question: *what should I eat?* You will gain an easy-to-implement, creative, and colorful strategy to help refine your daily food plan. Along the way, you will learn to create culinary works of art at each meal that celebrate the pleasure that is an inherent and a necessary part of the dining experience. The only "side effects" of embracing this approach will be an enlightened appreciation for real food, a reduction in body fat, and reduced risk of chronic disease. Those among you with special nutritional restrictions will learn that this approach can easily be adjusted to accommodate your needs. I will also arm you with the tools to create a nutritional safe haven within your home, and show you how to shop smart, prepare foods in a manner that enhances their nutritional value, and even how to entertain guests and dine out without sacrificing the joy of eating well. I will empower you with healthy habits that will allow you to sustain your new manner of eating *for life*.

We will also delve into another fundamental activity shared by all humankind: movement. I will redefine what activity means to our health and well-being, and will shatter the notion that the only way to get strong and shed fat is with a health club membership and designer spandex. You will discover that the world is your gym and begin to uncover the endless movement possibilities and strategies to help sustain and reap the pleasure and benefits of a lifetime of activity.

This book will also explore how to cope with stress, emotional eating, physical pain, and other challenges that are often viewed as obstacles in the journey toward optimal health. These hurdles can cause even the most dedicated and well-intentioned person to veer off course and are often the reason that for so many, the quest towards wellness is met with failure and frustration. But not for you! I will help you learn strategies for managing pain, and for unraveling the emotional complexities that often lead to unhealthy eating behavior patterns in the first place. I will provide tricks and insider tips to help you overcome out-of-control indulgences and conquer cravings. I will reveal how to stay in control of your life in the face of adversity to help respond to life's challenges so you can remain empowered and triumphant, regardless of the obstacle.

From bodily functions to food sensitivities, the book will also address additional real life, practical matters that impact our day to day *manner of living*. Some of these concerns are universal in that they are shared by all of us; others are unique to only a few. Regardless, since they influence our heath and the health of our loved ones, we will learn to take command of them. You will learn the basics about human bodily functions, what 'normal' is, and learn how to stay in control of your health. You will learn how to identify possible food sensitivities, and about essential screening tests that can serve as a veritable crystal ball for your future health. After all, *knowledge is power.*

The final chapter of this book brings it all together by outlining a practical, step by step approach to putting the information you have learned into daily practice based on your personal priorities and goals. I also share with you a day in my life so you can see how I practice what I preach in the pages of this book. Additionally, I have assembled a wealth of additional resources and references that you can access for added support at any stage of your journey.

A Final Word

What does it mean to be on a slippery slope? It is an endeavor that once started, cannot easily be reversed. Once the first steps are taken no matter how small, there is no direction to travel other than *forward* along the slope. I trust that you will find the trajectory of this book leads us to a slippery slope; but it is a slippery slope that you will delight to be on! Here's how it works:

First you eat better... then
You will have more energy... then
You become more active and more engaged in life... then
You do more, see more, and have a better outlook on life, work, and relationships

Once on the slope, the momentum will propel you! You will be more, and offer more to those you work with, care about, and love, since you have filled yourself up with, what the French brilliantly call, *joie de vive*! You will prolong the quality of your health and your vitality, regardless of your age. You will live life to the fullest and prevent the onset of disease that we wrongfully attribute exclusively to aging. You will not merely be living; you will be *thriving.* This is one slippery slope that I am on and I hope you will join me.

My goal when writing this book was to offer the world a new way to approach health and a new way to look at life. In doing so, I aspire to give you the inspiration, the motivation, the support, and the tools to live your most exceptional life possible, to revel in and take pleasure in the world around you, and to prolong the quality and quantity of your time here on this glorious planet.

Enjoy the journey ahead.

Chapter 1

Destiny is not a matter of chance; it is a matter of choice. It is not a thing to be waited for, it is a thing to be achieved.
— William Jennings Bryan

Nature vs. Nurture

It has long been believed that our future is written in our genes. We all know that our genetics dictate our hair and eye color; but are we genetically programmed in the same way to develop heart disease or type 2 diabetes? Since the sequencing of the human genome, scientists have continued to elucidate the interaction between our genes and our health. The conclusion has long been maintained that our genes dictate our susceptibility to disease. While there is an indisputable degree of truth to this, an important variable has been missing from this conclusion. But recently, cutting edge research has shattered this limited view of human genetics. Scientists have discovered that there is a critical variable influencing the relationship between our genes and our health, and that variable is *you*. This revolutionary new understanding of genetics shows us that while our genes do influence our health; *we* can influence our genes.

To understand this novel way of looking at genetics, and more importantly to understand why it matters to you and what you can do about it, we must first have an understanding of the basics. Genetics is a remarkably complex subject; but, the fundamentals are actually rather uncomplicated. Simply stated, genes are codes. These codes inform (and are informed by) every facet of our body's current state, and of what the body will become. The codes communicate with every cell in our body through the expression of particular proteins, each of which has a very specific function. Thus, each part of our body does what it is told by the combination of proteins that are made. Some of the products of this gene 'expression' are easily seen, such as our eye color; others we cannot see, including our vulnerability to disease. Genetic codes are passed through families through the generations. That's how you can have your mother's lovely blue eyes and your dad's thick, wavy brown hair. That's also how you can have your mom's tendency towards heart disease, and dad's risk of Alzheimer's disease. Until a few decades ago, this was essentially where our understanding of the connection between genetics and disease ended. It's amazing how things change.

Scientific research is an ongoing quest in search of answers to unresolved questions. The more we learn, the more questions we have. With regard to genetics, as our understanding of genes evolved, scientists then wondered whether or not it would be possible to control gene expression. And if so, could we impact *what* our genes dictate to each part our body in order to help prevent disease? Remarkably, we now have the answers to these questions.

First, consider that our genes account for only a small part of our health as we age. In fact, most experts have long maintained that only about 30% of our health as we age is dictated by genetics, while 70% is based on our lifestyle choices. This fact alone earns huge points for the power of lifestyle over genetics, or nurture over nature. Yet, the seemingly small genetic effect that remains can still have a profound impact on health. A common mistake people make is to rationalize that even this 30% "genetic effect" can thwart our best attempts at rewriting our fate through healthy lifestyle choices. If your father, brother and grandfather all suffered heart attacks, and if it is coded in your genes that you too are predisposed to having a heart attack, then (whether or not you passed on the second serving of sugar coated deep fried bacon your whole life), surely suffering a heart attack is your destiny too. Or is it?

2

Contrary to what we have always believed to be true, the real answer may be a resounding "No." It now appears we have much more control over that 30% then we ever thought.

A Genetic Light Switch

As previously described, it is well established that genes determine the color of our eyes, our *real* hair color, and the shade of our skin. It is also clear that certain inherited genes may predispose us to cancer, heart disease, diabetes, and even obesity. But what if I told you we have a figurative "light switch" that can turn on or turn off these genes? More remarkably, what if I told you that you may be able to *control* whether that "light switch" is turned on or off? Would you take the necessary steps to assume control of the "light switch"?

If you responded yes to the question above, then you are going to delight in the facts that follow! Through the emerging and revolutionary scientific fields known as epigenetics and nutrigenomics, we learn that these genetic "switches" *do* exist. Even better, we know that in certain cases we *can* turn them on and off. In other words, no longer do we need to passively rely on our genetic destiny; we now know that in many cases we can control whether our genes express themselves or not. This changes everything!

Epigenetics

Epigenetics is a relatively new field. In essence, it informs us as to how we can communicate with our genes. It focuses on the *epigenome*, which has essentially been identified as a layer of biochemical reactions that function to turn our genes "on" and "off." In simple terms, the epigenome can be thought of as an instruction manual for one's genes. Epigenetics helps us understand how to figuratively *speak* to our genes in a language they understand; like a mother to her child, the epigenome tells our genes what to do and what not to do.

To appreciate the implications of epigenetics, consider two identical twins. Now imagine that they were separated at birth; given up for adoption and raised separately by two different families in two different environments. The fascinating thing about identical twins is that they are genetically identical. Therefore, with the traditional understanding of genetics, we would expect that as they age, regardless of their environment of lifestyle choices, they would succumb to the same aging patterns and fall victim to the same chronic diseases as written in their genetic code. If one twin had heart disease, we would expect the other to have heart disease as well. But this is NOT what we see.

Twin studies are some of the best ways to tease out the effects of nature (genetic predisposition) and nurture (the environment, including lifestyle choices) on our health. For example, researchers at the Spanish National Cancer Center in Madrid published some groundbreaking results. They looked at forty identical twins between the ages of 3 to 74.[1] The young twins that were growing up together were not only genetically identical, but were virtually identical epigenetically as well. Yet, when they looked at the genetic profiles of *older* identical twins, the researchers found that epigenetically they were dramatically different.

The epigenome is vulnerable to the choices we make as we live our life, including whether or not we smoke, whether we eat processed bacon on white toast with margarine or instead choose the poached wild salmon and organic broccoli. What we eat, what we drink, if we smoke, our exposure to pollutants, and how we manage stress, all have been shown to influence our epigenome.[2,3,4,5] As our epigenome changes, so does the expression of our genes. The communication between our epigenome and our genes therefore changes based on our environment. Because our epigenome informs our genes to either be silenced or to be activated, lifestyle factors that affect our epigenome can influence whether diseases like cancer and heart disease should be triggered; or, whether the same diseases should be kept at bay.

A number of behaviors and environmental factors have been shown to play an important role in human health by affecting the epigenome. Some examples of such factors that are often under our control and that may "turn on" or "turn off" our genes include:

1. What we eat
2. Activity and movement (or lack of)
3. How we respond to stress
4. Smoking, drug abuse, or excessive alcohol consumption
5. Exposure to environmental toxins

As you might imagine, there are also some environmental factors that influence our epigenome over which we have no control. Examples include select environmental pollutants and toxins, exposures during prenatal development, and traumatic (physical or emotional) stresses particularly those experienced during neonatal, childhood, and adolescent development.[6] We also inherit epigenetic patterns from our parents based on *their* environment and lifestyle. Fortunately, as we learn from the twin study mentioned previously, many of these epigenetic patterns appear to be amendable by the choices we make during our own lifespan.

Nutrigenomics

Nutrition is one of the most exciting epigenetic factors that we have the ability to control. The best part? We get to remedy any poor choices we make at least three times a day, with every meal! Thank goodness our bodies are so forgiving! Nutrigenomics is the study of how the nutrients we consume interact with our genes. Since the late 1990s, scientists have been learning more and more about how the foods we eat influence our genes. This has profound implications. Consider that historically, nutritional researchers have focused on how food choices can help prevent nutritional deficiencies and excesses, and thereby promote health. In this new era, where we are gaining insight into the effects of epigenetics and nutrigenomics, we now know that this focus is far too limited and short-sighted. Food needs to be considered as much more than just complex matrices of nutrients. Instead, food should be considered as information; information that tells our genes what to do. Think about that for a moment.....the food you eat can change the function of your genes. Really!

It is extraordinary when you think about it, perhaps even hard to believe; but this is the new reality, and it is time we all become aware of the astonishing effects food has on our genes and our health. As you read this, amazing and game-changing research is taking place around the globe looking into diet-genome interactions and how this understanding can be used to prevent disease and improve human health. Admittedly, our understanding of how to fully apply nutrigenomics is still limited, however the field is rapidly advancing and fascinating strides have been made in the area of cancer research in particular, which we can look to as a model of things to come.

As an example of what is happening in cancer research, let us first consider a simple stalk of broccoli. Since what seems like the dawn of time, mothers have made their kids clear their plate of this tree-like veggie. Being green and a vegetable, it has always been assumed to be the epitome of health food. Recently, however, broccoli has been celebrated for more than its greenness; today it is promoted as a dietary ally in the fight against cancer[7], but why? Through epigenetics and nutrigenomics we finally understand that it is not just because of the vitamins and minerals it contains.

Broccoli is part of the cruciferous vegetable family. Broccoli's relatives include cauliflower, cabbage, kale, and the delicious, but often underrated, Brussels sprout. One thing that this family has in common is that they all contain a compound known as sulforaphane. This compound appears to be worth its weight in gold in terms of cancer prevention. You see, studies have shown that though epigenetics pathways this compound with the fun-to-say name, is actually able to effectively prevent cancer cells from expressing themselves by altering the epigenetic patterns on the genes that regulate them. To date, sulforaphane has been studied for its preventive role in breast cancer, prostate cancer and colon cancer.[8,9,10] And the best part? We have only scratched the surface of its benefits. Even better, it is only one of potentially thousands of food components that can improve our health though epigenetic mechanisms. So mom was right after all; eat those greens. And don't stop there, in the coming chapters I will reveal many of the other wonderful foods you can eat to help you be well and stay well, for life.

You Are What Your Grandparents Ate

While the foods we eat clearly impact our own health, they also appear to impact the health of our offspring and the generations that follow. Randy Jirtle, PhD, the Director of the Laboratory of Epigenetics and Imprinting at Duke University, led one of the most groundbreaking studies in the field of epigenetics.[11] To understand his study, one needs a little deeper understanding of how epigenetics works – not to worry; the brief scientific primer is worth the reward!

Here it goes: one of the most well-known processes of epigenetics is called methylation. In most instances, if a gene is highly methylated it is turned "off," and if it is un-methylated (or in some instances, less methylated) it is turned "on." You can consider methylation as a process that puts little epigenetic tags on genes to signal whether or not to turn on or off the genetic "light switch".

Dr. Jirtle studied a gene found in both mice and humans, called *agouti*. When a mouse's agouti gene is *unmethylated*, (turned "on" in this case), the mouse has yellow colored fur, is obese and is prone to diabetes and cancer. When the agouti gene is *methylated*, as it is in most normal mice, the mice have brown fur, normal weight, and a low risk for disease. Obese yellow mice and skinny brown mice are genetically identical, but epigenetically they are clearly very different due to their different methylation patterns.

Many nutrients that we are familiar with, like folic acid and B vitamins, are necessary for methylation to occur. Therefore it makes sense that deficiencies of these nutrients may affect a person's methylation status. Dr. Jirtle wanted to see what would happen if he fed pregnant yellow mice a methyl-rich diet, specifically containing the nutrients folic acid, choline, vitamin B12, and betaine. His findings were remarkable. The offspring of these overweight, yellow mice were brown and healthy, and remained that way for life! It appears that it not only matters what *you* eat, it matters what your mother ate too. And it doesn't end there: it may even matter what *her* mother ate.

Animal studies suggest that epigenetic changes can remain in families for generations! Studies in humans have also provided evidence that epigenetic inheritance through generations can occur, and are affected by our external environment, including our food supply and exposure to stressors like trauma or smoking. Men take note; this time it is not only about mom – the epigenetic patterns found in the father may also contribute to these trans-generational epigenetic inheritance patterns.[12]

Should you be worried that nobody told your mother to eat methyl-rich foods? Should you fret and be fearful that you are now cursed because your mom's diet may have been desperately lacking particular nutrients while you were *in utero*? Absolutely not! Stress has been demonstrated to be another factor that can negatively alter our epigenome[13] so no need to add insult to injury. Also, remember that while our genes are fixed, our epigenome is not. It is never too late to make choices that will favorably impact your epigenome and reduce the risk of disease. Whether you are looking to optimize your own health (at any stage of your life), or whether you are pregnant and want to optimize the health of your child, the key is to eat foods that provide the correct information to your genes. In the chapters to come, I will share with you which foods these are so you may incorporate them into your new *manner of living*.

The Bottom Line:
Our dietary and lifestyle choices have profound implications on our health far beyond what we once thought to be true. Food is more than just a source of energy and nutrients. Food is information that communicates with our genes. It is not only what we eat that has this power; how we choose to live our life, whether we manage stress, maintain healthy activity, and avoid harmful exposures, all influence our genes and in turn, influence our health. No matter what your past personal or family history may be, no matter what your age, you are now informed that the fate of your health is not fixed.[14] The decisions you make each day about how you live your life *do* matter and will alter your future health from today on... for better or for worse. *The choice is yours.*

Chapter 2

Our bodies are our gardens to which our wills are our gardeners.
— William Shakespeare

Change Your Body Composition, Change Your Life

The title of this chapter was inspired by the famous line "if you build it, they will come" from Kevin Costner's classic 1989 fantasy baseball film, Field of Dreams. But this alliteration is not just a gratuitous reference to ride Mr. Costner's catchy literary coat-tails; quite the contrary. The fact is, just like in the movie, it is true! If you change your body composition, you *will* change your life.

A healthy body composition can be defined in part, by a healthy ratio of muscle mass to fat mass coupled with an optimal waist circumference measurement. In other words, it is not only the amount of muscle and fat we have, but where on our body the fat it is located. So my dear reader, the scale is no longer the only tool we need. I apologize in advance if I sound harsh, but I really do not care that you want to weigh the same as you weighed during your senior year of high school. In fact, I don't care much at all what your bathroom scale says, and neither should you. Here's why: from both an aesthetic and health standpoint, it is not only our total body weight that matters, but the composition of that weight. As you read this chapter it will become clear why an arbitrary total body weight should <u>not</u> be our primary goal. It is time to step off the scale and stop worrying so much about our weight, and instead start looking at what we are made of: our body composition. To do this, from now on there are two important numbers that you need to be tracking:

1. Your waist circumference, and
2. Your body fat percentage.

To appreciate the profound importance of this, let us start from the beginning by understanding what our bodies are made of. In the simplest terms we can divide the body into two components: fat mass and fat-free mass.

Fat -free mass: This refers to all *non*-fatty tissue in our body such as muscle, bone, organs, blood and water. Fat-free mass contains virtually all the body's water, all the metabolically active tissues, and is the source of all metabolic caloric expenditure. Our fat-free mass and our muscle in particular, acts as the body's natural fat-burning engine! Therefore, it is important to maintain, or gain, muscle mass during our lifespan particularly when we are looking to shed body fat. Adequate muscle mass is also critical for supporting our health as we age, but more on that later.

Fat mass: The fat in our body can be further divided into two types: essential and non-essential fat.

a. **Essential fat:** This is the fat that is critical for normal biological function. It includes fats that are incorporated into our nerves, brain, heart, lungs, liver, and mammary glands. We require this fat for basic survival and function. Women have a slightly greater requirement for this type of fat than men primarily to support their reproductive needs.

b. **Non-essential fat (storage fat):** This refers to the fat reserves of the body. It is also where the majority of body fat is contained. Adipose tissue, made of fat cells, exists primarily below the skin (subcutaneous) and around major organs (visceral). This fat is the most variable constituent of the body, in that it can come and go without affecting our basic survival and reproductive functions.

10

Again, women are able to store more than men, particularly to support reproductive needs.

When we test body composition in a living organism, it isn't possible to differentiate between essential and non-essential fat. However, when one is over-fat or obese, they are considered to have an excess in the non-essential storage form of fat. It is this type of fat that we aim to restore to within a healthy range when we set out to improve our body composition. (Methods for testing and interpreting our body fat percentage are described at the end of this chapter.)

Together, our fat mass and fat-free mass makeup our total body weight. So, when we are just monitoring total weight on a scale, we don't know whether the weight we are losing is coming predominantly from our fat mass or our fat-free mass fat; in other words, we don't know if the weight loss is from water, fat, or muscle. A major problem is that in most cases the mass we are losing is not from the storage fat but rather from the fat-free mass. The best case is that we are losing water, but often the worst case is true: we lose muscle mass. It makes sense, then, that we need to monitor the type of weight we are losing, so that if we see the wrong kind of loss we can intervene as soon as possible to reverse it.

So why does the body instinctively tend to shed muscle more than fat? The answer is fascinating, and surprisingly logical. When we decide to reduce our intake of calories with the intent of losing weight, the body is forced into a state of energy deficit; more energy is being expended than being consumed. While you might think this is exactly what you were trying to do, and you see the result on the scale, this caloric deficit forces your body into "survival mode." The body must quickly determine how to retain the same functions with less energy. Your tissues are not concerned that you have an upcoming reunion or beach vacation, it is concerned with efficiency. Therefore, the body will look to shed tissues that are least efficient. In other words, tissues that use the most energy to survive are the first tissues sacrificed. Fat has very low energy needs. Muscle, on the other hand, is a veritable energy drain so, is the first to go.

Our body is always striving to function at a state of maximal efficiency. When there is a surplus of energy, it is stored (usually as adipose/fat tissue). When there is an energy deficiency, high-energy tissues are sacrificed in conjunction with the release of stored energy. Thus, in a state of energy restriction that defines most diets, the body instinctively reverts to a primitive protective response that will be least damaging to its physiological needs. Keep in mind that the immediate goal of the body is not long-term healthy body fat loss, but rather short-term survival until 'regular' energy intake is resumed.

Here is the paradox: muscle is our fat-burning engine and yet it is the first to go! Muscle has a very high metabolic demand which means it uses a lot of energy. Muscle burns excess energy and body fat, but from the viewpoint of the body during "survival mode" (such as with most commercial dieting), it sees the muscle as depleting precious energy resources. So, in a time when energy intake is minimized, the body sheds the tissue that is burning up the most energy: muscle. But, the body retains its fat. This is why most people end up reducing their muscle mass when they embark on a typical weight loss plan. Sure the number on the scale drops, but at what cost? The long-term consequences are severe both from an aesthetic and a general health standpoint. When most of these people resume their normal eating patterns, body fat is quickly put back on.[15, 16, 17] Worse than that, often even *more* fat is gained than was lost in the first place because with the loss of muscle came a decrease in the ability to burn excess energy and body fat. And so, the yo-yo phenomenon begins. The good news is, if you have been, or are currently one of these people caught in the yo-yo cycle, then not to worry; it is never too late to adopt a new *manner of living* and halt the yo-yo phenomenon, for good.[18]

Let us now consider the opposite, ideal situation of losing *fat* while preserving muscle. We get lean, we look slender and firm, and by retaining our muscle mass, we optimize our ability to burn fat. As we become more efficient at burning energy we are less likely to regain the fat. Did you know that those who retain lean muscle as they age are more resilient to illnesses contracted later in life?[19] Instead of weight loss, our focus is therefore fat loss. Specifically, we want to decrease body fat while increasing or maintaining lean muscle mass. So how do you do this? How do you shift toward fat loss instead of muscle loss?

The advice in this book arms you with the tools to support an optimal body composition, and to preserve or gain lean muscle mass and keep body fat within an optimal range. In general, engaging in activity that gets your heart racing (e.g. dancing, walking, playing, biking, and running) will help decrease fat mass, while strength training activities (e.g. lifting weights and resistance activities) will help maintain or increase lean muscle mass. Because muscle needs more calories to be sustained than fat, those who have more lean body mass have higher metabolisms, expend more calories, and need more calories to maintain muscle mass. This is the optimal body composition that your new *manner of living* outlined in the chapters that follow will help you achieve and sustain.

Skinny Fat

Once we shift our focus towards achieving a healthy body composition, and not merely a "healthy" body weight, a fascinating reality becomes clear. When it comes to body composition, appearances can be deceiving. We all recognize that someone who is 5 feet 2 inches tall and weighs 297 pounds is considered obese, but, did you know a 5 foot 10 inch tall supermodel weighing 125 pounds might also be considered obese? Did you know a 4 foot 10 inch tall grandma weighing 85 pounds might *also* be considered obese? Who knew a grandma and a supermodel could have so much in common.

Healthcare practitioners use the Body Mass Index (BMI) system to classify each of us as either underweight, normal weight, overweight, obese, or morbidly obese. You may have seen a BMI chart in your healthcare provider's office. It compares your weight relative to your height.

ACTION STEP: Determine and interpret *your* BMI.

Calculate your BMI using the following equation:

BMI = (weight in pounds / [height in inches]^2) X 703

Example:
      Weight = 150 pounds, Height = 5'5" (65 inches)
      BMI: [150 ÷ (65)^2] x 703 = 24.96

Interpret your BMI using the following chart:[20]

BMI	CATEGORY
Below 18.5	Underweight
18.5 - 24.9	Healthy
25.0 - 29.9	Overweight
30.0 - 39.9	Obese
Over 40	Extreme or high risk obesity

While the BMI is a good instrument to use as a general screening tool for body weight, it is often inadequate when we want to consider the real impact of body weight and body composition on our health.

According to the BMI, a person classified as being of "normal" weight is considered to be healthy, but in reality, in some cases this may be the farthest thing from the truth. Even if a person fitting this classification appears to be of "normal" weight, they may still have what is called *sarcopenic obesity*. The examples of the thin supermodel and grandma are classic illustrations of this type of obesity.

Sarcopenic obesity, or sarcopenia, describes a condition when someone's body fat is excessive relative to the amount of muscle mass and strength that they possess.[21] In fact, the word sarcopenia comes from the Greek words *sarx,* meaning flesh, and *penia,* meaning loss.[22] You may have heard this referred to as being "skinny fat," which is an appropriate, albeit strange, description. Although most people who appear obese also have sarcopenia, often times someone with sarcopenic obesity appears thin, and may even be underweight by standards established by the BMI. This is because their ratio of muscle to fat is very low, or in other words, they have excessive body fat compared to muscle even though they may look "skinny."

What causes sarcopenic obesity? Studies inform us that everything from excessive calorie intake, physical inactivity, low-grade systemic inflammation (steps to prevent this type of inflammation are presented later in this book), changes in hormonal balance, and even the aging process itself all may lead to the development of this condition.[23] Of these, aging and reduced activity are among the greatest culprits. In fact, if we were to maintain a sedentary lifestyle, our muscle mass and strength would progressively decline beginning around the age of 30 years.[24] Interestingly, an unhealthy manner of weight loss also accelerates the development and progression of sarcopenia.[25] This is another critical reason why we need to stop focusing on the number on our scale, and instead focus our attention and efforts on reducing body fat loss and maintaining or increasing lean muscle mass as we age.

So, you may be wondering, what is the big deal if someone is skinny fat? They still can look thin, perhaps just a little less toned. Isn't being "skinny fat" still better than being just fat? Maybe not.

In the process of developing sarcopenic obesity, fat tends to accumulate around the midsection (more on this later) and also begins to infiltrate muscle, resulting in decreased strength.[26] Worse than this, and perhaps because of it, sarcopenic obesity may also increase the risk of developing chronic diseases like heart disease, hypertension or type 2 diabetes.[27,28] If that doesn't provoke sufficient concern, consider this: sarcopenia has been identified as a significant cause of frailty, disability, and loss of independence as we age.[29]

It is important to mention that excess body fat is not the only culprit contributing to the health consequences of sarcopenia or general obesity. Scientific researchers have been stumped trying to figure out why some people with excessive body fat show no additional risk factors for disease, whereas someone with even just slightly elevated body fat can play host to chronic diseases such as type 2 diabetes, or cardiovascular disease. Evidence now informs us that the issue is not just about the total amount of fat you store, but *where* you store that fat.

Waist Circumference

We used to think fat was just a passive blob of tissue that did nothing more than loiter on our bottom, and belly, and chin, and arms, and… well, you get the point. Interestingly, we now know that fat cells are anything but lazy: fat cells work overtime secreting hormones and other chemicals that are released into our body. Can you guess which fat cells are the busiest in the body? That's right, the fat cells that make up our belly fat.

It appears that the fat cells deposited around our midsection are very different from the fat cell deposits on our bottoms, or anywhere else on our body. These belly fat cells, collectively known as Visceral Adipose Tissue or VAT, (named for this fat's proximity to our abdominal organs which are collectively referred to as the abdominal viscera) are a veritable hormone factory. Working overtime, the fat around our midsection actively produces hormones and chemicals that trigger inflammation throughout our body.[30] Excessive amounts of these circulating inflammatory chemicals have been linked to a variety of chronic diseases, including heart disease,[31] Type 2 diabetes,[32] Alzheimer's disease,[33] and cancer.[34]

Another reason why excessive VAT is considered dangerous to our health is the proximity of this fat to our vital organs. VAT is not only deposited at our midsection, but also near our heart, lungs, and liver.[35] Even in the absence of other risk factors, excessive abdominal fat independently places you at greater risk for developing obesity-related conditions.[36] According to the National Institutes of Health, a person who has an increased waist circumference, *even if they have a normal body weight*, has increased risk of hypertension, heart disease, and type 2 diabetes.[37]

The good news is that we are in control of our VAT and have the power to restore it to a healthy amount! While belly fat is the most dangerous fat, it also appears to be more readily shed than fat found elsewhere on the body. In order to estimate your VAT, begin by measuring your waist circumference.

The figure that follows shows you what your maximum waist circumference should be depending on your gender.

Waist Circumference Measurements

Gender	Waist Circumference Goal	Health Risk *	Increased Waist Circumference	Health Risk *
Men	Less than 40 inches (102 cm)	Decreased	Greater than 40 inches (102 cm)	Increased
Women	Less than 35 inches (88 cm)	Decreased	Greater than 35 inches (88 cm)	Increased

* Reflects relative risk of developing hypertension, heart disease, and type 2 diabetes.

Source: Adapted from National Heart, Lung, and Blood Institute (NHLBI)
http://www.nhlbi.nih.gov/guidelines/obesity/e_txtbk/txgd/4142.htm

It's Time to Make This Personal

Thus far in the book we have been discussing matters from a rather generic point of view. It is time to make this personal. It is now time to begin implementing *your* new *manner of living*.

Let's get started.

Throughout this book, you will encounter GOALS, TIPS, and ACTION STEPS to take, to improve your health and quality of life. The goals I am recommending are ones that are universal; ones that we all can share in during our mutual quest towards better health. The action steps are designed to help you achieve these, and other goals. The tips are offered to make taking each step easier or in some cases, more pleasurable! You have already encountered your first actions step in measuring your BMI, and below are your first suggested goals. These are particularly important, as they will establish a baseline from which you can monitor your improvement. NOTE: For some of us, these goals may take longer to achieve than for others. Remember that it often takes years to put the fat on, therefore you should expect that it will also take some time to lose the fat in a healthy manner – but rest assured that as you stay the course, it *will* happen.

GOAL: Achieve and/or maintain a waist circumference below 40 inches if you are a man and below 35 inches if you are a woman.

ACTION STEP: Measure your waist circumference. Knowledge is power!

To accurately measure your waist circumference:

> ➢ Place a tape measure around your bare abdomen just above your hip bone. Make sure that the measuring tape is snug, but not too snug; it should not compress your skin. It should also be parallel to the floor. Relax, exhale, and measure your waist.

Now that you have measured your waist circumference, another easy and helpful number to learn is your **waist to height ratio** (WHtR). The WHtR is your waist circumference divided by your height. It is another valuable measurement to be mindful of as it not only allows you to personalize you waist circumference measurement and relative risk further, but it has also been shown to be an even better predictor of diabetes and cardiovascular disease risk than BMI or waist circumference alone.[38,39,40] To minimize your risk, the goal is to limit your waist size to less than half of your height or in other words, keep the ratio at less than 0.5. For example: For a 6 foot tall man, this would mean having a waist size less than 36 inches, while a 5 foot 4 inches tall woman should have a waistline no larger than 32 inches. The nice and simple thing about the WHtR is that it appears to be equally applicable at assessing risk in women, men, different ethnicities, and even in children.[41]

GOAL: Limit your waist size to less than half of your height.

ACTION STEP: Measure your waist to height ratio.

$$WHtR = \frac{waist\ circumference\ (inches)}{height\ (inches)}$$

Waist to Height Ratio (WHtR)	Relative risk
Less than 0.5	Low risk
Greater than or equal to 0.5	Increased risk
0.58 or greater	Substantial risk increase
0.42 or less	Increased risk (underweight)

GOAL: Achieve and/or maintain optimal body fat percentage as described in the chart below.

ACTION STEP: Measure your body fat percentage.

To measure your body fat percentage many options exist. Below are a few suggestions.

> ➢ The simplest is to invest in a home scale that measures body fat and not just weight. Look for one that *combines* both a handheld *and* lower body measurement. In the Additional Resources section at the back of this book I have listed some of my favorite, cost effective home units.

NOTE: *Do not worry too much whether or not the scale you purchase is the most accurate product on the market. The key is to get a baseline measurement. As long as you perform subsequent measurements using the same equipment, you can get a good indication of relative changes in your body fat and lean muscle mass.*

> ➤ Alternatively, you may ask your doctor or local gym if they are able to measure your body fat for you. The best option for regular monitoring is **Bio-Electrical Impedance Analysis (BIA).** It is both a convenient and highly accurate means of measurement and the one I generally recommend and used in my own clinical practice. It works by having a low-level electrical current run through the body and measuring how that current reacts to different tissues in the body. In this way it can determine the amount of fat relative to lean muscle mass in the body. Most home scales that measure body fat use this technology, however, your doctor will generally use a higher quality BIA device and therefore offer more precise and accurate monitoring than the typical home unit.

> ➤ A **Caliper Pinch Test**, also known as the skin-fold pinch test, involves using a caliper to measure body fat by pinching the skin at various areas on the body. While this can be quite accurate as well, make sure it is performed by an experienced individual as there is significant potential for error in inexperienced hands.

> ➤ While a technique called **Hydrostatic Weighing** is one of the most accurate ways to measure body fat, it is also costly and inconvenient as it requires expensive equipment, technicians and submerging yourself in a tank of water. This is generally used more for research and high level sport performance than regular body fat monitoring.

> ➤ **MRIs** and **CT Scans** are also highly accurate means of measuring body fat but these are neither convenient nor cost effective for regular monitoring.

Body Fat Percentages for Adult Females:

Age	Increased Risk	Healthy	Increased Risk	Greatly Increased Risk
	(BMI less than 18.5)	(BMI 18.5-24.9)	(BMI 25.0-29.9)	(BMI 30.0 +)
20-39	Less than 21%	21% to 32%	33% to 38%	39% +
40-59	Less than 23%	23% to 33%	34% to 39%	40% +
60-79	Less than 24%	24% to 35%	36% to 41%	42% +

Body Fat Percentages for Adult Males:

Age	Increased Risk	Healthy	Increased Risk	Greatly Increased Risk
	(BMI less than 18.5)	(BMI 18.5-24.9)	(BMI 25.0-29.9)	(BMI 30.0 +)
20-39	Less than 8%	8% to 19%	20% to 24%	25% +
40-59	Less than 11%	11% to 21%	22% to 27%	28% +
60-79	Less than 13%	13% to 24%	25% to 29%	30% +

Source: Adapted by Shape Up America! Gallagher, et al.. Am J Clin Nutr. 2000;72: 694-701.

A final word about body fat percentages

As you can see from the charts above, not only can too much body fat be harmful, but too little body fat may also increase one's disease risk by interfering with the normal healthy functioning of the body. Often when fat levels are too low, our energy levels decline. But that is not all: our tolerance for cold is diminished, and excessively low body fat can lead to musculoskeletal problems, including osteoporosis, and can result in hormonal imbalances in both men and women. In women of childbearing age, excessively low body fat can lead to loss of menstruation and problems with reproduction. But how low is too low?

Some athletes safely maintain levels of body fat that would be considered low (less than 8% in men and less than 21% in women). At this time, it is generally agreed by most experts that in certain cases, such as in the well-conditioned athlete, low body fat does not *always* pose an increased health risk. However, all bets are off if someone with a low body fat begins to experience fatigue, reduced resistance to cold, and decreased athletic performance, and/or hormonal imbalances such as those leading to loss of menstruation in women. These are all signs that body fat levels have become too low and the body is no longer able to adapt. In such cases steps need to be taken to safely increase levels of body fat to prevent long term and potentially irreversible health consequences.

Too much body fat increases the risk of many diseases including type 2 diabetes, high blood pressure, stroke, heart disease, and certain cancers. When the fat is located around the abdomen, the risk of acquiring these diseases increases even further. The good news is that whether you have too much body fat or too little, when your body fat returns to within acceptable ranges the risk for developing these diseases progressively decreases. So, it never too late to make changes, and there is no better moment to begin then *right now*.

ACTION STEP: Complete the chart that follows to determine *your* current health risk based on your current body fat percentage, waist circumference measurements, and your waist to height ratio.

Today's date:	
My waist circumference	
My associated health risk	□ Increased risk □ Low risk
My waist to height ratio	
My associated health risk	□ Increased risk □ Low risk
My body fat percentage	
My associated health risk	□ Increased risk □ Low risk

Beauty Inside Out

If everything I have described so far does not serve as sufficient incentive to motivate you to make a positive shift in your *manner of living* and stick with it for life; perhaps this reality check will...

To have radiant skin and luscious locks, it is often helpful to step away from the cosmetic counter and move into the kitchen. Before you scream blasphemy, consider this: the cells that make up our heart, liver, muscles, and bones depend on proper nutrient intake to optimize their function. Maintaining proper internal organ and tissue function, proper epigenetic communication, preserving lean muscle, and minimizing VAT are all critical for maintaining even the most superficial aspect of our body: our appearance. Our hair follicles and skin require the rest of the body to function properly. In other words, to look good on the outside, you must be healthy on the inside! Be assured that the same foods and lifestyle factors that promote healthy heart and lung function also promote healthy hair and skin.

Consider salmon and nuts as examples to illustrate how food impacts our health both on the inside, and out. Salmon is an abundant source of omega 3 fatty acids that nourish the scalp and may delay wrinkling of the skin.[42] Nuts, like cashews and almonds, are a great source of zinc, which may prevent shedding of hair.[43] These same foods also support immunity, heart health and can help prevent cardiovascular disease. See how this works? By adopting a healthy lifestyle you get to slay many dragons with just one sword!

Conversely, if you maintain unhealthy dietary habits such as repeatedly eating poor quality foods, eating too much or even too little, or if you adopt other destructive lifestyle habits like smoking or choosing to lead a sedentary life, your body will pay for it, inside and out. Often, such behaviors can manifests in esthetic changes including the graying or the loss of hair, premature wrinkling and dryness of the skin and/or brittle, peeling nails. These same damaging lifestyle choices may also lead to heart disease, cancer, disability, and even premature death.

The good news is that again, our bodies are wonderfully forgiving. (Thank goodness!) Regardless of where you are starting today, as you adhere to the healthy *manner of living* discussed in the coming chapters, you will begin to feel better, gain strength and energy, you will reduce your risk factors for disease and disability, and you may even see improvements in your skin, nails, and hair. Before you know it, you will be celebrating your new *manner of living* with radiant health on the inside and out and the best part is; it all begins with some great food!

Chapter 3

One of the very nicest things about life is the way we must regularly stop whatever it is we are doing and devote our attention to eating.
— Luciano Pavarotti and William Wright.
Pavarotti, My Own Story

Diversifying Your Food Plan

Whether you realize it or not, we are all adhering to a food plan. Your plan may have been influenced by countless books, articles and experts that have promised you the secret to weight loss or longevity by eating (or not eating) certain foods. Your food plan may have been shaped by your acceptance or rejection of your mother's words of dietary wisdom as you were growing up. Or maybe your food plan is simply to you eat whatever is convenient when you are hungry. Even then, your willingness to consume select convenience foods is often a product of past influences. Each of our individual food plans has been molded by our culture, our upbringing and our memories of foods that we associate with home, comfort, and family. They have been influenced by the restaurants in our community and by the products and foods choices available in our neighborhood grocery stores. Our food plans have also been influenced, often profoundly, by the savvy marketing of deceptively delicious processed "foods" made by commercial food manufacturers. Thanks to clever advertisements and sometimes questionable ingredients, these junk foods or artificial, highly processed foods often permeate our subconscious, tantalize our taste buds and render us blissfully 'addicted'.

A myriad of other factors affect our food plans as well. Many among us have opened our minds and mouths to unfamiliar foods thanks to the growing popularity of celebrity chefs turned television personalities. The hipsters among us might have done the same, motivated by the desire to be associated with the trendy, contemporary cult of "foodies." Our food plans are also influenced by our schedule: the amount of time we have to eat, the hours of the day that we dedicate to meal time, the locations where we choose to consume food, and the companions that join us each day on our culinary journey. Let us not forget that our emotions have a powerful effect on when, where, and what we eat. In fact, for many of us, emotions can be the predominant influence. My point is that for better or for worse, intentionally or not, we are all adhering to a food plan that is influenced by an extraordinarily diverse and complex array of factors. That said, it is now time to subject your food plan to some *intentional* refinement with your health in mind.

Making new choices with regard to the food we eat may seem like a daunting challenge, one that is often easier said than done, but remember three things:

1. You can do this.
2. You will not feel deprived with the strategy I propose.
3. We are in this together! Through the pages of this book, I am here to help and support you throughout this journey. Rest assured that I have made every attempt to make the transition into your new *manner of living* as seamless as possible. I have also anticipated potential obstacles and offer you the support and solutions for overcoming them on your path to success.

So, take a deep breath,

Inhale.................................... Exhale...

Now, let us clear the plate (figuratively and literally) and start from the beginning.

There are no good foods and bad foods. There are, however, *real* foods and *not real* foods.

<u>GOAL</u>: Eat only whole, real food; the food that your body was designed to use.

The first step in refining your food plan is to choose to eat only *real* food. What does this mean, and how do you make this distinction? The esteemed food journalist and bestselling author Michael Pollan described this with brilliant simplicity in his book *In Defense of Food.*[44] He wrote, and I paraphrase, that anytime you go to a grocery store, imagine you are there with your great, great grandmother. If she would not recognize a food ingredient as being *real* food, then chances are it is not.

The science of food manufacturing has evolved over the past few decades to produce edible products that are affordable, convenient, and taste good. But, as is commonly said in professional nutrition circles, the ingredients in most highly processed foods that prolong *their* shelf life, shorten our own.

The reason for this is that highly processed, artificial food products are often not "food" as nature intended. To once again cite the wise words of Michael Pollan, these are not food but rather are "edible food-like products"[45] that merely provide energy to human beings. The ingredients that make up many of these highly processed edible products are manufactured in laboratories, not in nature. In fact, many of the ingredients used in such products did not even exist 100, 50, or in some cases even just 10 years ago (remember olestra?). It is my opinion, and the opinion of many other nutritionist experts, that these ingredients are not the food that our bodies were genetically designed to use. I subscribe to the school of thought that when it comes to food, nature provides for humanity quite well. In chapter 8, I identify some specific food additives commonly found in artificial, highly processed foods that are known health hazards. In the meantime, from now on choose to fill your pantry and body with whole, *real* foods.

Before I proceed, allow me to clarify that food processing and synthetic food manufacturing is not *always* a bad thing. There are some processed foods that may be healthy, but you have to know what to look for (and by the time you finish reading this book you will!) Not to mention that, in developing nations when food is scarce, food processing is a reasonable solution for maximizing a food's energy and nutrient density to prevent starvation and malnutrition. The problem is that when these same types of highly processed foods are consumed by people who have abundant access to food, the result is that the consumer often ends up *over*-fed and, at the same time, under-nourished. This can be seen in the fact that the overwhelming influx of processed "edible food-like products" that have permeated the kitchens and drive-thrus of America has bred a generation of children that are overfed and, in many cases, obese. Remarkably, similar to their third world counter parts, these obese children are often also suffering from malnutrition. It seems unbelievable, but it is true.

ACTION STEP: In taking steps toward refining your food plan, begin by staying as close to nature as possible when choosing what to eat. Choose to eat minimally or unprocessed, whole, real foods such as vegetables, fruits, nuts, seeds, legumes, grains, meats, fish, oils, herbs, spices, and dairy. These are the foods that we as human beings were designed to eat. Each of these foods contains essential nutrients that without them our bodies would cease to function. I will suggest ways to personalize and refine this recommendation further in the pages to come.

Before getting into more detail, some of you may be surprised to see me encourage you to eat dairy or even meat and oils. You may have pegged these foods in the past as "bad" ones that you should limit and only consume occasionally. I now challenge you to remove the "bad" stigma from these, and all real foods. That's right; don't call that cheese *bad*!

All *real* food is good food. We just need to be mindful not to indulge in too much of a good thing. Even when we enjoy the wonderful goodness of whole real foods we still need to pay attention to quantity, so that we do not overdo it. Fortunately, it is much harder to overeat when consuming whole, real foods then it is when consuming artificial, refined, highly processed foods. Furthermore, when we define food as being good and bad we also tend to evoke emotions that correspond to our consumption of that food. We feel good eating the good foods and bad when we eat the bad ones. This is a dangerous practice because when we deprive ourselves of the "bad" food, psychologically this creates a sense of restriction which often turns into a craving. After all, do we not always want what we cannot have? This is the classic conventional dieter's experience. If we do too much of this, the pleasure of eating disappears and instead a sense of deprivation begins to rule. We crave the bad foods, and even worse, our success is defined by merely settling for the good/healthy ones. Not only does this mindset eliminate the joy of eating, it is simply not sustainable, just ask any chronic dieter. Worst of all, it implies that healthy eating involves the sacrifice of pleasure, which is simply false.

Forsake labeling food as either "good" or "bad." Focus on the delicious diversity and exciting new flavors that a novel or improved food plan can offer! Food should never be approached with guilt, disdain, or a sense of deprivation. Instead, shift your way of thinking and look at creating a food plan with boundless food choices; choices that have always been available to you but that may have been hindered by your past food exposures and experiences up until now.

Now, I respect that some of you are accustomed to a fast food drive-thru or a microwaved boxed meal after a busy day at school or work, and the shift to whole, real food may appear challenging at first. For those of you who feel a little daunted, consider the experience of learning to swim for the first time. At first, the water is cold and, naturally your first inclination is to jump back on land where it is stable, warm and comfortable. In fact, you may need to get back in the pool several times before getting used to the water. But when you allow your body the chance to acclimate to the water long enough, the water no longer feels piercing cold, but instead feels almost warm and comfortable. You then try to take your first swim stroke; of course you would struggle at first, but you wouldn't give up so quickly and retreat to the security and stability of dry land. It is with persistence that you begin to find your balance, and with time and repetition the strokes begin to come naturally.

Making refinements to your current food plan is no different. At first you may be hesitant to make new food choices. You may miss the comfort of old food patterns, habits, conveniences, and dietary addictions. You may feel a little uncomfortable at first. Believe me that your palate will, perhaps slowly, become accustomed to new food taste sensations, novel preparation methods and intriguing new food choices – your palate will delight in the real foods your body is designed to enjoy and thrive upon. There may be times when you revert back to old habits, which is okay, but your stick-to-it-iveness makes it easier and more satisfying to stay with your new food plan. Eventually, eating real foods becomes natural – like swimming – it no longer requires major conscious intent... it just becomes your new routine – your new *manner of living*. With your new understanding and approach to foods, you will not have the sense of restriction or missing out, only pleasure, enjoyment, and vitality – all the wonderful benefits that comes with eating the foods your body has been designed to use.

Which leads us to the next question: "What, exactly, should you eat?"

At this point I can simply give you a list of foods to eat and call it a day, but doing that would be doing you a disservice. I want you to learn how to choose what to eat; to empower you with the understanding of how to make the right choices with regard to your health. Consider the old adage that *if you give a man a fish he eats for a day, if you teach him to fish he eats for a lifetime*. There are few instances where that sentiment is more appropriate than when it comes to eating well for life. As a professor of Clinical Nutrition, I would be remiss not to take this opportunity to teach you a thing or two about nutrition. Therefore, dear pupil, prepare for class.

Chapter 4

All truths are easy to understand once they are discovered;
the point is to discover them.
— Galileo Galilei

Nutrition 101

To understand how to make the right choices when deciding what to eat, it is important to first start with the basics. My years in clinical practice helping patients shed unwanted fat has convinced me that it is critical to build a strong foundation of healthy eating habits in order to be successful. I have found that patients who understand the basics about food and nutrition have an easier time developing good eating habits and make better choices as to what foods to eat, and which ones to avoid. So, to help you build your new nutritional foundation, I now will don my Professor of Clinical Nutrition hat and begin:

Students, welcome to Nutrition 101.

Nutrition is quite complex, yet there are some fundamental concepts that are easy to grasp and allow us to appreciate what our body truly needs. I have broken these concepts down into eleven short easy-to-understand lessons that we will cover in this chapter.

Lesson #1: Macronutrients and Micronutrients

All foods without exception can be described by their two components: micronutrients and macronutrients. Macronutrients (*macro* meaning large) are the large, measurable components of our foods, and they are the nutrients that our bodies need a lot of. There are only three macronutrients (not counting water, which we also need a lot of); they are protein, fats/oils, and carbohydrates. We measure macronutrients in grams (the weight) and calories (the measure of the amount of *energy* the nutrient provides). All foods contain at least one, and in some cases all three, of these macronutrients.

Micronutrients (*micro* meaning small), are the vitamins and minerals found in foods. They are called micronutrients because our bodies do not require very much of them. Although they are not a source of energy (they do not have calories) and our need for these nutrients is small, they are immensely important and are inextricably linked to our ability to survive and to thrive.

Lesson #2: Essential and Non-Essential Nutrients

The human body is amazing. If you feed the human body one type of fat, it can convert it into another type of fat that it needs. What this means is that you do not have to eat _all_ the types of fat that are found in your body as there are some the body can manufacture on its own. The same holds true for the other macronutrients as well as some of the micronutrients. However, while this remarkable backup redundancy mechanism exists for many nutrients, it does not exist for all of them. There are some nutrients that we need and can only get from what we eat; these are called "essential" nutrients. These nutrients that we cannot make on our own are required precursors of important molecules that support essential body functions. If we do not consume them in sufficient quantities we will begin to demonstrate signs and symptoms of nutritional deficiency. Categories of essential nutrients include certain vitamins (including vitamins C, and B_3), minerals (including potassium and magnesium), fatty acids (such as alpha-linoleic acid an omega 3 fatty acid) and the amino acids that we get from consuming protein.

There are also some micronutrients that we call "non-essential". These are pretty much all the other nutrients. Do not let the name fool you; these nutrients are just as important for human health as the essential ones. The difference is that our bodies can generally make these non-essential nutrients on its own so, we do not need to consume these nutrients in abundance or in some cases, at all. Examples of non-essential nutrients include cholesterol and select amino acids like alanine or taurine.

Finally, there is a third group of nutrients that are considered "conditionally essential". Conditionally essential means that as the name suggests, under some conditions we may require a greater intake of these nutrients. For example, if my intake of an essential fatty acid is low, then I cannot make the rest of the fats that my body needs. I would therefore need to increase my intake of some of the fats that I am not making. In this example, a non-essential nutrient becomes essential (since I'm not making it) and is called "conditionally essential." Other instances when an increased intake of select nutrients might be required are when we are not producing enough to meet our needs due to an interaction with a medication, or due to the presence of a disease that is leading to rapid depletion of a nutrient, or in some cases, our natural production of certain nutrients may decline with age. Vitamin D is a good example of a nutrient that our body can normally produce on its own through sunlight exposure (non-essential) but, as we age or due to select health conditions, our body may not be producing enough and thus, we need to increase our intake of it through food and/or nutritional supplementation.

Lesson #3: Vitamins

Vitamins are a class of micronutrients that support and/or facilitate every single biochemical reaction, and even the structure, of our body. Simply put, we need them to survive.

Much of what we know today about vitamins started with a crew of sailors who had bleeding gums. True story. It was in 1747 when a Scottish physician name James Lind, serving on the Royal Navy ship the H.M.S. Salisbury, carried out experiments on sailors who were suffering from scurvy. Interestingly, this was the first ever documented clinical trial in the history of medicine![46] Lind proved through his study that citrus fruits cured scurvy. We later learned that scurvy is a disease that results from a deficiency of vitamin C. Vitamin C is necessary to maintain the integrity of the connective tissue, especially collagen, in our body. Without vitamin C the sailors were unable to generate new healthy collagen-rich tissues (including their blood vessels) and blood leaked out of their capillaries and their gums. As you might expect, sailors with scurvy also had many bruises. If vitamin C levels are not restored, this deficiency will lead to death.

This experiment demonstrated that while the body is largely self-sustaining, we do depend on our environment and our food to maintain optimal health. The body can heal itself but in order to do so, it must be provided the right resources. The example above illustrates that vitamin C is necessary for maintaining the integrity and health of the human body. Yet, as critical as it is, the body can only store a limited amount of vitamin C and these stores are quickly depleted if fresh supplies of this vitamin are not consumed. Vitamin C is therefore an essential nutrient. We must get it regularly from the food we eat *each day*.

There are only two vitamins that we produce endogenously: niacin and vitamin D. There are two others that healthy bacteria in our gut make for us, biotin and vitamin K. Together these four vitamins are generally deemed non-essential vitamins. However, there are times when we do not produce enough of them, or our physiologic need for them increases. For this reason, it is more appropriate to consider these vitamins as conditionally essential. In general, however, we need to get the rest of the vitamins (including vitamins C, B6, folate, thiamine, riboflavin, etc.) from our food sources every day. If not, in time we will begin to show signs of deficiency just like the vitamin C deficient sailors.

Conversely, if we consume too much of some vitamins, we can show signs of excess; so again, it is possible to have too much of a good thing. Problems with micronutrient excess are typically limited to minerals and fat-soluble vitamins. The vitamins that are fat soluble, namely vitamins A, D, E, and K require fats and oils to be absorbed into the body and excessive amounts can be stored for extended periods of time in our fatty tissues, including the liver. Therefore, consuming too much of these vitamins can lead to organ toxicity.

Water soluble vitamins, like vitamin C, are not stored in high concentrations and generally remain in the blood. If we intake too much, the excess is typically just filtered by our kidneys and expelled from the body in our urine. Fortunately, when vitamins are consumed from natural food sources (in reasonable amounts) they rarely result in pathological excess. Nearly all case studies of vitamin excess or toxicity are from excessive consumption of dietary supplements, not from excessive consumption of the nutrients from whole, real foods.

Lesson #4: Minerals

Minerals are like vitamins in that they are micronutrients required by our body in relatively small amounts to function and survive. Without them, basic biochemical processes and structures cease to function properly (or at all). The minerals that we require the greatest amount of are calcium, magnesium, potassium, sodium, zinc, and iodine. However, there are about thirty more that we require to some degree.

Minerals are like fat soluble vitamins in that they are stored in our tissues. For example, we all know that calcium is stored in our bones. However, calcium is also required for other functions in our body; if our levels of calcium become too low to support these other functions, the body leaches calcium out of bone. It is therefore important that we get an adequate intake of minerals from the food we eat. In general, only small amounts of dietary minerals are required, but they are essential nonetheless. That said, just like fat soluble vitamins, consuming too much of certain minerals like iron can be dangerous.

Lesson #5: Phytonutrients

Separate from macro- or micro-nutrients, it has recently been discovered that plant foods contain an additional dietary component known as phytonutrients, sometimes called phytochemicals. Similarly, some animal foods have been found to contain components called zoochemicals. Currently, these components are considered nonessential. However, as our understanding of these food components evolve, we are beginning to appreciate that while they are not essential for preventing overt nutritional deficiency, they may be essential for *optimizing* health and function. Scientific research has only begun to uncover the identities and the hidden value of these nutrients but they have been reported to wield profound benefits to human health ranging from preventing oxidative diseases such as cancer and Alzheimer's to delaying the aging process itself. In chapter 1, I mentioned the compound sulforophane, which is found in broccoli. This compound with known anticancer activity is an example of a phytonutrient, illustrating that phytonutrients have profound implications for optimizing human health and preventing disease.

Lesson #6: Antioxidants

Rather than being a distinct type of food component, antioxidants essentially describe a particular function of certain micro- and phyto-nutrients. Antioxidants neutralize free radicals that oxidize and damage healthy cells. Although these damaging oxidant molecules (free radicals) are harmful to cells and tissues, many are produced as natural byproducts of normal reactions taking place in our body. Free radicals also accumulate as a result of our external environment, with higher concentrations resulting from exposure to smoke and other pollutants. They can also accumulate in response to excessive physical activity. Although activity is beneficial in a myriad of ways, it imposes a great demand on the human body resulting in increased free radical production. It is for this reason that as our activity level increases so do our antioxidant needs and as with all micronutrients, whole, real foods are the optimal source.

The one thing that all the nutrients we have discussed up until now have in common is that none of them contain calories. They are sources of nutrition, but not of energy. Let's look now at the macronutrients, the three nutrients that provide energy, namely protein, carbohydrates, and fats/oils.

Lesson #7: Carbohydrates

Carbohydrates have endured quite a figurative beating over the past few years. But carbohydrates are not as bad as they have been made out to be. They are essential for our survival. In fact, one of the nutrients of choice of our brain is glucose which is the fundamental building block of all carbohydrates. We need carbohydrates; we just need to eat the right kind and the right amount.

Carbohydrates are generally referred to as either simple sugars or complex carbohydrates. A great way to understand the difference between these two types of carbohydrates is by considering how they get into the blood. A simple sugar is essentially straight glucose and is found in "foods" such as candy, cookies, sugary sodas, many processed breakfast cereals, pasta, bagels, and white breads. Eating these simple sugars is tantamount to an injection of sugar! The body has very little work to do to digest these refined sugars and they are easily and immediately absorbed into our bloodstream. Complex carbohydrates, on the other hand, found in foods such as vegetables, legumes, fruits, nuts, seeds, and whole grains, are like eating a time-release capsule of sugar. Our bodies must first digest the long glucose chains, releasing the individual glucoses before they can be absorbed into the body. This results in a slow steady stream of sugar into the blood instead of the spikes of glucose that result from intake of simple sugars.

There are times when you may want an onslaught of simple carbohydrates, such as when running a race. However, for everyday nutrition your body prefers a slower dose of glucose and therefore you should primarily consume complex carbohydrates. As a general rule, food sources of complex carbohydrates are also generally rich in fiber, vitamins, minerals, and phytonutrients. Simple carbohydrates, on the other hand, are ready made for the body to absorb, but aside from offering a quick energy fix, they have very little to offer. In fact, they are often referred to as "empty calories" since they generally provide calories/energy without offering any significant additional nutrients. Simple, refined sugars are found in most processed snack foods, and in some whole, real foods such as honey. However, most whole, real foods tend to be sources of complex carbohydrates.

In recent years, many popular dietary fads have advocated for the complete elimination of all sugars or carbohydrates from our diets. However, our understanding of biochemistry and physiology informs us that this approach is inherently flawed, if not dangerous. We need sugar. In fact, our brain utilizes glucose and relies on it for optimal function. Have you ever noticed how exhausting thinking can be? Just ask any student that has spent hours studying! Sugar is one of the foods of choice for our brain and our brain uses up our sugar supply rapidly during mental activity.[47,48,49] In fact, just being alive, the brain uses up significant amounts of sugar during *all* types of activity. In a given day, the 1.5 kilogram (3.3 pound) human brain utilizes 100 to 150 grams of glucose simply for survival![50] So sugar itself is not the enemy; but excess *added* sugar is.

A Word about Added Sugar

Added sugars refers to the sugars we consume each day *above and beyond* the sugars attained from eating balanced servings of vegetables and other complex carbohydrates from whole, real foods. Specifically, it refers to *any* sugars or caloric sweeteners that are added to foods or beverages during processing or preparation. Common foods with added sugars include snack foods like cookies, bagels, muffins, candy, sweet rolls, pastries, sweetened yogurts, soda, and even sweetened fruit juices. Added sugar also includes the sugar we add to our coffee or berries, or the honey we add to our tea. Because many natural whole foods are a great source of carbohydrates (sugars), <u>your body does not need to get *any* carbohydrate from added sugar</u>.

The American Heart Association (AHA) recommends that **women should not consume more than 100 calories per day of added sugar (about 6 teaspoons or 24 grams of sugar)** and **men should not consume more than 150 calories per day (about 9 teaspoons or 36 grams of sugar)**.[51] Other experts have simply recommended that refined sugars be kept as low as possible.

You might think that this is a lot of added sugar, after all you do not add 6 teaspoons of sugar to your coffee in the morning, but you may be surprised at how much added sugar is in the foods we eat every day. A Pepsi® cola or Coca-Cola® contains 10 teaspoons or 42 grams of sugar! That means that by drinking one cola you exceed the AHA's recommended amount of added sugar *for an entire day* for women or men. If you think fruit juices are lower in sugar, think again. There is almost an identical amount of sugar in Minute Maid® Orange Juice (48 grams of sugar per 16 ounces!) and lemonade[52] as there is in that cola.

TIP! For less sugar and more fiber, vitamins, minerals, antioxidants, and phytonutrients, consume *whole fruit* instead of fruit juices.

Your juice may not be the only thing high in added sugar at the breakfast table. A typical bowl of frosted flakes has about 25 grams of added sugar and sweetened, fruit-flavored yogurt has anywhere from

11 to 27 grams. If you enjoy the occasional cocktail, consider that per ounce, crème de menthe has 14 grams of added sugar and coffee-flavored liqueur has 16 grams of added sugar. If you gravitate toward baked goods, consider that a single average-sized chocolate chip cookie has 2 teaspoons of sugar, a 4-ounce iced cupcake has 6 teaspoons, and a 4-ounce piece of angel food cake contains 7 teaspoons. If you enjoy sweet sauces, 1 tablespoon of ketchup has 4 grams of sugar and 2 tablespoons of honey barbeque sauce has a whopping 13 grams of sugar. Stop for a moment and think about the foods you consume; are you exceeding the daily added sugar recommendation?

In general, to determine if a food is high in added sugars, take a look at its nutrition label:[53]

> ➤ If there is *over* 15g of total sugars per 100g serving of that food it is <u>HIGH</u> in sugar.

> ➤ If there is 5g of total sugars *or less* per 100g serving of that food it is <u>LOW</u> in sugar.

> ➤ If there is *between* 5g and 15g of sugar per 100g serving of that food it has a <u>MODERATE</u> amount of sugar.

At this time, food labels are quite confusing when it comes to sugars. While plans are in place to one day require food manufacturers to clearly identify added sugars on labels, currently the label only reveals the amount of "total carbohydrates" and the amount of "sugars." **Total carbohydrates** refer to the amount of complex carbohydrates and dietary fiber in a food along with the amount of natural sugars (such as lactose in milk products or fructose in fruits), added sugar sweeteners, and the non-digestible additives such as stabilizers and thickening agents in a food. **Sugars** refer to the amount of natural sugars and added sweeteners in the food.

If a food has no fiber, fruit, or milk products in it, then the <u>total</u> amount listed beside "sugars" comes entirely from *added* sugars. For example: a can of Coca-Cola® contains 42 grams of total carbohydrates and 42 grams of sugars. Since Coca-Cola® has no naturally occurring fibers or sugars, this is *all* added sugar. Reading the ingredient label we can verify this and sure enough, "sugar" is the second ingredient on the can of Coca-Cola® right after water. Yogurt on the other hand has some naturally occurring sugars (lactose), so in a typical serving we can generally expect to see anywhere from 3 to 5 grams of sugar even in plain unsweetened yogurt. Anything more than that is coming from added sugars. As mentioned earlier, some sweetened yogurts can have upwards of 26 grams of sugar! To put that into perspective, one Twinkie® has 19 grams of sugar.

Reading the ingredient list on a packaged food offers us even greater insight in helping us determine if a food product contains added sweeteners. Keep in mind that food manufacturers can add natural (such as lactose) and artificial sweeteners (such as high fructose corn syrup) to processed foods and in such cases, both are considered "added sugars". Look for additives like: *corn syrup, high fructose corn syrup, honey, fructose, glucose, fruit juice concentrate, raw sugar, agave nectar, molasses, and various syrups*. The earlier these ingredients appear on the ingredient list, the greater the amount of that sugar in the food. A smart action step is to avoid or at least minimize the consumption of foods with any sugars listed as one of the first three ingredients.

So why the major concern about added sugars? As mentioned previously, the body does not need these sugars *at all*, and the potential for harm from excessive consumption is significant. In addition to increasing the propensity for weight gain, excessive consumption of added sugars may contribute to depression and dementia[54] and may even impact our ability to consolidate and retain memories, which detrimentally impacts our ability to learn.[55] Furthermore, excessive added sugar consumption particularly when part of an overall unhealthy dietary pattern, may contribute to detrimental alternations in the composition of our gut flora (the bacteria and other microbes that reside within us) which has been linked to obesity and other chronic disease.[56] Excessive sugar consumption may also alter the body's glucose metabolism, resulting in insulin resistance, metabolic syndrome, and type 2 diabetes mellitus.[57] In turn, those conditions increase the risk of heart disease and early mortality.[58] Prolonged consumption of added simple sugars essentially puts us at risk for diseases that can be challenging to reverse.

Still not convinced that it is worth choosing the raw almonds instead of the candy bar? Consider this: added sugars have also been shown to dull the signals in the brain that tell us to stop eating.[59] When this mechanism is dulled, we are more likely to reach for seconds and thirds, and even crave those late night snacks. Perhaps this is another reason why we see increased rates of weight gain and obesity in those that consume excessive amounts of added sugars.

Need even more convincing? A 2014 study published in the Journal of the American Medical Association found that overconsumption of sugar may increase your risk of dying from cardiovascular disease even if you have a normal BMI ("normal" weight). The researchers found that greater sugar consumption doubled the risk of death and the more sugar one consumed over the course of the 15-year study the more their risk of dying increased regardless of their age, weight, or amount of physical activity.[60]

If you experience cravings for added sugars, the next chapter is for you! Together we will explore a solution to stop those cravings once and for all. Eating in a manner that slows the release of sugar into the blood stream will curb your cravings and satisfy your hungry brain and belly.
The take home message is to choose sources of complex carbohydrates primarily from vegetables, nuts, seeds, and fruits. Not only will all these carbohydrates provide the preferred slow release of glucose, but these foods provide fiber and are rich in vitamins, minerals, antioxidants, and phytonutrients.

As we come to the end of Lesson #7, you may wonder why whole grains and legumes were left off of the list of carbohydrates described in the previous paragraph. Aren't they also smart choices when it comes to carbohydrates? The answer is unequivocal: it depends.

Lesson #8: The Whole Grain Controversy

Grains and legumes are rich in complex carbohydrates, and like the other complex carbohydrates described above, they too are excellent sources of fiber, vitamins, minerals, antioxidants, and phytonutrients. So what's the problem? Grains and legumes in their raw, unprocessed forms contain a compound called phytic acid (or phytate) which has been the subject of much controversy. Those experts who advocate against consuming foods rich in phytate cite evidence that it essentially "grabs on to" or chelates, essential minerals such as iron,[61] manganese,[62] calcium,[63] and zinc[64] in the intestines.[65,66] Not only is the chelated mineral prevented from being absorbed into our bodies, but other studies also suggest that phytic acid inhibits digestive enzymes in our gut leading to *even more* problems with our digestion and subsequent ability to absorb essential nutrients.[67] Thus, it may be advisable for some of us to reduce our intake of grains and legumes, or at least consume them more mindfully.

However, like every good controversy, there is another side to this story. While phytic acid does have some questionable effects on our health, it also appears to offer some significant benefits. Studies have suggested that phytic acid found in grains and legumes can actually be considered a phytonutrient in that it not only has significant antioxidant properties, but also has potential anticancer benefits as well.[68] Another argument supporting the consumption of this controversial compound is that the chelating ability of phytic acid may actually be beneficial in some instances. Phytic acid may prevent excessive absorption of minerals like iron, which can potentially be harmful to our health when consumed and absorbed in excess. Furthermore, it appears that even if phytic acid does cause a decrease in mineral absorption, it may only be temporary; over time our body appears to adjust to the mineral imbalances they impose. As an example, several studies show that subjects given high levels of whole wheat at first excrete more calcium than they take in, but after several weeks, they appear to adapt and no longer excrete excess calcium.[69]

To eat phytic acid or not to eat phytic acid? That is the question! While Hamlet may never have asked that precise question, I bet you just did. What is a well-intentioned eater supposed to do? Foods that contain phytic acid are generally considered healthy. In fact, legumes and whole grains have long been celebrated for their nutritional benefits. So here are three important considerations:

1. **How we prepare food matters**. It matters so much that I have dedicated an entire chapter of this book to food preparation. For now, know that the manner by which we prepare our food can significantly affect the phytic acid content. For example, heat used to cook a food will reduce its

phytic acid content. Soaking legumes or whole grains prior to cooking will reduce the phytic acid content even further. Soaking them in acidic mediums such as yogurt, buttermilk, or water with lemon juice or vinegar will reduce the content *even* further.[70] The figure that follows shows different preparations of the grain quinoa and the effect on phytic acid levels in the food.

Example: **QUINOA PHYTIC ACID REDUCTION**[71]

Process	Phytic Acid Reduction
Cooked for 25 minutes at 212 degrees F (100°C)	15-20 percent
Soaked for 12-14 hours at 68 degrees F (20°C) then cooked	60-77 percent

2. **A well-balanced diet is the best solution to support adequate mineral absorption and healthy digestion.** If you are adhering to a food plan that is well-balanced, as you most certainly will be by the time you finish this book, incorporating foods sources of phytic acid is not a problem. Studies have shown that dietary patterns that are abundant in vegetables rich in vitamin C, like kale and strawberries, or foods that are rich in beta carotene, like carrots, may actually counter the inhibitory effect of phytic acid on iron absorption.[72,73,74] It is therefore, not necessary to completely eliminate phytic acid from our diet; we simply should keep our intake at a reasonable level while consuming a diet abundant in vegetables, proteins, and healthy fats.

3. **Trust your gut.** Literally. Did you know that an estimated 100 trillion microorganisms representing more than 500 different species inhabit the normal healthy bowel? These beneficial gut-dwelling bacteria are essential for supporting optimal health. These microbes keep pathogens (harmful microorganisms) in check, aid in digestion and absorption of nutrients, support our immune function, and even provide nutrition by synthesizing vitamins. They also produce an enzyme called phytase, which actually helps break down phytic acid.[75] Thus, if you possess good digestive health and normal

gut flora, your body is well suited to consuming foods containing phytic acid without suffering significant consequences.

NOTE: phytic acid in grains is different from gluten, which is a protein that is also found in many grain products. Gluten sensitivities and gluten allergies will be discussed separately in chapter 18.

Because we are all a little different, there are some people that do need to limit their phytic acid consumption more than others. In practical terms, this means properly preparing phytic acid-rich foods in a manner that reduces the phytic acid content and restricting consumption to two or three servings per day while adhering to a well-balanced, nutrient dense manner of eating.

Those that may need to be most mindful of phytic acid intake include:

1. **People with a food allergy, intolerance, or sensitivity:** You may know someone who is allergic to peanuts or gluten. When someone is **allergic** to a food or food component, their body perceives that food as an invader and mounts an immune response against it. Some food allergies are mild with symptoms ranging from itchiness to hives, others are severe and can even be life threatening.

   Food intolerances are different. These are far more common than food allergies and are the result of the inability to effectively digest a certain food. As a result, food intolerances often result in gastrointestinal disturbances like bloating, gas, nausea, or diarrhea. You may know someone who is lactose intolerant; this is one of the most common dietary intolerances worldwide.[76] People who are lactose intolerant lack the enzyme lactase, which is required to break down lactose, a sugar found in many dairy products. Someone with lactose intolerance will therefore experience digestive disturbances when they consume foods that contain lactose such as milk or certain cheeses.

   Food hypersensitivity is not as well understood as food allergies or intolerances. This is when someone simply has a negative reaction to a certain food or food component such as gluten, soy, or monosodium glutamate (MSG). Food hypersensitivities can be inconsistent and variable, even in the same person. Symptoms often present as gastrointestinal problems but may also present as headaches, joint pain, weakness, or fatigue.

If you suspect that you have an allergy, intolerance, or hypersensitivity to grains or legumes, please see your doctor, a certified nutritionist specialist (CNS), or a dietician. Food allergies can be diagnosed with blood tests and intolerances can be diagnosed with blood tests and a dietary food journal. An "elimination diet" can often be an effective way to identify food intolerances or sensitivities. (The "elimination diet" is discussed further in chapter 18).

2. **Vegans:** When adhering to a vegan dietary pattern (where no animal products are consumed), people often rely heavily on grains and legumes as dietary staples. While these foods are excellent sources of nutrition, through the effect of phytic acid it is possible that excessive consumption may increase vulnerability to mineral deficiencies in vegans, specifically iron deficiency. This is of particular concern since many vegetarians already find it challenging to consume iron in adequate amounts. Anemia may result with inadequate iron consumption and/or absorption. Anemia is a condition marked by fatigue and weakness that occurs when the body does not have enough healthy red blood cells to carry oxygen to body tissues. If left untreated, the consequences can be severe. Low levels or iron, folic acid, and vitamin B12 in the vegan diet place vegans at high risk for this condition. To prevent anemia, vegans should monitor iron and other nutrient levels periodically though routine blood work that can be ordered by any doctor. In fact, this simple blood test should be a part of every vegan's regular preventive health plan. Vegan or not, *always be an advocate for your own health.* Ensure you communicate your needs to your doctors as not every doctor will inquire about your eating habits, unless you initiate the dialogue. In a later chapter I will present some additional suggestions on how you can refine your manner of eating if you

choose to adhere to a vegetarian food plan and still ensure a nutritious and abundant diet.

3. **People with compromised gut health.** If you are at risk for or suspect you may have dysbiosis (abnormal gut flora caused by an overgrowth of undesirable microorganisms or the absence of the protective good bacteria) you may benefit from limiting your intake of phytic acid.

It is important to note that dysbiosis is more common than you might think. Dysbiosis may be caused by prolonged antibiotic use either as a child or adult. Additionally, conditions including, but not limited to, irritable bowel syndrome, inflammatory bowel disease, rheumatoid arthritis, and even chronic physical and/or emotional stress, and you guessed it – a manner of eating that is consistently high in simple sugars and overly processed foods - have all been linked to detrimental changes to the composition of our intestinal microflora.[77,78,79]

But that is not all. Recent studies have suggested that alternations in our gut flora compromises our immune function and can also be seen with and/or contribute to diseases as diverse as obesity, diabetes, atherosclerosis, colorectal cancer, nonalcoholic fatty liver disease, and even select mental health conditions including depression, anxiety, and autism.[80,81,82,83,84]

To help restore digestive health, begin by talking to a certified nutritionist or other licensed healthcare provider. They will often begin by identifying the underlying cause of the dysbiosis and then create a plan to help remove or minimize the causative factors and restore normal balance to the gut microflora. To accomplish this, often practitioners will recommend supplementing your manner of eating with *lactobacilus acidophilus* and other healthy bacteria. Foods and supplements that contain certain kinds of beneficial live bacteria are known as **probiotics**. Probiotics can be consumed as dietary supplements, but they can also be found in foods such as unsweetened yogurt, a drinkable cultured milk called *kefir*, and a cultured black tea called *kombucha*. Probiotics are also often found in fermented foods like sauerkraut, *miso* (made from fermented soybeans and used to make soup and other Japanese dishes), and the popular common Korean side dish *kimchi*.

It is also important to supply the body with sources of **prebiotics.** Prebiotics are food ingredients we cannot digest but that beneficially stimulate the growth and activity of the healthy gut bacteria. They are essentially the food for the probiotics. Examples of dietary sources of prebiotics include: insoluble fiber sources like apples or oats, and foods such as onions, asparagus, Jerusalem artichoke (sunchoke), and jicama. (By the way: jicama happens to be one of my favorite crunchy replacements for chips when I enjoy a dip. Try it!) Finally, an overall healthful dietary pattern like the one described in this book, will further support the maintenance of a healthy gut flora. [85,86]

Lesson #9: Fats and Oils

Let us shift our attention now to fats and oils. Similar to carbohydrates, fats and oils have also long been misunderstood and as a result, often receive a bad rap. Allow me to eliminate all misconceptions once and for all. Fat is not the enemy; fat is good![87] Just a few pages ago we discussed essential and non-essential nutrients. Well, some fats and oils are known as "essential fatty acids." As their name states, these fats are essential. Approximately two thirds of our brain is made up of fats. Fats are also essential for making up the membranes of every cell in our body and supporting healthy cellular functions; they are critical for maintaining the integrity of our skin, hair, and every organ in our body. They are also necessary for our body to absorb the fat soluble vitamins A, D, E, and K. Whether we like it from an aesthetic point of view or not, we also need fat to store energy, protect our organs from friction and jarring, and insulate us from the cold. We need fats and oils; we just do not need them in excess. Unfortunately, in modern western society we often consume too much and not the right kinds.

As with all things in nutritional biochemistry, understanding fatty acids is a complex business. However, when it comes to what we eat, we really only need to focus on three forms of fatty acids: unsaturated, saturated, and trans (partially hydrogenated) fats.

Alright students… POP QUIZ time!

Which of the following fats has been shown to have absolutely no health benefit, and may actually be harmful?

a. Unsaturated fats, like those found in avocados, fatty fish, and nuts
b. Saturated fats, like those found in coconut, poultry, beef, and eggs
c. Trans fats, like those found in processed baked goods such as cookies, chips, and crackers

ANSWER: c

If you got that right, congratulations!

Did you know that in addition to the more obvious places like processed and packaged cookies, chips, and crackers, trans fats can also be found in cans of tomato paste and in soups? Trans fats are sometimes found in the most unpredictable places, so make sure you read the ingredient list on all food labels. Keep in mind, there is no biochemical or physiological need for trans fats. In fact, our body does not know what to do with them! It is almost like eating a plastic toy. Trans fats may be edible, but they are not real food. Do not eat them.

On the other hand, contrary to what you may have been told, we *do* want to eat saturated fats… in moderation. While *excessive* intake of saturated fats has been linked to inflammation,[88] myocardial infarction,[89] and cancer,[90] moderate amounts are important, nay *essential*, for our health. In fact, a 2014 study published in the prestigious Annals of Internal Medicine, boldly concluded that "current evidence does not clearly support cardiovascular guidelines that encourage …low consumption of total saturated fats".[91] Now, before you reach for the bacon, butter, and fatty steak consider that while the study reported that just reducing saturated fat alone does not appear to confer health benefits, it did not declare that eating *more* saturated fats will. The take-away message from this study is that if your overall manner of eating is inadequate (high in sugar and artificial, processed foods), then it is not the saturated fat that should be your primary concern. Similarly, as part of a healthy overall manner of eating, saturated fat in moderation does not pose a problem and should be included as part of a healthy manner of eating. Choose saturated fats sources such as grass-fed meat, full and low-fat dairy products including cheese, and tropical oils including coconut oil. Since pesticides are fat soluble, when possible opt for organic sources of these high fat foods.

Last but most certainly not least, unsaturated fats are the main fats our bodies were designed to use. These are the fats that should make up the majority of the dietary fats in our food plan and can be found in foods such as nuts, seeds, olives, and olive oil, and fatty fish.

Omega 3 Fatty Acids: Believe the Hype!

One type of unsaturated fatty acid is the ever popular omega-3 fatty acid. One specific omega-3 fatty acid falls into the category of "essential" since our body cannot manufacture it: alpha linoleic acid, often abbreviated ALA. We need ALA and other omega-3 fatty acids to survive, and the best way we can get them is from the bounty that *Mother Nature* has provided. Fish is the best source of these fats; vegetarians will be pleased to know that they can also be found in plant foods such as flax seeds, chia seeds, and walnuts.

Much hype has surrounded omega-3 fatty acids and rightfully so; we need them. Actually, that's doesn't do them justice. We REALLY need them! Omega-3 fatty acids are required to build the membranes of literally every cell in our body; from our skin, to our heart, to our bones, every part of us depends on this fat for healthy functioning. The saying *you are what you eat* has never been as true as when considering essential fatty acids.

When we eat omega-3 fatty acids, our body uses them to build the membrane that surrounds every cell in our body. But the membranes of cells do more than just protect the cell; the membranes store the different types of fat we eat. When cells are subjected to stress or injury, the cells use the stored fats to make other important compounds. If we do not eat the right fats, (and the right amount of the right fats), the body will still manufacture the cell membranes but instead of using the right fats as the building blocks, it is forced to use whatever alternate type of fat is available. So, the simple truth is that if you only feed your body trans fats and saturated fatty acids from chips, burgers, and fries, your cells will not have enough of the omega-3 fatty acids needed to function properly.

When reaching for fats, be sure to choose mostly sources of unsaturated fats like avocado, almonds, walnuts, and olive oil; opt for fatty fish like salmon, herring, sardines, mackerel, and tuna over ground beef. If you eat meat, choose only grass-fed meats (as opposed to grain-fed meats) which are naturally higher in health promoting omega 3 essential fatty acids.

Lesson #10: Protein

All proteins are long chains of amino acids, and amino acids are the building blocks of all our muscle tissue. When we consume protein, enzymes in our stomach and small intestine break these chains down into their component amino acids so they can become accessible to our body. Therefore, when we aim to lose fat and preserve or gain lean muscle, it is critical that we have sufficient levels of amino acids available. But amino acids have other very important functions in the body besides building lean muscle. We require amino acids to produce a number of hormones and neurotransmitters, including serotonin which allows us to feel a sense of well-being and happiness. Furthermore, studies have shown that a modest relative increase in daily protein intake can help improve satiety, facilitate body fat loss, and support maintenance of a healthy body composition.[92,93,94,95,96]

There are twenty different nutritional amino acids required for human health. Our body is able to produce ten of them, so those ten are deemed "non-essential" because we do not need to get them from the food we eat. The other ten, the ones that we cannot produce, are "essential amino acids" and therefore, must be obtained from food. Unlike fats and sugars, the body does not store excess amino acids for later use, so we need to replenish our supply daily. If we do not, and even if we are short just one of those ten essential amino acids, this can lead to the improper formation of *new* muscle tissue, along with a decrease in cellular and tissue function, and compromised synthesis of hormones, neurotransmitters, and cell membranes.

Fortunately, there are many delicious foods sources of essential amino acids! Animal proteins (chicken, eggs, and fish for example) contain all the essential amino acids. Some vegetable protein sources, such as soy and quinoa contain all the essential amino acids as well. But, most other vegetable protein sources do not contain all ten essential amino acids in adequate amounts. Beans, for example, contain adequate amounts of a few essential amino acids while rice contains adequate amounts of the others. Therefore, to get a complete set of all essential amino acids, vegetarians need to eat food sources of complementary proteins, like rice *and* beans, every day. It is worth noting that contrary to what was commonly believed in the past, complementary proteins do not need to be consumed during the same meal. As long as they are consumed during the same day you will still meet your nutritional need and gain a complete set of all essential amino acids.

When choosing the type of protein to eat, we must not only consider sources of essential amino acids but we must also consider everything else we are consuming at the same time. Take red meat, for example. While it is a complete protein source, meaning it is rich in all the essential amino acids, it also seems to have some less desirable nutritional qualities that with each bite of red meat, we introduce into our digestive track.

An interesting study exploring the issue of red meat and mortality was conducted by researchers at Harvard University and published in a January 2012 issue of the Archives of Internal Medicine.[97] The researchers observed more than 110,000 adults over 20 years, and found that consuming just three ounces of *unprocessed* red meat per day resulted in a 13% greater likelihood of death during the course of the study. Even worse, those study participants that ate an additional serving of *processed* meats, such as hot dogs or bacon, saw their risk of death increase by 20%! The good (and not so surprising) news was that choosing healthier sources of protein resulted in lower mortality risk. For example, choosing poultry, dairy, legumes, or fish all resulted in a significant reduction in mortality risk for the men and women participating in the study.

If it is not the protein and amino acids, what is it about red meat that might cause an increased risk of mortality? As I suggested earlier, the blame can be laid on those additional undesired dinner guests that accompany the essential amino acids with each bite of red meat. Excessive amounts of nitrites (used to flavor and preserve processed meat) and iron have been implicated as possible contributing factors.[98] If the potentially damaging effects of excessive consumption of these compounds is not enough, other harmful chemicals are also produced as a result of common meat cooking methods, which may be adding further insult to injury. I will discuss the matter of food preparation in detail in chapter 9.

So, in order to get all your essential amino acids while limiting your intake of less healthy foodstuffs, choose healthful complete protein sources such as fish, shellfish, eggs, plain Greek yogurt, poultry, and if you eat beef, choose organic, grass-fed beef. If you prefer a vegetarian diet, complete proteins sources include quinoa and soybeans. Remember that most other vegetarian protein sources, like brown rice and legumes such as lentils and kidney beans, contain incomplete proteins. To ensure that you consume adequate amounts of all ten essential amino acids when adhering to a vegetarian manner of eating, make sure you choose complementary vegetarian protein sources during the same day.

ACTION STEP: To improve satiety, and to support a healthy body composition, aim to consume some *healthy* protein source (animal protein or vegetarian protein) with *every* daily meal and snack.

Lesson #11: Does Counting Calories Add Up?

It is well accepted that fat contains nine calories per gram, and carbohydrates and proteins have four calories per gram. Fiber is often placed in a separate category as having two calories per gram. These values inform the calorie counts listed on food labels that many among us have grown to depend on as our guide to track our overall caloric intake each day. However, recent scientific evidence has revealed that this practice may not be as foolproof as once thought.

Outside of our body we can accurately measure the energy or calorie value of any given food. But once we eat them, things change. Complex, whole foods are more challenging for our body to break down. So while in the lab we may be able to measure the amount of energy that food contains, the complex composition of the food makes it difficult for us to access all the available energy in that food when we consume it. Some foods even require us to expend significant energy to digest them, thereby reducing the net caloric impact of that food. Good examples of this include fibrous plant foods. The cell walls of certain plant foods are tough! They require us to expend significant energy as part of the digestive process to break through them and access the nutrients and the energy they contain.[99] Some whole foods are so tough to access that they may pass through our body completely intact! This means that not only are we unable to access all the energy (calories), we also lose out on the nutrients.

A 2012 study at the USDA shed some light on this phenomenon by investigating the calories in almonds. Researchers found that when the "average" person eats almonds she receives just 128 calories per serving rather than the 170 calories per serving listed on the label.[100] The issue was not that the label was wrong. The issue was that almonds are an example of a food that requires significant expenditure of energy to digest and absorb, so the net calorie intake is less than the actual calorie content of that food.

During our lesson on carbohydrates earlier in this chapter, I described how eating simple sugars is like an injection of glucose directly into our bloodstream. Because simple sugars in candies or white bread require very little energy to digest and absorb, the number of calories on the label of such foods is likely identical to the amount of calories we obtain when we eat them; the processing of the food has done most of the work for us already! Almonds, on the other hand, are an example of a whole food that requires significant energy for the body to digest and absorb. The added energy expended breaking down almonds and complex whole, real foods like it, (including vegetables, fruits, other nuts, seeds, complex whole grains, etc.) is not reflected on the calorie count listed on a food label.

An interesting 2010 study illustrates this concept. Participants in one group were provided either 600 or 800 calories of whole wheat bread with nuts and seeds served with cheddar cheese. Another group of participants were provided the same number of calories in the form of white bread with a "processed cheese product." The findings were remarkable: those in the whole wheat group expended twice as much energy digesting the food as those in the white bread group.[101] Twice as much!

It appears that the more we process a food, the easier it is for us to access the energy it contains.[102] Even the process of cooking affects the amount of energy we gain from the food. This is because the heat ruptures plant and animal cells in the food which reduces the amount of work our body has to do when we eat that food. While this seems like an argument in favor of eating raw foods, keep in mind that some whole foods (including many vegetables) are so complex that our digestive process is ineffective at gaining access to all the nutrients the food contains without a little help from the cooking process. Therefore, when working to improve your body composition, it is smart to often choose to eat whole raw foods but do not avoid cooking altogether; like most things in life, a balance provides the best result. Just keep in mind that the more a food is processed before we eat it, the easier it is for us to digest it and in turn, the more likely its calorie label is accurate. If you process your food enough, you will actually gain as many calories as the packaging says.

There is one additional consideration: as humans we are all beautifully unique. Not only do we have different personalities, eye color, and hair color, but as it turns out we metabolize and digest food differently as well. Some of us need to do more work than others to digest and absorb the same foods. Even if two people eat the identical food that has been prepared in an identical way, they will not obtain the exact same number of calories. This is because we all have different amounts of enzymes in our digestive track and different microbes in our gut that contribute to the digestive process. The anatomical size of our digestive tracks may even have subtle but meaningful differences. Using lactose as an example, someone that lacks the enzyme lactase will gain less energy from milk as one that possesses that enzyme. Without this enzyme, lactose goes through the body undigested, retaining many or all of its calories on the way out.

The Bottom Line:

What does this all mean? It means that we need to be careful not to focus too much of our attention on counting calories. Monitoring calorie intake is helpful only as a *guide* of our overall intake. There is no point in becoming obsessive over every single calorie consumed. Furthermore, this also means that we now understand that not all calories are created equally. From a genetic standpoint, a nutritional standpoint, and now from an energy standpoint, we see that our body reacts differently to different types of foods. Quality matters. The foods that consistently promote heath and optimize body composition are those foods that are unprocessed or minimally processed, whole, real foods.

Graduation

Congratulations! You have officially passed Nutrition 101. You now have a foundational understanding of nutrition that will help you make smart decisions when deciding which foods to eat. In the coming chapters I continue to share with you additional important information about food and nutrition that will make it even easier to make informed decisions about eating well, for life! But first, come join me for the next stage of our journey as we dine on the Mediterranean.

Chapter 5

One cannot think well, love well, sleep well, if one has not dined well.
— Virginia Woolf

Dining on the Mediterranean

Imagine you are along the Mediterranean coast with crystal blue water gently caressing the white sand beaches as the warm sun blazes down upon your skin and a gentle, cool wind tempers the warmth of the air making it the most perfect climate you have ever experienced. After completing a stroll along the coast, you take a seat among friends and family at a table with a feast overflowing with colorful vegetables and fruits, perfectly cooked fish and meats delicately seasoned with fresh herbs and spices, and legumes glistening as the sun hits the extra virgin olive oil that gently blankets their façade. Two glasses are positioned adjacent to each table setting, one filled with water and the other filled with a ruby red wine shimmering like a gemstone. This, dear reader, is the type of food plan you are going to be on; inspired by the Mediterranean dietary pattern, this is a glimpse of your new manner of eating. While the warm sun, cool breeze, and ocean views may not be available to everyone, the rest is. This food plan is not about going without; this food plan invites you to delight in all that you may have been missing.

The main inspiration for the food plan that I will be sharing with you in the pages to come is the Mediterranean dietary pattern. This manner of eating reflects the *traditional* nutritional habits of the people of Crete, Greece, Southern Italy, Spain, Southern France, Portugal and parts of the Middle East. It includes foods such as olive oil, fresh vegetables, legumes, nuts, seeds, whole grains, herbs, spices, eggs, yogurt, cheeses, lean meats, and fish all topped off (if you like) with a great glass of wine; all delicious, satisfying, whole real foods.

You may wonder why, among all the dietary patterns across the globe, does this one stand out; what is so good about the traditional dietary habits of people from around the Mediterranean Sea? To appreciate the value of this manner of eating let us begin by meeting Dr. Ancel Keys, the physician that first shed light on the benefits of adhering to this dietary pattern.

During 1945, while stationed in Salermo, Italy, an American physician named Ancel Keys observed that, despite poverty and limited access to medical care, rates of chronic disease in the region surrounding the Mediterranean Sea were among the lowest in the world and life expectancy was among the highest.[103] These facts led Dr. Keys and his team of researchers to study the lifestyle of those residing in this region to unlock their secrets. Their inquiry led them to the conclusion that dietary pattern was the key.[104]

Since that time, well over 40 scientific studies have shown that adhering to the Mediterranean dietary pattern can keep you alive and healthier, longer than virtually any other manner of eating. The results of a 10-year study published in the Journal of American Medical Association demonstrated that adherence to a Mediterranean dietary pattern and a healthful lifestyle were associated with more than a 50% lower rate of all-cause mortality and cause-specific mortality.[105] Translation: Your risk of dying from the diseases that can kill you is reduced by more than 50% just by living well and eating some delicious foods.

This manner of eating has been shown to lower your risk of dying from heart disease, cancer, and from developing type 2 diabetes, high cholesterol, and high blood pressure. As if that isn't enough, it has also been shown to prolong the *quality* of life, and not just the quantity of life. The Mediterranean dietary pattern has been linked to reduced rates of depression, lower risk of dementia and developing Alzheimer's disease, and a reduced risk of becoming obese. It has also been shown to be effective in aiding in the loss of body fat and in supporting the maintenance of a healthy body composition. [106,107,108,109,110,111,112]

To date, one of the most exciting studies demonstrating the profound benefits of this manner of eating was published in 2013 in the Journal of American Medical Association.[113] To test the benefits of the Mediterranean dietary pattern, a team of researchers in Spain used the same study design that is used to test the efficacy of new drugs. They performed what is called a *randomized controlled trial*, which is considered to be the gold standard of clinical trials, and many experts have called the findings of their study "game-changing".

Why, you may ask?

Here's why:

Over 7,000 men and women between the ages of 55 and 80 participated in the study. *Before* entering the study, each of these 7,000 participants had either type 2 diabetes or at least three of the following major risk factors for heart disease: smoking, high blood pressure, elevated LDL (bad) cholesterol levels, low HDL (good) cholesterol levels, overweight or obesity, or a family history of premature coronary heart disease. Each participant was randomly assigned to one of three different diets groups, received counseling to help support their assigned diet, and was monitored for 5 years.

This is where it gets good.

The researchers found that those participants who adhered to a Mediterranean dietary pattern were 30% less likely to have a heart attack, stroke, or death related to cardiovascular disease than those on a low-fat diet.[114] To offer some perspective, these benefits are similar to the benefits seen in patients taking cholesterol-lowering statin drugs,[115] *without the side-effects.*

Game-changing.

The best part? *It's never too late to start reaping the benefits.*

Remember the study I referred to above that showed this dietary pattern is associated with lowering death rates by more than 50%? This finding was for individuals aged 70-90 years of age![116] The other study that showed this dietary pattern is just a good as a statin drug for decreasing cardiovascular disease risk and death? If you recall, the study participants were up to 80 years of age and *already* had signs of and risk factors for cardiovascular disease before joining the study! Pretty powerful stuff.

Among all the ways of eating that has been the subject of scientific investigation and research, the Mediterranean approach consistently stands out as a leader. So what is it about the foods and the people of the Mediterranean that makes it so exceptional? There are three principle factors that set it apart from most other dietary patterns:

1. Food choices tend to have a low glycemic index/load
2. Phytonutrient rich plant foods are emphasized
3. Foods choices tend to have anti-inflammatory properties

Let us look at the importance of each of these three qualities.

The Glycemic Index and the Glycemic Load

The **Glycemic Index**, (*glyco* – sugar, *emia*-blood), often abbreviated GI, is a ranking of foods that contain carbohydrates that is based on their effect on blood sugar levels. This index reports how much your blood sugar increases in the two to three hours after eating a particular food.

Foods with a *low* GI produce only small fluctuations in our blood sugar and insulin levels.[117] This slow, steady rise, without much blood sugar fluctuation, acts a lot like a time-release capsule of sugar. This is beneficial to our body in that all our cells need to be fed with sugar, so a slow release is perfect for

Glycemic Index (GI)
GI of 70 or more = high
GI of 56 to 69 = medium
GI of 55 or less = low

optimum function and utilization. In contrast, foods with a *high* GI produce wild fluctuations in our blood sugar and insulin levels. These foods act more like a sugar injection which pushes our body to extremes, which, over time, leads to increased risk of a variety of chronic diseases, including obesity.

While the GI provides us with a frame of reference for how quickly a carbohydrate is turned into simple sugar and enters our bloodstream, the **Glycemic Load** (GL) gives us a better picture of the overall impact of a particular food. This is because it takes into account the *serving size* of a food, the actual amount of the food you would consume. For example, watermelon has a high GI ranking of 76, but its GL is a relatively low at 8 per 1 cup serving. Most nutritionists agree that we should not be exposing our body to a GL of greater than 50 each day. To

Glycemic Load (GL)
GL of 20 or more = high
GL of 11 to 19 = medium
GL of 10 or less = low

understand the impact of food on our blood sugar and why it matters to our health, let us look at what happens each time you consume a simple cookie.

Your Body on a Cookie

There it is, taunting you; calling your name with the promise of a delectable delight to tantalize your taste buds and satisfy your hungry belly. Its sweet aroma seduces your senses. You simply cannot resist and so it happens; your brain sends the signal. You reach for the cookie and place it into your mouth. While a cookie may look like a tasty delight to you, to your body it is merely another source of energy and your hungry body wants access to it. Because the cookie is essentially pure sugar, it has both a very high Glycemic Index and a high Glycemic Load. Beginning in your mouth, you start breaking down that cookie using digestive enzymes in your saliva. This cookie lacks significant amounts of protein and fiber and is just simple carbohydrates. Your body is able to break it down very easily into the simple sugars (glucose) and just as easily, absorb the sugars from your digestive tract into your bloodstream. Immediately, this huge influx of glucose causes your blood sugar levels to skyrocket. You perceive this response as a satisfying rush of energy; however, this it is not a state of being that is most healthful for your body. Instead, you satisfied your hunger with a quick fix.

If you have not eaten in a few hours, eating such sugary snacks certainly raises your blood sugar levels back to their normal range. However, these same sugary snacks, because of their high Glycemic Index and Glycemic Load cause us to overshoot the normal blood sugar levels. Although you may initially feel satisfied, the body does not like this state of excessively high blood sugar. In order to restore a more balanced blood sugar environment, the body goes on high alert. Signals are sent out to activate the release of insulin to quickly cause your tissues to take in the excessive glucose and restore some semblance of order to your physiology.[118] Insulin works to transport the glucose from the blood stream into our cells. But, the excessive glucose that is now in the bloodstream demands the release of excessive amounts of insulin to manage it. However, the result of this high level of insulin secretion is that cells and tissues now gather up too much glucose. Have you ever felt the feeling of coming down from a sugar high? What happened is that the massive release of insulin caused your blood levels of glucose to drastically drop! This resulted in your feeling sluggish and fatigued.

Naturally, your instinct is to restore the high you were feeling right after eating that cookie so instead of reaching for some grilled salmon and broccoli, which takes way too long for the body to break down, you reach for another cookie. How can you resist? And so the roller coaster ride begins. Blood sugar goes up and down, up and down. Some call this phenomenon the *vicious cookie cycle*! This is exhausting for your body. Over time, day after day, year after year, your system slows down its ability to respond to your extreme manner of eating. The pancreas, which secretes insulin, gets tired and the tissues that respond to the high levels of insulin become exhausted. The result is that the insulin signals stop working. A condition known as insulin resistance develops. Systemic inflammation and weight gain occur, and ultimately, if this persists, it leads to the eventual onset of type 2 diabetes. As you might have suspected, this state of affairs is not limited to the cookie and foods like it; we also see this same response when you repeatedly eat excessively large quantities of food at one sitting.

That is your body on a cookie. Any questions?

A low Glycemic Index or low Glycemic Load food (such as an avocado, green leafy vegetable, almonds or lentils) has a very different effect in our body when we consume it. These foods contain complex carbohydrates, and it takes time for the body to break them down into individual glucose molecules. This results in a far slower release of glucose into the blood stream, which you perceive as a prolonged energy level. No more 3:00 PM sluggish feeling! Your energy level remains stable throughout the day. Furthermore, your insulin levels remain in control and constant. All remains well within your physiological world.

Foods with a low Glycemic Index (GI) and low Glycemic Load (GL) have consistently been shown to benefit our health and support the maintenance of a healthy body composition. Consider a 2013 study completed at Harvard which compared the effect of consuming meals with the same number of calories, but different GI. The researchers found that the *higher* GI meals not only resulted in greater increases in blood sugar, they also found that it led to increased hunger and even caused an activation of the same regions of the brain associated with reward and craving, that are activated in response to addictive substances like alcohol and drugs.[119] This important study shows us that eating simple carbohydrates like a cookie or white bagel can actually lead to increased cravings, making it even harder for us to adhere to a healthful manner of eating, and further reinforcing the fact (if it is not yet abundantly clear) that the *quality* and not just the quantity of what we eat matters. Lowering the GI or GL of our daily meals has also been shown to help improve cholesterol levels, blood pressure, and even reduce systemic inflammation. [120,121] The best part is that it is also an easy and delicious strategy to incorporate into our food plan.

The Virtues of a Plant-Based Dietary Pattern

Another characteristic of the Mediterranean manner of eating that makes it so good is the emphasis on plant foods. Before you think that we have reached the part of the book where I start unabashedly praising vegetarianism, please understand that contrary to popular belief, vegetarians are not always healthy. Case in point: While my brother was studying for a semester at my alma mater, McGill University in Montreal Canada, he had a roommate who was a proud vegetarian; no meat, no fish, and no eggs, only select dairy was acceptable. The funny thing is that all I ever saw this guy eat was grilled processed cheese sandwiches on white bread, and macaroni and cheese! Sure no cows were harmed, but he sure was! The meals were devoid of most essential nutrients – he was a classic example of someone that was well fed but malnourished; and he was a vegetarian.

This brings up a very important point: vegetarianism appears to be among the healthiest way of eating, if it is done right. The problem is that often amateur vegetarians focus more on what they are *not* eating than what they *are* eating (or what they should be eating). Because there are a few essential nutrients that are challenging for vegetarians to attain, it is important that if you do choose to become a vegetarian you do so in a healthy and responsible way. I discuss many of the special considerations for vegetarians in chapter 6. The reason I bring this up at this stage of our journey is that while vegetarianism is not for everyone, we can all benefit from establishing a plant-based foundation to our food plan.

Well-planned vegetarian diets are often associated with health advantages including lower blood cholesterol levels, lower risk of heart disease, lower blood pressure levels, and lower risk of hypertension and type 2 diabetes.[122] In fact, a 2013 study in Journal of the American Medical Association reported that adherence to a vegetarian dietary pattern has been associated with a reduction of all-cause mortality.[123] Remember those essential micronutrients we discussed in chapter 4? Well, they are almost exclusively found in the domain of plant foods. Incorporating a variety of richly colored vegetables and fruits into our meal plan ensures that we are consuming a wealth of vitamins, minerals, antioxidants, and phytonutrients. Keep in mind; I am not advocating an all-or-nothing dietary change. A vegetarian dietary pattern is not for everyone and you most certainly do not need to eliminate meat and fish from your dining repertoire to be well. What you should do is use vegetables as your primary source of nutrients, the foundation of your manner of eating, and include the animal proteins as the "cherry on top."

Anti-Inflammatory Foods

Most of us think about inflammation when we are injured. We have a cut or a sprained ankle and it becomes inflamed - warm to the touch, red, painful, and swollen. Believe it or not, this type of inflammation is good. It is a protective feature of our body that allows for healing after we have sustained some sort of trauma. This is known as *acute* or short term inflammation. The problem is when inflammation is *chronic* or persistent. Can you imagine your sprained ankle being red and swollen forever? As part of normal life processes, we accumulate micro-traumas in nearly every part of our body. Exposure to environmental pollutants, radiation from the sun, and even the air we breathe, all contribute to these micro-traumas. Naturally, our body responds with acute inflammation at the site of damaged tissues. These damaged tissues can be the arteries, our gastrointestinal tract, and even our brain. The problem is compounded when inflammation is not just limited to one part of the body, but instead is affecting the *entire* body, and is unremitting. This type of inflammation is referred to as *systemic* inflammation.

So what is the relationship between inflammation and food? Systemic inflammation appears to be caused by a variety of factors including what we eat. As described previously, certain preventable factors like obesity and an increased waist circumference can result in the production of chemicals that promote inflammation throughout our body. Excess consumption of select foods such as simple, processed sugar, deep-fried foods, and grain-fed red and processed meat appear to trigger these same pro-inflammatory effects.[124] Mounting evidence is revealing how unhealthy daily food choices are linked to cardiovascular disease through the generation of pro-inflammatory chemicals.[125] But, it is not only about cardiovascular disease. Chronic, systemic inflammation has also been linked to a variety of other health conditions including type 2 diabetes,[126] Alzheimer's disease,[127] and cancer.[128]

In recent years, this recognition that certain foods have anti-inflammatory properties has inspired a new dietary pattern. Popularized by Dr. Andrew Weil, one of the first prominent integrative medicine physicians, the anti-inflammatory dietary pattern encourages the consumption of foods known to reduce inflammation in our body (such as dark green leafy vegetables, salmon and other fatty fish, and raw nuts) while limiting the intake of foods with pro-inflammatory effects. In turn, the reduction of systemic inflammation has been shown to decrease the occurrence and progression of a variety of chronic diseases. In chapter 19 I include a detailed list of all the foods that may promote inflammation, and all the foods that may reduce inflammation in our body.

So how do you know where you stand with regard to systemic inflammation? One way is to analyze the foods you eat; the other more objective way to measure it is by a simple blood test. Ask your doctor to test your **high sensitivity C-Reactive Protein (hs-CRP)** levels. This biomarker is an indicator of systemic inflammation. There is now extensive published scientific literature demonstrating that increased levels of hs-CRP in otherwise healthy individuals may predict future risk of heart attack, sudden cardiac death, stroke, and peripheral arterial disease, even when cholesterol levels are low.[129]

High sensitivity C - reactive protein (hs-CRP) levels and relative risk of cardiovascular disease (CVD):

Relative Risk of CVD:	Low Risk	Intermediate Risk	High Risk
hs-CRP Level:	Less than 1.0 mg/L	1.0 – 2.9 mg/L	Greater than 3.0 mg/L

The majority of the foods found within the Mediterranean manner of eating have natural anti-inflammatory properties.[130] This may help explain why we have observed so many benefits in terms of disease prevention and disease management by people that adhere to this manner of eating. In fact, adherence to the traditional Mediterranean diet is associated with a reduction of hs-CRP[131] even in the absence of weight loss.[132] Therefore, the good news is that no matter what your hs-CRP level is today, you can improve it - thereby reducing your risk of chronic disease - simply by adopting a healthy *manner of living*.

A Word on Wine

When we discuss the Mediterranean manner of eating, sitting outdoors near the sea with a vineyard nearby, it may be hard to imagine having a meal without a glass of rich, beautiful red wine. After all, if a glass of

66

red wine is a staple of their evening meal, and the people of the Mediterranean are generally healthier, it would stand to reason that there may be some benefit. In fact, it has been suggested that there are antioxidant and phytonutrient compounds in red wine which may contribute to the healthful benefits of this dietary pattern. The antioxidants in red wine may help prevent heart disease by increasing levels of HDL cholesterol (our "good" cholesterol) and protecting against artery damage. However, there is still no clear evidence that red wine is better than other forms of alcohol when it comes to possible heart-health benefits. Beyond this, red wine contains a phytonutrient called resveratrol that has been the subject of much attention in recent years. Studies suggest that resveratrol might help protect us from obesity, heart disease and diabetes, reduce systemic inflammation, and even promote longevity. However, most studies on resveratrol have been conducted in mice, not in people, so while the prospect of potential benefits is exciting, the true effects in humans remain unknown at this time.

Overall, the benefits of red wine consumption particularly with regard to supporting our heart health, look promising. So, if a little is good, more is better, right? No! The recommended daily limit of alcohol intake is no more than one drink (12 ounces of beer, 4 ounces of wine or 1 ounces of spirit) for women, and no more than two drinks for men based on body mass and innate ability to metabolize the alcohol. That said, *if you do not drink, this is no reason to start.* And for those of you who do, keep in mind you cannot save up the number of glasses per day and rationalize that "I didn't drink Monday through Thursday so Friday I can have 4 extra glasses!" Nope. It does not work like that. In fact, consuming more than the above amounts in one day, is considered binge drinking, and has dire health consequences.[133]

Simply eating grapes, or eating other food sources of resveratrol such as blueberries and cranberries, has been suggested as one way to get resveratrol without drinking red wine. Being physically active is another way we can get the same HDL boosting benefits that have been observed with consumption of red wine. Also, if you have problems controlling your alcohol intake, then do not use this as an excuse to drink. We can only derive the benefits of red wine if we manage to stay on a plan of low to moderate consumption. Even a little too much intake shifts the scales from a benefit to heart health to exponentially *increasing* our risk for disease and death.

It is worth noting that the American Heart Association <u>does not recommend</u> drinking wine or any other form of alcohol to gain potential benefits. Drinking *too much* alcohol can raise triglycerides, may lead to high blood pressure, heart failure, not to mention an increased calorie intake. Furthermore, we all know that consuming too many calories can lead to obesity and a higher risk of developing type 2 diabetes. Excessive drinking and binge drinking can lead to stroke, cardiomyopathy, cardiac arrhythmia, and even sudden cardiac death.

ACTION STEP: If you do drink wine and are trying to shed body fat, here is a tip to help you still enjoy the wine without overdoing your caloric intake. Wine can be considered as being similar to a fruit in terms of its caloric and nutritional value. Let me clarify that this is by no means an assertion that wine is a viable substitute for eating fruit but rather that this is the closest way to classify it so we can understand how to incorporate it into our food plan. Therefore, on days when you enjoy a glass of wine, choose the wine instead of a serving of fruit that day *and* have an extra serving of vegetables instead. Also, be sure to avoid any other added sugars that day. By making that small substitution, you are maintaining the same caloric intake without losing out on beneficial micronutrients and phytonutrients. Cheers!

Dietary Patterns of Other Cultures

I would be remiss if I neglected to mention that the Mediterranean manner of eating is certainly not the only dietary pattern that has been shown to have profound health benefits. If we look to other traditional dietary patterns around the globe, we see that there are others that also exemplify principles of smart nutrition while supporting the prevention of disease. For example, many herbs and spices used in traditional Indian foods have potent anti-inflammatory properties. In addition, the traditional Japanese dietary pattern contains an abundance of cruciferous vegetables that have been shown to have powerful anti-cancer properties. The traditional Japanese dietary pattern also contains an abundance of fish that are rich in anti-inflammatory omega-3 fatty acids.

So why focus on the Mediterranean dietary pattern? For many of us accustomed to a standard American type dietary plan, it incorporates many foods with which we are familiar. This is an important consideration when deciding to change your dietary pattern. Familiarity with the food types and preparation methods increases your chances of sticking with it. Another, but no less important, reason is that most of the scientific nutritional studies have focused on this manner of eating. That said, there are many delicious and health promoting features of other cultural dietary patterns from across the world that I encourage you to incorporate into your own food plan. To make it easy, I have compiled most of this information for you. I have incorporated the best features from each of these global dietary patterns into my specific recommendations for your new manner of eating outlined in the next chapter.

The chapter that follows will give you the tool to put all the information and recommendations discussed thus far into practice. So dear reader, I now present to you, *the art of eating well.*

Chapter 6

To eat is a necessity, but to eat intelligently is an art.
— La Rochefoucauld

The Art of Eating Well

The moment you have been waiting for! This chapter provides you with a list of the cornucopia of beautiful and delectable food options selected to tantalize your taste buds, satisfy your hunger pangs, and optimize the quality and quantity of your life. That's right; the list of foods that follow will allow you to put into practice all the great stuff that we have discussed thus far.

You are about to see the foods that represent the best from across the globe. These foods are more than just nutrient rich: they possess anti-inflammatory properties, and have a low or moderate glycemic index and load that keep your blood sugar and energy levels steady. These are the foods, herbs, and spices that speak to your genes in the right way, maintaining cellular health, and are rich in vitamins, minerals, and phytonutrients allowing your body to thrive. These are the foods the human body was designed to use. The list is intentionally extensive and therefore adaptable to your taste preferences or to allergies or sensitivities you may have. Most importantly, these foods taste great and are going to fuel you in the way your body needs to be fuelled on the journey that is your new *manner of living*. (Remember, if a particular food is not on the list it does not mean you should never eat it again, it simply means with a few exceptions, it should not be a part of your *usual*, every day manner of eating)

Before we look at *what* to eat, (I promise, we are almost there!) there is one final critical piece of information that you need to be mindful of: *when* and *how much* to eat.

Here are nine ACTION STEPS to help you get the most from your daily menu.

1. **Listen to your body.** Become familiar with cues that signal hunger and satisfaction. Your body takes good care of you when you feed it whole, real foods. If you are from the school of thought that depends on taking a calorie inventory of all you eat, remember to be careful not to put too much trust into calorie counting. As we learned in Nutrition 101 in chapter 4, calorie counting is not yet a perfect science and not all calories are created equally. Use calories as a guide to inform your daily energy needs, and do not rely only on your eyes to guide the amount of food you consume; listen to your gut when it comes to determining how much to eat. If you suspect you have lost the ability to heed your body's hunger and satiety signals, do not worry. In an upcoming chapter I will teach you how to become reacquainted with these cues. In the meantime, just **aim for three meals and two snacks each day.**

   While calorie counting is not foolproof, being familiar with an estimate of one's daily caloric needs can still be a helpful guide to provide you with a general idea of how much energy your body needs. In reality, portion distortion common to modern society has left many of us out of touch with what quantity of food our body actually requires.

   In general, daily caloric needs for most people will range from approximately 1,200 kcals to 2,200 kcal per day. Petite, small framed women typically fall on the low end of this range, while taller, larger framed men are on the higher end.

Depending on your size, aim for meals to range between 300-600 kcals and snacks to range from 150-200 kcals.

To arrive at a more precise estimate of your daily energy needs, break out your calculator and use the following simple equations:

a) **Calculate your Basal Metabolic Rate (BMR)**
   The basal metabolic rate (BMR) is the amount of energy/calories your body uses at rest. The following equation (known as the *Mifflin St. Jeor* equation) will provide a good estimate of your BMR.[134,135,136]

   Note: To convert your weight to kg, divide your weight in pounds by 2.2. To convert your height to cm, multiply your height in inches by 2.54.

Women:	BMR= (10 X weight in kg) + (6.25 X height in cm) – (5 X age in years) – 161

Men:	BMR= (10 X weight in kg) + (6.25 X height in cm) – (5 X age in years) + 5

My BMR	kcal

b) **Adjust your energy needs based on your activity level:**
   Add activity calories[137] by multiplying your BMR from above by the appropriate activity factor (BMR x activity factor) based on your *current* level of activity as described in the chart that follows.

Your Current Activity Level	Activity Factor	Details
Sedentary / Minimal Daily Activity	1.20	Minimal daily physical activity, desk job
Mild / Low Daily Activity	1.37	Physical activity for less than 30 minutes, 5 times per week/or light activity 1-3 days per week
Active / Moderate Daily Activity	1.55	Physical activity 30-60 minutes (or less time but high intensity) 3 - 5 times per week/or mild activity 6-7 days per week
Very Active / Strenuous Daily Activity	1.72	Physical activity more than 60 minutes (or less but high intensity) 5 or more times per week/or activity 2 times per day
Extremely Active	1.90	Twice daily exercise and physically active job

My Activity Adjusted BMR	kcal

c) **If your goal is to *maintain* your current body composition:** The resulting value above is an estimate of the amount of energy/calories your body requires to maintain healthy functioning each day at your current weight.

NOTE: if you want greater simplicity, lack math skills and a calculator at this moment, then the following formula can be used to determine a *very rough* estimate of your daily energy needs based on your current weight. In other words, it offers a general estimate of the number of calories you need to consume each day to *maintain* your current weight based on your current level of activity.

IMPORTANT: Please keep in mind the chart that follows often *under* estimates daily caloric needs. Only use it to get a quick and very rough estimate of daily energy needs. The equation outlined above will be far more reliable. Skip this one if you already calculated your estimated energy intake using the equations previously outlined.

Number of workouts per week	Multiply current weight by:	Example: 120 pound adult
0	10	1,200 kcals/day
1-2	12	1,440 kcals/day
3-4	14	1,680 kcals/day
4-5	16	1,920 kcals/day

My estimated daily calorie needs (maintenance)	Kcal

d) **If your goal is to *reduce* body fat:** It is estimated that to lose one pound a week, you need to reduce your calorie intake by approximately 500 calories each day. (Keep in mind this reduction in calories can come from reduced daily food intake and/or increased daily activity.)

Gender	slightly increased body fat	Significantly increased body fat (BF) (>30% BF men, >35% BF women)
Men:	Subtract 200-500 calories/day	Subtract 300-700 calories
Women:	Subtract 100-300 calories	Subtract 200-500 calories

My daily calorie needs for healthy BF loss	Kcal

For example:
Weight Loss Calories = Maintenance calories - Weight loss calories
1,625 – 250 calories (for 1/2 lb weight loss/week) =1,375
Round to 1,400 calories

e) Now, to determine an estimate of the number of calories to aim for at each snack and meal, divide your final energy/calorie needs into 5. As a guide, estimate roughly 3 meals each day at between 300-600 kcals for each meal, and roughly 2 snacks per day at between 150-250 kcals for each snack.

For example:
Calorie needs of 2,000 kcal/day: each snack (2/day): 200 kcal, each meal (3/day) 450 kcal

Calorie needs of 1,350 kcal/day: each snack (2/day): 150 kcal, each meal (3/day) 350 kcal

2. **Find portion control in the palm of your hands:** There is simple, free, and portable way to estimate how much food to consume at every meal and it is literally in the palm of your hands. Consider that the size of your palm without fingers is roughly equivalent to one 3 to 4 ounce serving of an animal protein such as fish or meat. Your closed fist is roughly equivalent to one cup, so *half* the volume of your fist is one serving of grains or legumes such as rice or beans, respectively. A loose, open handful is a perfect gauge of one serving of fruit or nuts, while two open handfuls should be the minimum amount of vegetables you enjoy at each meal. The volume of your entire thumb is roughly equivalent to a tablespoon and therefore, serves as an estimate of one serving of nut butter such as almond butter or a serving of cheese. Finally, the volume of the tip of your thumb is roughly a teaspoon; the perfect estimate of a serving of fats such as olive oil. Granted, each of us have different sized hands so the relative size of a serving for a petite person is different from that of a very large framed person but alas, so is the quantity of food they need to consume. So, use your *own* hand - not someone else's - to gain perspective on the portion sizes that can satisfy your needs.

3. **At *each* meal and snack, consume food choices that incorporate protein, carbohydrates, and a little fat.** The body's needs are surprisingly simple. In addition to vitamins, minerals and water, the body requires carbohydrates, protein, and fat... and that's it. Getting a little of each of these macronutrients ensures

that your blood sugar is kept steady throughout the day, your belly and brain are satisfied, and you get maximal nutrition and nutrient absorption. Remember, protein is essential for satiety so **ensure you incorporate some protein into *all* meals and snacks**. Thus, if any macronutrient group has to be compromised one day during a snack or meal, *do not* let it be protein. This is often easy with meals but make sure you apply it to snacking too. A good rule to adhere to when choosing snacks is the following: anytime you consume a carbohydrate, make sure you also consume at least a little protein with it. For example, instead of just having an orange (carbohydrate source), enjoy the orange with a few almonds (protein source which also contains healthy fats).

4. **Eat your first meal within 30 to 45 minutes of first waking.** There is a great quotation by Josh Billings the 19th century American humorist, which reinforces this recommendation perfectly: *"Never work before breakfast; if you have to work before breakfast, eat your breakfast first"*. Countless studies have convinced how important this first meal of the day can be. Do not allow more than 30 to 45 minutes of your morning to pass without adding some fuel to your metabolic flames.

5. **Eat something every 3 to 4 hours.** Never go more than 4 hours without a small, balanced snack or a meal. Remember how important it is to maintain stable blood sugar levels throughout the day. If you go too long without eating, your blood sugar will bottom out and your body will tire and become lethargic. Waiting too long between meals also encourages the onset of overwhelming hunger pangs that can make it much harder to make healthy food choices. That overwhelming hunger can tempt you into reaching for a quick fix sugary snack to bring on instant yet transient gratification… don't do it!

6. **Your last meal or snack should be consumed at least 2 hours before bedtime.** Eating close to bedtime is often due to boredom or habit rather than due to true hunger. Although we will discuss this later, it should make sense to you that if you have eaten less than two hours ago, you should not be truly hungry.

7. **Eat breakfast like a king, lunch like a prince, and dinner like a pauper.** Believe it or not, there is now scientific evidence to add credence to this old adage.[138,139,140] Most recently, a 2013 study found that even though all study participants consumed the same type of foods, the same number of calories, has similar energy expenditures, similar appetite hormones (leptin and ghrelin), and similar sleep duration, those eating the majority of their calories earlier in the day (prior to 3:00 pm) lost more body weight than those study participants that consumed the majority of their daily food intake after 3:00 pm. To add insult to injury, the late eaters were also found to have lower insulin sensitivity, which has been shown to increase the risk of developing type 2 diabetes.[141] This suggests that our body may be better equipped to deal with the sugar in our food in the morning rather than in the evening.

8. **Savor your meals and snacks!** Avoid rushed and distracted eating and instead, find pleasure in your meals. In an upcoming chapter I will share with you some of my favorite recipes that are easy to prepare and very delicious to eat making it even easier to find joy in your meals! Later on I will also discuss the importance of eating mindfully, being truly present and undistracted at mealtime so you can enjoy the food in front of you without overdoing it.

9. **Your manner of eating is about quality, quantity, and style.** I hope I have made it clear by now that what you eat, how much you eat, and *how* you eat, all matter. This may feel like a lot to consider for every bite of food, but as you implement your new *manner of living* one a step at a time, this will all become second nature; instinctive, like brushing your teeth. Remember that wonderful "slippery slope" I promised you within the preface of this book? You are now ready to embark upon it.

Creating Your Daily Culinary Masterpiece

Whole, real food when well selected and well composed, is one of civilizations most magnificent works of art. The best part? We get to indulge our senses in its delightful beauty and delicious flavors repeatedly, every day of our lives! Good food, like good art, nourishes the mind, body, and soul. And just like when composing art, one's needs, tastes, and preferences should all be taken into account when we compose out plates.

To simplify your daily composition of culinary works of art, I have grouped foods together by colors. Consider this your culinary artist's palette. As the artist you get to decide how you wish to design each snack and meal each day. Visualize the primary colors red, blue, and yellow represent our macronutrients: proteins, carbohydrates, and fats. I have further grouped plant foods by their actual colors representing the distinct phytonutrients they offer. To maximize our daily nutrient intake, our goal each day, is to create a culinary picture using the most diversity of color on our plate. Remember, variety is the spice of life! In a given day, be sure to select your daily fats, carbohydrates, and proteins from different food sources and when possible, from a variety of different colors. For example when it comes to protein, at breakfast choose whole grains and legumes as your protein source, for a snack choose a Greek yogurt, for lunch have seafood, and for dinner choose poultry or edamame. This will guarantee the greatest accumulation of health promoting nutrients each day. Finally, as with art, remain mindful that there *is* such a thing as too much of a good thing. So make smart choices, embrace diversity, innovation and creativity, but avoid excess.

And now I present to you, a feast for the eyes and the palate. The delicious, delectable, and nourishing foods that are to become your newly refined food plan, your new manner of eating.

Your Culinary Palette

Choose 1 source of Protein (P), Carbohydrates (C), *and* Fat (F) at each snack or meal

To help navigate the culinary color palette:

1. *Individual foods that contain substantial amounts of more than one of each macronutrient (fat, carbohydrate, and protein) are noted with a combination of (P), (C), and/or (F). These foods alone can satisfy more than one of these macronutrient needs at each meal or snack.*

2. *Vegetarian protein sources are marked with a (v)*

3. *Gluten free grains are marked with a (gf)*

4. *Serving sizes are included to help inform your choice of how much to eat. Estimated caloric value per average serving of each food or food category is also indicated.[142]*

5. *Foods listed in the flavor enhancer column, and in the unlimited carbohydrate category should also be enjoyed in unlimited abundance! Choose foods from each color category as each color represents another healthful phytonutrient.*

6. *When it comes to oils, look for those that are "expeller-pressed" and "cold-pressed". Expeller-pressed (naturally pressed) refers to a chemical free, mechanical process that extracts oils form nuts and seeds, and cold-pressed refers to oils that are expeller-pressed in a temperature controlled environment that preserves the aroma, flavor, and nutrients. While I generally do not recommend it, if you use Canola oil, only choose those that are certified organic since conventional processing methods often involve genetic modification and use pesticides in production.*

Carbohydrates (C)

Vegetables and Fruits
(1 serving = 80 calories)

Purple and blue

Blueberries, blackberries, 1 cup

Grapes, 15

Plum, 3 small

Beets, 4 medium

Pomegranate seeds, ½ cup

Orange, yellow, and red

Strawberries, raspberries 1 ½ cups

Cherries 15

Cranberries, 1 ½ cups

Peach, 2 small

Orange, 1 large

Nectarine, 2 small

Apple, 1 medium

Banana, 1 small

Watermelon, 2 cups

Cranberries, 1 ½ cups

Grapefruit, 1

Carrots (4 small raw, 20 baby; 1 ½ cup cooked)

Mango, ½ medium

Cantaloupe, ½ medium

Sweet potato, 1 small baked

Yam, ½ cup cooked

Butternut squash, 1 cup cooked

Acorn squash, ¾ cup cooked

White

Parsnips, 1 large

Turnip, 4 smalls

Green

Pear, 1 medium

Honeydew, ¼ small

Kiwi, 2

Grains
(1 serving = ½ cup cooked = 75-100 calories)

Spelt (v)

Barley (v)

Bulgur (v)

Whole oats (v)

Whole grain crackers, 3 (v)

Whole wheat tortilla or pita, ½ (v)

Brown rice(v) (gf)

Amaranth (v) (gf)
Sorghum, 1 ounce (v) (gf)
Buckwheat (v) (gf)
Millet (v) (gf)
Teff (v) (gf)
Wild rice (v) (gf)
Basmati rice (v) (gf)
Quinoa (P) (v) (gf)

Protein (P)

Fish and Seafood   **(1 serving = 3-4 oz = 150 calories)**
Sardines (F)
Salmon (F)
Mackerel (F)
Herring (F)
Scallops, 12 large
Rainbow Trout (F)
Shellfish (shrimp etc.)
Canned light tuna in water (skipjack, yellowfin or tongol), ¾ cup
Meats   **(1 serving = 3-4 oz = 150 calories)**
Grass fed beef (F)
Lamb (F)
Chicken (F)
Turkey (F)
Eggs, 4 whites
Eggs, 2 whole (F)
Soy *(choose organic)*   **(1 serving = 150 calories)**
Edamame (soy beans), 5 oz (C) (F)
Tempeh, 3 oz (C) (F)
Tofu , 8 oz or 1 cup (C) (F)
Dairy   **(1 serving = 6-8 oz = 80 calories)**
Kefir, ½ cup
Organic soy milk (v)
Rice milk (v) hazelnut (v) almond (v) hemp milk (v) (C)
Parmesan, (dry, grated) 4 tbsp
Feta cheese, 1 oz
Cottage cheese, 1%, 4 oz
Ricotta, part skim, 2 oz
Mozzarella, part skim, 1 oz
Greek yogurt (F)

Legumes (1 serving = ½ cup = 110 calories)
Garbanzo beans (chickpeas) (C)
Kidney beans (C)
Black beans (C)
Lima beans (C)
Cannellini beans (C)
Lentils (C)
Split peas (C)
Peanuts, 10 (F)
Hummus, 1/4 cup (C)

Fats (F)
Oils (1 serving = 1 tsp = 40 calories)
Extra virgin coconut oil
Extra virgin olive oil
Truffle oil
Hazelnut, almond, or walnut oil
Hemp oil
Avocado oil (high smoke point)
Sesame oil (high smoke point)
Light olive oil (high smoke point)
high-oleic sunflower oil (high smoke point)
Grapeseed oil (high smoke point)
Nuts and Seeds or 1 tbsp butters made of any of the following: (1 serving = 100 calories)
Pistachios, in shell, 25 (v)
Almonds, 12-15 (v)
Cashew nuts, 10 (v)
Brazil nuts, 3-4 (v)
Walnuts, 12 (v)
Hazelnut (Filbert), 10-12 (v)
Macadamia nut, 4-5 (v)
Pecans, 10 (v)
Chestnut, 5 roasted
Pine nuts, 80
Coconut, unsweetened shredded, 2 tbsp
Coconut, 1.5" x 1.5" piece
Pumpkin seeds, 70 seeds or 2 tbsp (v)
Sunflower seeds, 2 tbsp (v)
Vegetables
Avocado ¼
Olives, 8-10

No culinary work of art is complete without the rainbow of colors provided by the following to decorate your meal with <u>unlimited amounts, daily</u>:

Unlimited Carbohydrates	
(unlimited! at least 4 serving a day) 1 serving = ½ cup, unless otherwise stated	
Purple and blue	
Eggplant	Cabbage
Orange, yellow, and red	
Red, yellow peppers	Tomatoes
Spaghetti squash	Radishes
Artichokes	Bamboo shoots
Yellow zucchini	Radicchio, 1 cup
Green	
Kale, 1 cup	Broccoli
Spinach, 1 cup	Brussels sprouts
Okra	Green beans
Snow peas, sugar snap peas	Bok choy
Escarole	Celery
Collard greens, 1 cup	Swiss chard, 1 cup
Celery Dandelion, mustard, beet greens, 1 cup	Iceberg, butter, red/green leaf lettuce, 1 cup
Mesclun, 1 cup	Romaine lettuce, 1 cup
Endive, 1 cup	Arugula, 1 cup
Kohlrabi	chicory and watercress
Sea vegetables like kelp	Chives, onions, leeks
Cucumber and dill pickles	Green peppers
Asparagus	Zucchini
White and Brown	
Cauliflower	Bean sprouts
Jicama	Water chestnuts
All mushrooms	Cabbage
Sauces and Condiments	
Tomato salsa	Horseradish
Kim Chi	Sauerkraut
Mustard, Dijon mustard	Light soy sauce
Vinegars	Wasabi

Use the following to enhance your culinary work of art by including <u>unlimited amounts</u> to taste, of the following <u>daily</u>:

Flavor enhancers (unlimited!)	
Herbs and Spices	
Dill	Cilantro
Rosemary	Coriander
Oregano	Cinnamon
Basil	Chili peppers
Caraway	Chives
Mint	Curry
Saffron	Fennel
Cardamom	Lemon grass
Ginger	Nutmeg
Garlic	Pepper
Parsley	Paprika
Rosemary	Sumac
Sage	Thyme
Turmeric	Tarragon
Za'atar	Chaat Masala *(NOTE: often contains salt)*
Extracts (choose "pure" not "imitation" extracts)	
Vanilla	Anise
Almond	Lemon or peppermint

Choose the following to hydrate your palate throughout the day:

Hydration sources
Unlimited
Water
Unsweetened tea
Herbal teas
Unsweetened sparking waters
In Moderation
Coffee
Caffeinated teas

When a recipe calls for a sweetener to liven the palate, use one of the following in moderation:

Sweeteners
Raw cane sugar
Coconut palm sugar
Date sugar or paste
Maple sugar
Raw honey *(the darker the better)*
Muscovado
Sucanat

Putting It into Practice

Some examples of the foundation of a great culinary masterpiece meal or snack (with a little carbohydrates, proteins, and fats):

✓ Regular or low fat Greek yogurt (P) (F) with blueberries (C)
✓ Avocado (C) (F) and chicken (P)
✓ Sweet potato (C) and salmon (P) (F)
✓ Fat-free Greek yogurt (P), strawberries (C), and walnuts (F) (C) (P)

Some ideal standalone snack options that meet all macronutrient needs in one (This redefines fast food!)

✓ Almonds (F) (C) (P)
✓ Edamame (P) (F) (C)

To complete each snack or meal described above, add as much of you like of the unlimited carbohydrates and/or flavor enhancers. It is now a culinary masterpiece!

Finally, be sure to raise a glass and say "cheers" to each work of art you create six times daily, with any of the unlimited sources of hydration!

TIP! If you prefer getting started slowly, commit to beginning your new manner of eating with just one meal. And what better meal to start with the then first one, breakfast! For your first meal of the day, toss away that bagel and cream cheese, say good-by to that cereal and milk, and sayonara to the foodless, coffee on the go breakfast. Instead, welcome in an energizing vegetable and fresh herb frittata or a cold poached salmon filet with avocado over green leafy vegetables. You will be amazed how your energy levels skyrocket that day!

"I Do Not Like Green Eggs and Ham"

The foods that I have listed above are those that I recommend you make the foundation of your culinary repertoire. However, I suspect a number of you are looking at the food list above and thinking "what on earth is okra?" or perhaps you're thinking, "Brussels sprouts?! I hate Brussels sprouts!" Before you snub some of these unfamiliar or previously disliked foods completely, do I need to remind you of the ageless wisdom of Dr. Seuss and his green eggs and ham? [143]

I realize that a few of the foods listed may be new to you or may even seem undesirable to you at first blush. If that is the case, first, let me remind you that you do not need to eat everything on the list. The list is intentionally diverse, to satisfy all preferences and palates. That said, I now challenge you to try one new food each week! If in the past you have had a not–so-favorable relationship with one of these foods, I challenge you to try it again by preparing it in a novel and delicious way. As your palate naturally evolves through the processes of developing and refining your food plan, you may be surprised how much you like it!

ACTION STEP: If you share the "fast food meal plan" with the majority of Americans and you get your vegetables primarily from potatoes, iceberg lettuce, and pickle slices, the mere thought of introducing other vegetables might seem like full-on torture. To overcome any initial hesitation, the first week that you begin your new manner of eating, stick to foods that are familiar. For week two, choose at least one new food from the same family as those vegetables to which you are accustomed and each week after that, taste at least one more new food. Also, experiment with new preparation methods. You may be surprised by the delicious, flavor explosion that can come from a piece of broccoli or Brussel sprouts when well prepared. Be adventurous and most importantly, have fun with it.

The following are some suggestions to help expand your palate without making huge culinary leaps of faith:

- **If you like iceberg lettuce: try spinach.** It can be used in the same way as lettuce and adds a wealth of additional nutrients and flavor.
- **If you like white rice: try quinoa.** Prepare it and use it in the same way you would prepare and use white rice. You will enjoy the slightly nutty flavor it adds to your foods and your body will thank you for this high fiber, nutrient dense ingredient upgrade.
- **If you like white potatoes: try a sweet potato.** Prepare it in the same way you prepare white potatoes. You will be delighted by the sweet and savory balance it offers.
- **If you like carrots: try parsnips.** When cooked, it has the same sweetness and versatility as carrots but offers different nutrients and a sweet flavor.
- **If you like spinach: try kale.** Sauté it as you would spinach, it has a slightly more dense texture than spinach and a lovely bitterness that is balanced well when served with meats and fish. If you use it raw, remove the stem, drizzle with a little extra virgin olive oil and a pinch of salt, and then massage the leaves for a few minutes. This will help reduce any bitterness and bring out a delightfully sweeter flavor and silkier texture.
- **If you like white mushrooms: try crimini mushrooms.** Use them anywhere you would white mushrooms; there is very little difference in flavor but you gain an abundance of additional vitamins, phytonutrients, and immune enhancing benefits!

ACTION STEP: You would not eat steamed chicken without any seasoning, so why on earth would you prepare your vegetables in that manner? Of course you do not like Brussels sprouts if that is how you have had them before. Consider this: roasting almost any vegetable with a little salt and pepper and olive oil brings out its natural sweetness. Did you know roasted green beans and asparagus can be just as addictive as French fries? No kidding! How about pureeing any vegetable in broth over low heat and adding salt, pepper, and fresh herbs to create a vegetable soup that will have even the pickiest eater sopping up every savory drop of it! Bringing out delectable flavors in vegetables can be surprisingly easy and I encourage you to sample some of the simple recipes I have compiled in chapter 10. I suspect you will be pleasantly surprised and satisfied by what you taste!

General Dietary Modifications

For those among us that have special dietary preferences or needs, I have included here some recommended modifications that will help satisfy dietary preferences without compromising nutritional needs. Some of you may choose to maintain these as part of your regular manner of eating, some of you may opt to select these modifications simply on certain days when for example, you are at a brunch and wish to consume more fruit that day, or you have not made it to the grocery store all week so out of necessity are going to have to consume less nuts or seeds for a few days. Remember, one of our goals is to include variety into our daily *manner of living* and select fats, carbohydrates, and proteins from a variety of different food sources at each meal. However, if you opt to limit variety on select days by choice or by necessity, then below are some suggestions to ensure you do not compromise nutritional quality in the process.

Want to eliminate or consume fewer legumes?
- Replace legumes with nuts and seeds and increase unlimited carbohydrates by at least 1 serving each day to ensure adequate fiber and nutrient intake.
  OR
- Replace legumes with another protein source and increase unlimited carbohydrates by at least 1 serving each day to ensure adequate fiber and nutrient intake.

Want to eliminate or consume fewer nuts and seeds?
- Replace nuts and seeds with legumes, and increase unlimited carbohydrates by at least 1 serving each day to ensure adequate fiber and nutrient intake.
  OR
- Replace nuts and seeds with another protein source and increase unlimited carbohydrates by at least 1 serving each day to ensure adequate fiber and nutrient intake.

Want to eliminate or consume fewer grains?

- Replace with other carbohydrates or unlimited carbohydrates by at least 1 serving each day to ensure adequate fiber and nutrient intake.

Want to eliminate or consume fewer fruit?

- Replace with other carbohydrates or unlimited carbohydrates by at least 1 serving each day to ensure adequate fiber and nutrient intake.

Want to eliminate or consume less gluten?

- Under the category of carbohydrates, avoid consuming grains that are not marked with the (gf) symbol, and refer to chapter 18 for additional detailed information about a gluten free manner of eating.

Vegetarian and Vegan Modifications

For those of us adhering to a vegetarian or vegan dietary pattern whether it is a trial for one day or as our standard manner of eating for life, I have outlined some additional modifications to ensure your protein and micronutrient intake is not compromised.

✓ Choose high protein vegetables from the green color palate such as kale, spinach, broccoli, and Brussels sprouts.

✓ Enjoy complete vegetarian protein sources such as edamame or quinoa.

✓ Generally, the following food combinations together are equivalent in amino acid profiles to the one complete animal protein serving:

> ➢ Any grain and any legume serving such as rice and lentils
> ➢ Any seed or nut with any legume such as hummus made with tahini (sesame seed paste) and chickpeas
> ➢ Any seed or nut with any grain such as a nut butter, like almond butter or walnut butter with whole grain crackers

✓ If not vegan, choose eggs, Greek yogurt, and cheeses as additional protein options.

Potential deficiencies of micronutrients like iron, vitamin B12, vitamin D, and omega-3 fatty acids can be avoided by well-planned vegetarian diets. Below are some suggestions to ensure adequate intake of each of these nutrients for vegans. I have also included tips to help facilitate absorption of each of these nutrients since at the end of the day, when it comes to nutrients, *it is not what you eat that matters, but what you absorb.*

Nutrients at risk of deficiency for vegans	Select Vegan Food Sources	Special Considerations
Iron	Select dried fruit such as prunes, apricots and raisins, also peas, lima beans, spinach, asparagus, quinoa, and pumpkin seeds	Iron absorption is enhanced by nutrients such as vitamins A and C. Therefore, combine iron rich foods with foods high in these nutrients like citrus fruit, strawberries, or red peppers to enhance absorption. Avoid consuming iron at the same time as iron absorption *inhibitors* such as phytate or phytic acids (found in grains), tannin (found in tea and coffee), and calcium (found in dairy products).
Vitamin B12	Vitamin B-12 fortified foods, such as fortified organic soy and rice beverages, fortified nutritional yeast (try it on popcorn or over lentils or vegetables)	Vegans generally should consider taking vitamin B12 supplements because there are few vegan foods that provide an adequate source of this important nutrient.
Vitamin D	Porcini mushrooms, vitamin D fortified foods such as organic soy milk, and rice milk	Deficiency of this vitamin is common and there are very few good vegan food sources so vegans should generally consider supplementation.

Calcium	Broccoli, spinach, kale, almonds, sesame seeds, tahini, tofu, fortified organic soy and rice milk, pinto or kidney beans	If deficient, avoid consuming at the same time as grains, seeds, and nuts that contain phytic acid, which can inhibit calcium absorption. Recall: Phytic acids in these foods can be degraded through cooking.
Zinc	Nuts or nut butters (pecans, almonds, cashews, peanuts etc.), oranges, peas, dried figs whole grains, legumes, and soy products	Phytic acid in grains, seeds, and legumes, binds zinc and thereby decreases its bioavailability. Again, phytic acids in these foods can be degraded through cooking.
Omega-3 fatty acids	Ground flaxseeds, chia seeds, walnuts, oil from brown algae (kelp), and hemp seed–based beverages	Disease, stress, smoking or eating a diet high in trans and saturated fat and low in essential micronutrients, can impair the ability to convert many vegan sources of omega 3 fatty acids into the desirable forms of docosahexaenoic acid (DHA) and eicosapentaenoic acid (EPA). Microalgae is the most promising source of long-chain omega-3 fatty acids for people who do not consume fish and is available in supplement form.

A Word on Hydration

We often limit our focus to food when considering our manner of eating but proper hydration is a critical part of the equation. Adequate hydration is essential for life and to support our basic physiologic functions. Furthermore, thirst and dehydration can mimic hunger pangs. In fact, many times the signal of thirst is often misinterpreted and we reach for food when we should be reaching for a glass of water. As a general rule, when hunger pangs hit and if you have recently eaten, then first reach for a source of hydration before you reach for food. Also, do not wait until you are thirsty to reach for a source of hydration, by the time your body is transmitting the signal of thirst it is likely that you are already dehydrated.

Here are some easy and delicious ways to increase your daily intake of fluids:

• Eat more high water content foods. Most vegetables such as zucchini, bell peppers, jicama, cucumber, lettuce, eggplant, celery, raw broccoli, and raw spinach, fruits including tomatoes, strawberries, blueberries, cantaloupe, watermelon, apples, pears, navel oranges, mango, and even good old chicken soup; all these foods are tasty, nutritious, filling, low calorie *and* hydrating.

• Add fruits like berries, citrus, or melon to water or even add vegetables like cucumbers (think spa water). This simple trick gives the water an extra satisfying taste and as an extra bonus, it also adds antioxidants and other nutrients from the fruit to the water!

• Craving the fizz of soda? Try plain soda water with natural fruit essences (not sugar or artificial sweeteners) added.

• Make a Mint Water-jito! Add fresh mint and limes to spring water for a delicious calorie free, non-alcoholic, minty treat!

Cheers!

Chapter 7

We are all inventors, each sailing out on a voyage of discovery, guided each by a private chart, of which there is no duplicate. The world is all gates, all opportunities.
— Ralph Waldo Emerson

Do Not Go Grocery Shopping Until You Read This

The grocery store can be a perilous place; perilous because your intentions and the store's raison d'etre do not necessarily align. The store shines its bright lights illuminating colorful packages strategically placed and labeled to catch your eye and maximize their profit. The end of the aisle is prime real estate in grocery stores, and companies pay a premium to have their products placed there to entice and tempt even the most well-intentioned shopper. You are on a quest to find real foods, the ones that are nutrient dense and that support optimal health. The product labels call out at you: "Low fat," "High Fiber," "Low sugar," "Prevents heart disease," "Low sodium," Omega 3's! Omega 3's! Omega 3's! Whew!! It seems obvious that foods which bear such proud and prominent labels surely must be good for you. Right? *Is all that glitters really gold?*

Make no mistake about it: food is big business. The savvy shopper is aware that the motives of those that produce and distribute our food may not always be in line with those that consume it. The Latin expression *caveat emptor* meaning *buyer beware* has never been more true than when it comes to navigating the grocery store aisles. This chapter will arm you with the information you need to see through the glitz and glam and interpret food labels to make the best choices when it comes to the food you eat.

Deciphering the Code: Understanding Food Labels

While I am clearly an advocate for eating whole, real foods as mentioned previously, not all packaged foods are poor choices. In fact, some delicious and healthful foods are packaged both for our convenience and cost-effectiveness, and can absolutely be incorporated in our daily food plan. In fact, canned or frozen fish, legumes, and vegetables may be excellent and often cheaper sources of these healthful foods. We simply need to know what to look for.

NOTE: With canned foods always be sure to check sodium content. Sometimes sodium is increased in these foods to serve as a preservative. Look for low sodium versions or rinse the foods before eating to eliminate some of this sodium.

Labels can be deceiving. We often reach for a food because the label makes it sound like it is a smart choice when actually that food item may be more harm than good. To avoid making such mistakes, here is a quick and concise primer on deciphering food labels so you know what to look for when purchasing packaged foods.

Serving Size

The first thing I always look at on a food label is the serving size. I learned this lesson rather early on. Like most universities, there was a little snack shop on my school's campus that sold grab and go goodies to students. Everyone's favorite was the 'giant cookie.' I remember a friend of mine commenting on how this cookie tasted so good and was healthy too! I promptly went to the store and grabbed one of those giant five inch cookies. Always proud of the fact that I do my own due diligence (I was quite a health conscious eater even back then), I glanced down at the nutrient label on this cookie. Sure enough, the fat content and type was acceptable, sugar and calories were relatively minimal and ingredients all appeared to be from whole, real food sources. Had I found the holy grail of cookies? Here it was. I walked to the counter and paid. I could not wait to sit down in class, tear open its wrapper and enjoy this "healthy" treat. So that is what I did.

Mmmmm.... It tasted good.

As I glanced down again at its wrapper, filled now only with crumbs and small remnants of this delightful taste of heaven, I thought this is too good to be true; only 200 calories for a giant cookie like this. However, this time I noticed one important detail on the label that I previously overlooked: The serving size! The serving size described on the label was $1/8^{th}$ of the cookie! Who eats $1/8^{th}$ of a cookie?! My 200 calorie treat was actually a 1,600 calorie whopping indulgence – practically my daily caloric intake in one cookie!!

Needless to say, from that day forward I learned my lesson. So, my lesson now becomes your first lesson: The first thing to consider when reading a label is the serving size. Changing the number of servings in a particular package of food is one strategy food marketers use to make their foods seem more desirable than they really are. This is because the entire rest of the label, including all the nutrients and calories is based on a single serving. Thus, the serving size is probably the most important part of the label. Knowing how many servings are in a food package gives us an accurate understanding of the nutritional content of that food. In some cases, the serving size may be an accurate reflection of what one normally would eat in one serving. However, in other cases, like my cookie example, it can be absolutely arbitrary and in no way reflective of the nutrient intake you get from consuming a "reasonable" portion of that food.

Another reason companies may report small serving sizes on their labels is that it gives them flexibility in how they can label their product. There are laws that govern what can be placed on labels, and many of these laws refer to serving size. Let us use trans fats (a.k.a. hydrogenated fats) as an example. If one serving of a particular food contains less than 0.5 grams of trans fats, then by law the label can say it contains zero grams of trans fats. This is why some processed foods like macaroni and cheese and the 'giant cookie' has so many servings per container. Confusing? Yes it is. That is why then next thing we will look at is the ingredient list.

Ingredients

The ingredient list is always posted at the bottom or to the side of the nutritional label and describes in quantitative order which ingredients appear in that food. That is to say that the first ingredient on the list is present in the greatest amount and then each subsequent ingredient appears in progressively smaller quantities in that food.

I always recommend glancing at the ingredients list next since here we can see truly what is in that food. This is because here all the ingredients in a food must be listed, and there are no FDA laws that food manufacturers can creatively manipulate. You see, as I mentioned before, a food can list zero grams of trans fats on the label if it has less than 0.5 grams per serving. However, that does not mean there are no trans fats in that food, even though the FDA still permits a food like this to proudly and legally label itself as trans-fat free! This is especially helpful to us as consumers, because if a single serving of that food is less than what you would reasonably consume in one sitting, (such as in my cookie story), you may be consuming more trans fats then you think. So, if you look at the ingredient list, look for words like partially-hydrogenated or hydrogenated fats. If these words are listed then, even if the label says zero grams trans fats, there are still trans fats in that food.

And *do* look for it, since trans fats can pop up in the most unusual places. Take tomato sauce for example. It is the most basic food that really only needs to include tomatoes and perhaps some salt as a preservative. However, there are some brands that include hydrogenated fats and even high fructose corn syrup. Be sure to choose the brands that do not add these unnecessary ingredients, or better yet, get creative in the kitchen and make your own fresh tomato sauce from scratch. The point is to get in the habit of reading ingredient labels. If the foods you choose have undesirable ingredients, put them back and find a similar item. Nearly every time you will find a comparable product right next to it on the shelf made by another manufacturer (or sometimes even the same one!) but without those undesirable ingredients.

ACTION STEP: One good tip when reading the ingredient list is to assess whether it is a short story or a novel. Most healthy packaged food products are a short story. They will typically have anywhere between 4 to 10 ingredients and each one is recognizable (for the most part) and should make sense. Take yogurt for example. Here is the ingredient list from a real yogurt commonly found in your grocery store:

Grade A pasteurized skimmed milk, Live active yogurt cultures (L. Bulgaricus, S. Thermophilus)

For comparison sake, here is the ingredient list from another commercially available yogurt product also commonly found in your grocery store:

Nonfat Yogurt (cultured pasteurized grade A nonfat milk, modified corn starch, kosher gelatin, vitamin A acetate, Vitamin D3), Water, Chicory Root Extract (inulin), Strawberries, Modified Corn Starch, Citric Acid, Tricalcium Phosphate, Aspartame, Potassium Sorbate Added to Maintain Freshness, Acesulfame Potassium, Natural Flavor, Red #40. Phenylketonurics: Contains Phenylalanine.

If you ask me, the second example is a science project; it is *not* yogurt. (After you read chapter 8, come back to this ingredient list. You will be shocked to learn the effect some of these additives may have on human health).

Determine if that food you are eating is a whole, real food that has been packaged for convenience or a fake over-processed food like the "yogurt" above. Typically, if the ingredient list is more reminiscent of a novel by Tolstoy than a short, easily readable story by Dr. Seuss, then chances are the food is more test tube food than real food.

One more thing: as mentioned in chapter 4, do not forget to look at the amount and type of sugar in the food as well. Turn back to the section on *added sugars* in that chapter for a reminder of what to look for.

Percentages

Next, look at the percentages of Daily Value on the label. If we understand that you should receive 100% of a given nutrient over the course of a single day, then this gives you a simple way to get an idea how healthy the food is. (Don't forget, these values are represented for *each serving*). Here is a simple rule to gauge the nutritional value of each food. If the label reports:

5% or less of Daily Value:
The food is LOW in that ingredient

20% or more of Daily Value:
The food is HIGH in that ingredient

Between 5%-20% of Daily Value:
The food is a MODERATE source of that ingredient

Keep in mind one important caveat: not everyone has the same nutritional need for all nutrients. This is easily understood when you compare the needs of a short, small-framed woman to a tall, stocky man. So, instead of making labels incredibly complicated, (which would defeat the whole purpose of educating consumers), most food labels are based on recommendations established for a 2,000 calorie diet. But again, the value of the percentage is that it is a quick way to gauge whether that particular food high or low in each nutrient. For example, if a given food is high in sodium (as many canned goods are) you may want to choose another option if you have high blood pressure and are working to reduce your intake of sodium.

Label Claims

Heart Healthy! All Natural! Sounds good, doesn't it? The claims that food manufacturers and food marketers make are probably the most misleading aspects of food labeling. Many claims, such as "all natural," have no regulatory definitions set by the U.S. Food and Drug Administration (FDA), which makes them nothing more than meaningless marketing terms. For this reason, it is not uncommon to see foods rich in chemically-altered or genetically-modified ingredients being labeled as being "all natural." As a side note, do not confuse "all natural" with "organic." Foods certified as "organic" are subject to stringent regulations, which I will address in chapter 11. That said; keep in mind that just being organic does not make a food healthy. Did you know that you can get certified organic Mac and Cheese and Oreo cookies? I rest my case.

Even claims like "heart healthy" that *are* regulated by the FDA can be used in decidedly clever and deceptive ways. As a professor, to illustrate this point to my Clinical Nutrition students, I often share with them the packaging of a box of instant oatmeal. The oatmeal bears the logo of the American Heart Association and boldly claims in red type to be "Heart Healthy." Upon seeing this, who wouldn't think they are giving their child a healthy breakfast? However, inspection of the ingredient list and the percent daily values reveals that it has excessively high levels of added sugars (including high fructose corn syrup) and it is rich in trans fats, two factors known to contribute to heart disease. So how can this well-known food company get away with the FDA's stamp of approval *and* an endorsement by the American Heart Association? Simple: it is high in fiber.

You see, the FDA permits select food labels to promote a health claim providing the food contains an ingredient known to benefit a certain disease. In this case (each health claim has its own set of rules), as long as a single serving contains less than a specified level of fat, saturated fat, cholesterol, and sodium, and contains at least ten percent of the daily value of *either* vitamin A, C, calcium, iron, fiber or protein, it qualifies to promote a health claim.[144] So, the fact that the oatmeal contains a good amount of fiber, it is granted the privilege of bearing the "heart healthy" badge, regardless of what other "heart un-healthy" ingredients it contains. Pretty sneaky isn't it? For this reason, look at ingredient lists to see what is *really* in your food before being deceived by shiny marketing labels.

Sugar: The Sweet Controversy

One question that always comes up with both my patients and my students is the issue of when it comes to sugar is artificial or real better? This sweet controversy has been a topic of debate for decades. Here are my conclusions on this matter.

In chapter 4 we discussed the importance of limiting our consumption of *added* sugars. So, are artificial sweeteners a better option? The answer is *no,* and this is why: Artificial sweeteners are engineered food additives designed to give our taste buds the sensation of sweetness without the associated calories and spikes in blood sugar levels. While the premise seems solid, they are still chemicals with little to no nutritional value. Furthermore, they trick our brains into thinking that we are getting sugar into our body when we are not. In general, the data we have on artificial sweeteners and health is ambiguous and unclear, and the long term effects on health are still not known. Should our minds be put at ease because the FDA approves their use in foods? Studies have not demonstrated clear evidence of an association between these sweeteners and cancer in humans.[145] However, a 2005 European study found rats fed aspartame at comparable levels per body weight to humans had a higher risk of developing brain tumors, lymphoma and leukemia.[146] While findings from animal studies do not always translate to humans, they still do raise cause for concern. Keep in mind there are several food additives approved by the FDA that have been banned in other countries due to concern of *potential* dangers in humans. (I will describe these specifically in the chapter that follows.) Artificial sweeteners have also been linked to weight gain and adverse effects on blood sugar control and diabetes. They have been associated with obesity, type 2 diabetes, metabolic syndrome, and cardiovascular disease.[147] Most recently, a study by Israeli researchers published in the prestigious journal Nature, linked artificial sweeteners to obesity and metabolic disease. The researchers found that artificial sweeteners may contribute to these diseases by inducing harmful changes in our gut bacteria.[148] While these studies are compelling, the FDA maintains that existing data remains insufficient to clearly refute the use of artificial sweeteners in our food supply. That said, to me there is nonetheless sufficient concern to warrant avoiding their use.

Even some "natural" sugar substitutes are subject to debate regarding their impact on human health. Stevia has been purported to be the safest and best "natural" sugar substitute, yet it still has not been around long enough, nor has it been the subject of enough studies, for me to conclusively recommend it or use it regularly with peace of mind. Even agave nectar, which has been reported to be a safe "natural" sweetener, is the source of some controversy these days. Agave contains between 70 and 90 percent fructose by weight. Fructose appears to responds differently than glucose when we consume it. Fructose does not cause our blood sugar to spike the way glucose does and thus, it gives agave nectar its low glycemic index, which is part of the reason it became such a popular sweetener. However, the tradeoff is that while fructose many not increase blood sugar, instead it may increase energy intake and weight gain by not triggering these same insulin signals or the same satiety hormones (leptin) that are involved in appetite regulation, as glucose does. Not to mention, due to the manner by which fructose is metabolized there is additional concern that it may over time, contribute to fatty liver disease and heart disease.[149] However, one of the key reasons this is controversial is that since fructose is generally consumed as part of a more complex food or meal, studies that look at consumption of fructose in isolation may not be reflective of realistic consumption patterns. Furthermore, critics argue that the link between fructose and disease is correlative only and suggest that the consumption of fructose containing foods as part of ones manner of eating is no different than the consumption of any other type of sugar.[150]

The Bottom Line:

At this time, we simply are not clear about the effect these artificial or select novel natural sweeteners have on our health. Quite frankly, I am not comfortable using my body, or you using your body, as the test tube. My default position on undecided nutritional controversies? When in doubt, do not become the guinea pig.

My recommendation is therefore to choose tried and tested *real* sweeteners, and just use less. Keep in mind that even the whole, real food source sweeteners I list below are still added sugars and therefore should only be consumed in minimal amounts and on rare occasions.

I recommend choosing whole, real sweeteners such as:

- ✓ **Maple sugar**
- ✓ **Raw honey** (the darker the better; darker generally means more phytonutrients and more antioxidants)

✓ **Date paste** (made by blending dates in water to a honey like consistency) Much sweeter than regular white sugar so less is more! Start by using half as much date paste as you would white sugar. *Refer to chapter 10 for my easy recipe for homemade date paste!*

In addition to the options above, when baking, some good sweetener choices particularly when a recipe calls for granulated sugar, include:

✓ **Coconut palm sugar**
✓ **Sucanat** (whole cane sugar, a contraction of "**Su**cre de **can**ne **nat**urel")
✓ **Muscovado** (unrefined brown sugar from sugarcane juice with a strong molasses flavor)
✓ **Date sugar** (made by drying dates then pulverizing them!)

NOTE: Date sugar will not dissolve well in water, and since it doesn't melt it will remain as a slight brown fleck in foods. It is still great in baked goods or sprinkled atop Greek yogurt or ricotta cheese with berries! Keep in mind this tends to be much sweeter than regular white sugar so use half as much date sugar as you would white sugar.

These choices all are whole, real sources of sugar that impart a delicious sweetness to foods without any artifice. Another benefit is that a little goes a long way. These often have a strong natural sweetness so you can use less than you would need to with bleached, white table sugar. Nevertheless, it bears repeating that even when choosing whole, real natural sweeteners keep added sugar to a minimum; enjoy the sweetness but do so infrequently.

ACTION STEP: Baking allows us to be even more creative about ingredients we can use to sweeten our foods. Just like how you would use date paste, try baking with bananas, fig purée, or apple sauce to replace some of the added sugars (and added fats) in baked goods. These real sugar substitutes not only provide the additional sweetness your recipes demand but also impart natural moisture to the food so you can use less fats and oils as well. In addition to the nutrients they add to your baked goods, they also lend a delicious and subtle flavor that you can call your "secret ingredient!" Learn more tasty and healthy cooking tips in chapter 10.

Chapter 8

As I ate the oysters with their strong taste of the sea and their faint metallic taste that the cold white wine washed away, leaving only the sea taste and the succulent texture, and as I drank their cold liquid from each shell and washed it down with the crisp taste of the wine, I lost the empty feeling and began to be happy and to make plans.
— Ernest Hemingway, A Moveable Feast

Home as a Nutritional Safe Haven

In helping my patients get healthy, I find there is one important piece of advice that is paramount to their success; *make your home into a nutritional safe haven.*

It is natural that when we eat out at restaurants, at the homes of friends and family members, at a work meeting, when we are travelling, or at a party or reception, our food options can often be limited. Such situations force us to decide to either compromise some of our preferred dietary practices or, go hungry. Later on in this chapter I will share with you some of my personal strategies and suggestions for dealing with these types of situations. However, before we address strategies for dealing with the outside world, I encourage you to first take control over the one environment that is your own: make your home a nutritional safe haven.

What does this mean? Simple; it means that if it is not the type of food that your body needs and thrives on do not keep it in your home. The foods that you have at home should be those that you enjoy but not crave; those that offer you pleasure while also adding years to your life and life to your years! Home as a nutritional safe haven also means that you should not store foods in the back of your cupboards and simply rationalize that the Oreo® cookies are for the "guests" or the "kids".

Keep in mind:
1. The guests and the kids also benefit from the nutritional safe haven you will create and,
2. Who are you kidding! It's not about the guests or the kids! You know that the first time you have the slightest urge, those Oreo's® will be calling your name! So I ask, why expose yourself to unnecessary challenge? (Interestingly, you will see that as you stay the course with your new *manner of living*, you will be surprised how the Oreos® seem to have forgotten your name and how easily you will be able to turn a blind eye to these former culinary temptresses). In the meantime, avoid the unnecessary temptation by transforming your home into a safe culinary sanctuary.

The Extreme Makeover

Alright soldier! Now this is moment when I say jump! And you say, how high?

First, get into your kitchen. Next, open the pantry. Look at all the packaged foods it contains.

If you see any of the following additives in the list of ingredients printed on those packaged foods, throw those packaged foods out.

1. **High fructose corn syrup (HFCS)**
   While many concerns exist, HFCS most recently has been linked to increases in belly fat, inflammation, blood pressure, blood sugar, and pre-diabetes in adolescents.[151,152] Furthermore, this low cost sweetener is also a good marker for unhealthy, low nutrient density, highly processed foods. Get rid of it.

106

2. **Trans Fats: also referred to on food labels as hydrogenated fat and partially hydrogenated fat**
   There is indisputable scientific evidence of the potential harm to our health imposed by trans fats and there is no known benefit.[153,154,155] Get rid of it.

You are not done yet…

While the jury is still out on the health effects of several of the food additives listed below, most experts still agree that it is advisable to avoid their consumption. There is certainly no benefit to their consumption; only potential harm. Furthermore, the presence of one or more of these additives in a food item is most often a marker of an unhealthy, processed food anyways. Therefore, continue looking in your pantry and if you find foods that contain any of the following additives within their ingredient list, throw them out.

1. **Artificial food dyes:**
   Including Blue No. 1 and Blue No. 2, Red No. 3, Red No. 40, Yellow No. 6 and Yellow Tartrazine (Yellow No. 5). This is especially important if you have children. The greatest concern is with Red No. 40, Yellow No. 5 and Yellow No. 6. These dyes are commonly used in many food products targeting children even though they have been linked to hyperactivity and Attention Deficit Hyperactivity Disorder (ADHD).[156,157] Several of these dyes have also been linked to anxiety, migraines, and even cancer.[158] For this reason, many European countries have banned their use altogether or have mandated strict warning labels for products that contain them.[159] Yet, their use is still permitted by the FDA. They are most often found in candy, cookies, snack food, beverages, and baked goods. Some can even be found in pharmaceuticals and in poor quality dietary supplements.

2. **Sodium benzoate:**
   While considered safe in small amounts by the FDA, like the artificial food colorings described above, there is concern of potential as a carcinogen[160] and that it may promote hyperactivity and ADHD in children.[161] This additive is commonly found in soft drinks, fruit juices, and salad dressing.

3. **Potassium bromate:**
   Considered to possibly be carcinogenic to humans and therefore has been banned for use in food in Europe, Canada, and other countries including China. In the United States it is *not* banned and can still be found in baked goods including breads.[162]

4. **Butylated hydroxyanisole (BHA) and butylated hydrozytoluene (BHT):**
   The FDA permits consumption of both in small amounts even though the U.S. governments own National Toxicology Program states: "BHA is reasonably anticipated to be a human carcinogen based on sufficient evidence of carcinogenicity from studies in experimental animals"[163] and concerns exist for toxicity and carcinogenesis with excessive consumption of BHT.[164,165] These are often found in chips, chewing gum, some cereals, and candy.

5. **Propyl gallate:**
   Although the FDA considers propyl gallate to be safe and permits its use in the United States, this preservative is sufficiently suspect as carcinogenic that it has been banned in other countries.[166] This additive is commonly found in processed meat products and chewing gum.

6. **Monosodium glutamate (MSG):**
   Numerous anecdotal concerns ranging from headaches to fatigue and heart palpitations have been reported in individuals in response to exposure to MSG. Furthermore, a 2011 study found that adults in China that consume the most MSG are also most likely to be overweight.[167] The researchers suspect that MSG may interfere with leptin signaling which is the hormone that regulates satiety. However, a direct link between MSG and adverse reactions in humans has not been clearly established. It is reasonable to minimize intake of this food additive until a definitive conclusion is drawn especially if you have personally observed a sensitivity to this ingredient. In packaged foods, like other additives, MSG may also be a marker for otherwise unhealthy foods which is another justification for minimizing our intake until we know more. NOTE: MSG is a form of glutamic acid. If you are avoiding MSG then other forms of glutamic acid that should also be avoided

include: hydrolyzed soy/vegetable protein, autolyzed yeast extract, hydrolyzed yeast, and protein isolate. These additives are often found in soups, salad dressings, chips, and frozen entrees.

7. **Artificial sweeteners:**
   Including aspartame, sucralose, and acesulfame potassium (acesulfame-K). As previously described, many health concerns have surrounded the use of select artificial sweeteners[168,169,170] and they have also been shown to contribute to weight gain.[171] Furthermore, many experts agree that while the safety and effect on human health is still in question, more research is needed before we should permit their widespread consumption.[172] There is also an additional concern that using artificial sweeteners may make it harder for us to limit our intake and cravings for sugar. Even though they are artificial, the body still responds biologically to the intense sweetness which may be training our palette to crave foods with such extreme sweetness thereby making it harder for us to pass on the extra serving of dessert. Artificial sweeteners are often found in baked goods, "diet" foods, chewing gum, "diet" beverages, and packaged desserts. Furthermore, like many other additives described here, artificial sweeteners are also often a marker for a highly processed food.

8. **Carrageenan:**
   This one may surprise you since carrageenan is often found in many foods considered to be very healthy such as almond milk. However, there is sufficient concern surrounding this ingredient to at the very least minimize your intake of it until more conclusive research comes out to definitively implicate or exonerate it. Here is the issue: carrageenan is a food additive derived from seaweed and used as a thickening agent in foods like almond and soy milk, ice creams, cottage cheeses, and select processed foods. It is considered safe by the FDA however, recent studies have suggested that all forms of this additive can promote inflammation in the body particularly in susceptible individuals,[173,174] and as discussed before, chronic systemic inflammation can lead to conditions such as heart disease, Alzheimer's and Parkinson's diseases, and even cancer. Additionally, a 2012 study found that carrageenan can impair glucose tolerance, increase insulin resistance and inhibits insulin

signaling, all of which can contribute to the onset of diabetes.[175] Therefore, until we know more it is reasonable to at least minimize our intake of carrageenan, if not avoid it all together.

The one good news about carrageenan is that a few food manufacturers have recently reacted to concerns voiced by consumers about this ingredient and have announced an intention to remove carrageenan from their food products. The not so good news is they did not say when they would remove it or what they plan to replace this thickening agent with.

9. **Sodium nitrate/sodium nitrite:**
   I have intentionally left sodium nitrate and sodium nitrite for last on this list since the verdict is still not out on the impact that nitrites have on our health. I will discuss this further in chapter 19. In the meantime, know that while carcinogenesis has been seen in animal studies, there is minimal evidence of sodium nitrate and sodium nitrite playing a role in human carcinogenesis.[176,177] That said, when found in cured and processed meats, nitrates and nitrites are still considered to have the potential to pose a hazard to human health.[178,179,180] Nitrites and nitrates are often found in processed meats including processed bacon, hot dogs, and luncheon meats - which are advisable to avoid anyways - as well as in cured meats, and smoked fish for which at the very least, it is reasonable to minimize our intake. Nitrates and nitrates are also found naturally in vegetables, yet these sources do not appear to pose any problem and in fact, they may offer distinct health benefits.[181] At this time, it seems that not all food sources of nitrates and nitrites are equal with regard to their potential health benefits or risks.

Keep in mind, the simplest way to avoid these types of food additives is to stop buying processed food and choose to buy whole, real food instead. From now on when you go shopping take a copy of the foods listed in chapter 6 to use as your shopping list. And, if you do purchase packaged foods read the label first and choose foods without these unnecessary ingredients. In the meantime, in case you forgot, if you have foods in your pantry with these ingredients on the label, throw them out.

Finally, if you have any of the following items in that pantry, you know what to do; throw them out.

> ➢ White Bread, white pasta, and all other foods including crackers or breakfast cereals that have been made with refined, processed grains that are missing the fiber and nutrients found in their 100% whole grain counterpart. To identify refined grains in foods look for terms in the ingredient list such as: white flour, enriched wheat flour, or all-purpose flour.

I can imagine many of you are reading this page, paying attention to what I have written on it but, still sitting there reading. You may be rationalizing in your mind: *I cannot throw these things out because my husband, wife, son, daughter, cousin, uncle, dog, cat* (add your own people or pets here) *eats it.* You know what my response to that is? Get over it.

Remember, you are not doing this to accommodate a temporary period of food restriction and deprivation that you are on alone and making all your friends and family suffer through (a.k.a. "a diet"). You are developing a healthy meal plan and nutritional safe haven that will benefit the *entire* household including every guest that enters.

Let it go.

When disposing of the foods with ingredients that are described in this chapter, you may encounter food products that you have traditionally liked to always have on hand. Such foods may have been staples in your old meal plan. Do not let that stop you.

Let it go.

This is a moment of a renaissance to create that nutritional safe haven at home. This also means you do not need a stash of items "just in case company drops in" because your new food plan is great for them too! You do not need special foods for the kids because they will savor the same new manner of eating that you do. This step may be one of the most difficult ones you do, but as Nike® famously said: "JUST DO IT!"

And do it *now*.

Let it go.

ACTION STEP: If you feel uncomfortable throwing away food, consider donating it instead to a food bank. I have struggled with this since if the food is not good for you, it is certainly not good for someone that has less means then you do. That said when someone is starving and without food, then any food is better than nothing. In fact, this becomes a win, win situation. You achieve your goal while helping someone else achieve theirs.

Challenge! If you are trying to lose body fat, for every percent of body fat you drop, donate a bag of groceries to your local food bank. If you do not need to loose body fat you can still make it a habit once a month to donate one bag of groceries. Since your home from today on is a nutritional safe haven, from here on, the bags of food you donate will be filled with the good stuff so you will be paying forward a healthful *manner of living* to someone less fortunate.

Entertaining

Fortunately, you are not embarking on an isolating, restrictive food plan but rather one that is beneficial for everyone! Therefore, there is no need to alter your habits when company arrives. Your *manner of living* can be shared and celebrated with guests as well. If you have guests with shall we say, discriminating tastes such as a mother-in-law, learn how to prepare the foods she enjoys in a more healthful manner. She will hopefully, appreciate the effort and will be pleasantly surprised and delighted by how good it tastes! In the best case, she may even be inspired to put it into practice herself. What a wonderful way to pay it forward!

To help you succeed with this and with entertaining in general, in chapter 10 I have included some fantastic recipes for healthier spins on some traditional comfort foods and traditional cultural foods. I have also included some general tips of savvy substitutes that you can use to improve the quality of any traditional recipe without compromising flavor. You will also find some of my favorite recipes for everything from dips, snacks, and munchies to the most elegant of hors d'houvres. Entertaining will be a breeze!

Dining Out

At times, dining out can pose a challenge to most of us that are adhering to a healthful manner of eating. Menu choices can often be misleading; dishes can sound healthy such as a *filet of salmon over greens*, when actually, the salmon may be prepared fin deep in trans-fat laden oils, then coated with a sugar-based sauce, and the greens may be cooked beyond recognition; deplete of all the fragile nutrients they once possessed. When dining out and in doubt about how a food is prepared, simply ask the server. Most restaurants are generally willing to accommodate diners with special food preferences. If the food is prepared in an unhealthful manner, ask if other preparation methods are possible or ask the server to recommend an alternate menu option.

I must confess, I have a little sneaky tactic that I employ at times in restaurants to ensure my dietary request is taken seriously. I will tell the server that I have an allergy to the food item that I am trying to avoid. Yes, it is a gentle white lie but rather harmless, and having worked as a waitress while in college I have seen firsthand that when a waiter is busy, sometimes the allergy statement will be the only way your request is taken seriously.

Fortunately, these days many restaurants offer a variety of healthful options on their menus. Just keep in mind that it is easy to have too much of a good thing when dining out as portion sizes are often excessive are they are designed to satisfy the need for value held by most consumers. However, you can easily overcome this minor hurdle by eating mindfully; gauging your level of satiety with your gut; not with your eyes. It is not about clearing the plate but rather about satisfying your body's energy needs. Do not wait until you feel stuffed. Instead, when you feel comfortable and replenished that is when you should stop eating regardless of how much food remains on the plate. Do not allow external cues to dictate your body's needs. Whatever is leftover on the plate simply have it wrapped up and take it home to enjoy for lunch the next day or dinner that evening.

So, what about a situation when you are at a fantastic restaurant and an old culinary acquaintance appears on the menu and is calling your name? Yes, there are other healthy menu choices and yes, you can ask the waiter for an ingredient substitution but truth be told, on this occasion you actually just really want that menu item just as it is! What do you do? Do you reject that old friend?

If you dine out *infrequently* (four meals a month or less) then rejecting that old gastronomic friend can lead to a sense of deprivation. One thing I have always told my students and patients is that food is a pleasure! I never want to be responsible for taking the pleasure out of eating. For this reason, I have arrived at a solution for navigating through this type of situation.

When dining out for a special occasion, at times I will opt to employ what I call the **Choose Wisely Technique.** This simple technique allows me to indulge in decadent foods I enjoy while still maintaining control over my palate and not feeling any guilt or deprivation. To employ this technique, consider the following: When dining out, we are confronted with three major food choices that are not typically part of our regular dining experience at home. Specifically, we have options to eat bread that is served at the table prior to our meal. We have a choice to order a cocktail and, we have the option to select a delectable desert to end our meal. We also have the option of selecting a decedent entrée or appetizer.

When confronted by these choices especially if dining out is part of your normal culinary routine, enact the *Choose Wisely Technique.* Here's how it works. Each time you go out, choose to have EITHER the bread, the cocktail, the desert OR the decadent entree. The first three are all foods that tend to be high in added sugar and energy and therefore should be treated as sources of added sugar. Pick your poison or better stated, take pleasure in one indulgence, without being overindulgent. Today you may opt for the delicious homemade warm breads they provide; or you may choose to delight in the cool pina colada cocktail. Next time you may share in a decadent chocolaty dessert. The beauty in this technique is that each time you dine you can select which special food to have knowing that the next time you eat out you will enjoy the other one. There is no deprivation; just listening to what your discerning appetite is *really* craving on a given day. Enjoy it, savor it, delight in it and then, next time you dine out choose the other one. No deprivation, just delight, power, and control over your choices without a feeling of sacrifice; a new *manner of living*.

Dessert for Dinner?

On the rare occasion, there is nothing wrong with having dessert for dinner. Really! Allow me to explain. If you are craving a decadent dessert and you feel this is a craving that is overwhelming, then do not fight it; enjoy it! I would rather you go out, order a nice antioxidant rich tea and savor dessert as your dinner. I must emphasize this should not become a regular habit! It is not for every day, every week or even once a month. It is to respond to that once in a while inner voice, a few times a year when the craving, mood, and desire are overwhelming, and insatiable by any other means. In such occurrences, it *is* ok. In fact, it is good, as long as you truly savor it. No guilt, no regrets; just pure pleasure.

The reason this is justified, is that part of the process of refining your *manner of living* includes learning to *listen* to your body; paying attention to what it needs. If after implementing all these healthy strategies as part of your *manner of living* and one day you crave a particular culinary indulgence then by all means enjoy it. Savor it, revel in it! Then, for your next meal, simply resume your normal routine. No guilt, no feeling of self-sacrifice or punishment; just a healthful *manner of living*.

It is important to note that if this craving for desserts is *frequent* (daily or on most days), then most likely the craving is more of an emotional response (more on this in chapter 12) or habit, than a true craving. So, if you frequently have craving for sweets, try this technique: next time you crave that piece of cake first, wait 10 minutes. During those 10 minutes engage in some distraction from calling a friend, taking a bath, or reading a book. Is the craving still there? If so, reach for a piece of sweet fruit or berries. Does that sweetness satisfy the craving? Wait another 10 minutes to see. If the craving persists, then enjoy a small piece of that dessert. Many times, you will be surprised to see the craving for the dessert dissipate by practicing this simple technique. If the craving tends to persist despite this approach, then likely you are dealing with an emotional hunger rather than a true belly driven hunger. In chapter 12 you will learn how to regain control over emotionally driven food cravings.

Eating with Kids

With the exception of newborns and toddlers, children are designed to eat the same food as adults. Some parents argue with this point and claim their child will only eat food with Shrek® or some other cartoon character on the label. Yet, have you ever wondered why a child in China, Japan, or India can grow up eating the same traditional foods that their parents consume, but somehow the thought of serving "adult" food to our children in North America seems absurd?

The fact is, that children eat what their parents provide to them and we should be giving them the same high quality whole real food that we as adults are eating. The thinking that a child can only eat off a kid's menu is a tragic fallacy that has somehow permeated the collective consciousness of most North American parents. Have you ever really considered the type of food that is targeted towards our children? These 'kid friendly' foods and menus are often laden with fats, salt, sugar, artificial dyes, and other questionable additives and preservatives. In many cases these "foods" are so overly processed that one can argue that they are not even real food. Edible? Yes. Real food? No. In the best case, most of these kid friendly foods are high in energy but void of nutrients. In the worst case, they also contain many of the unnecessary additives that I described at the beginning of this chapter that actually have the potential to cause harm to human health. Either way, this is not the food we should be feeding our children.

In reality, children have fundamentally, the same nutritional needs as adults. The needs only differ as far as the *quantity* of nutrients and calories they need relative to adults but in general, there is no reason that you should eat poached salmon and roasted vegetables and serve your child a deep fried dinosaur shaped "chicken" nuggets and alphabet shaped French fries.

In 2005, The New England Journal of Medicine published a frightening report that revealed that the rapid rise in childhood obesity has led us to the first generation of American children that have a shorter predicted lifespan then their parents.[182]

116

The associated diseases and complications of obesity and being overweight (over-fat) including type 2 diabetes, heart disease, kidney failure, and cancer are predicted to strike people at younger and younger ages. A frightening fact is that previously type 2 diabetes was referred to as *adult onset* diabetes. It underwent a name change to type 2 diabetes since more and more children were being diagnosed with the disease. It was no longer appropriate to relegate the disease just to adults.

This problem has escalated to a point where in 2008 the American Academy of Pediatrics released controversial recommendations to begin high risk children on statin drug therapy in an attempt to decrease their risk of heart disease. The recommendation was made without sufficient evidence that this would benefit the children, but rather by extrapolating from data gathered in adult clinical trials and presuming that the same findings could theoretically be applied to children. Critics called this irresponsible. However, proponents of these guidelines argued that how can you blame them? Doctors are looking at dealing with unprecedented cardiovascular disease risk in young overweight and obese children; what else do you do with an 8 year old child that is presenting like a 57 year old overweight man?

Even though statin drugs are among the most prescribed drugs globally, no studies have ever looked at the side effects of these drugs when taken long term in children, particularly if taken for 40-50 years, or longer. Furthermore, there is no clear evidence either that this intervention is even benefiting the child.[183] This recommendation was clearly reactionary: if you can't beat 'em; join 'em. Children are getting sicker and fatter so instead of addressing the underlying cause, let's just work to lessen the consequences of these lifestyles. This thinking is all too commonplace in contemporary western healthcare. The approach of treating the symptom and not the underlying cause is easier; it limits a sense of personal and societal accountability. But the reality is in such situations, the cause in the majority of cases, is rooted in the poor choices we make about what we feed or do not feed our child. This requires reflection, accountability, and action. We <u>can</u> beat 'em. We <u>can</u> change the behaviors and lifestyle factors that have led to this problem in the first place. You can change these for your children and those children around you. The answer is simple; it is time to adopt a healthy *manner of living* for the children too.

The good news is there is no special program for kids. No new book to buy or app to download. As I have said countless times in this book thus far, the same principles of healthy living that apply to you apply to your children; regardless of their age.

You may think, so what if my child does not eat perfectly; he or she is not overweight, he or she does not have any risk factors for heart disease. Keep in mind that even if this may be the case, the dietary patterns and preferences that children adhere to as they age are greatly influenced by the manner of eating they are exposed to during early stages of their development. Therefore, childhood is a critical time for establishing healthful habits that will serve your children well as they grow.

While it is never too late to begin eating well, it is also never too soon to start developing healthy eating habits. Also, there is no better time than infancy to begin imparting these healthful habits. Food exposures during infancy have a profound impact on influencing an individual's lifelong food preferences. From the age of 6 months when table foods are first introduced, up until about 1 year of age, infants will develop a taste for almost anything you feed them. It may not be immediate, in fact often it can take between six and ten exposures to the same food for them to develop a taste for that food, but it will happen. It is common for a parent to pull a food item out of the repertoire if it is met with cries by the infant the first few times but do not give up on the good stuff. Keep reintroducing that healthy food item; it may take upwards of seven exposures to the food or more but generally, by the tenth time, the cries of dislike will often be replaced with giggles of delight!

If you missed the window of opportunity to develop a taste for broccoli in your infant, and you now are the proud parent of a picky eater, have no fear; hope is not lost! It is always possible to refine the taste preferences of a child, even for the pickiest eaters. Picky eaters may not be very adventurous right away when it comes to healthful, real foods and you may think they only have a small repertoire of food choices that they will even entertain on their palate, but with a little creativity, you can convert your picky eater into an open minded foodie.

Raising a Healthy Eater

So where do you begin? How do you convert a child that refuses to eat anything green or adamantly declines any food that does not resemble their favorite cartoon character, to eating and enjoying Brussels sprouts and spinach?

As with anything in life the best way to learn healthy habits is by actually practicing them. With children this is no different. Get them involved! Engage children in the shopping and cooking processes. Make it a fun game; have them seek out the delicious and healthful foods in the grocery store! Have them scope out the good ingredients on their own, have them find the most colorful array of vegetables and fruits. In the veggie section of the store, tell them to bring you the most delicious looking item they can find that is blue or red! Tell them that each color is another yummy and magical ingredient that will make them smart, tall, and strong! Tell them to find at least three different colors of vegetables to fill the cart. Be creative and have fun with it. Instill an understanding in your children of how to choose healthful foods based on their value and taste. Remove the stigma from foods as being good and bad. Don't even focus on calling it healthy; focus on the fun! Emphasize the delicious benefits of eating real food and forgoing fake, artificial products.

When you bring the food home, have the children help in the preparation. Have them help with mixing, washing, and if they are old enough, chopping. Have then set the timer, get them excited about how soon the food they prepared will be magically transformed through the cooking process into something deliciously wonderful. Who knows, you may even inspire a culinary spirit in your child and produce the next great chef as a result!

Here are six additional tips to convert your picky eater into a healthy, real food eater.

TIP#1: Expose seemingly picky eater to the same veggie *at least* six to ten times. You will be surprised how the first few times they may reject it but by the fifth or tenth time they may actually develop a taste for that food.

TIP #2: Engage children in the process of preparing veggies and healthful foods in creative ways. Remember, vegetables do not only have to be eaten raw or steamed. Have fun with the food! Check out my recipes suggestions for child friendly (and grown-up friendly!) items like cauliflower popcorn, sweet potato fries, or black bean brownies!

TIP #3: Don't tell a child to eat their carrots; tell them to eat "X-ray vision carrots"! Think your child will see through this? (Pun intended!) Consider these fascinating and playful studies by Brian Wansink, PhD, a Professor and the Director of the Cornell Food and Brand Lab at Cornell University. Dr. Wansink and his team of researchers invaded the lunchrooms of five ethnically and economically diverse schools and found that by calling carrots "X-ray vision carrots", the children consumed 66% of the carrots, as opposed to only 32% eaten when the carrots were labeled as "Food of the Day" and 35% eaten when they were unnamed. In their second study, Dr. Wansink and his team looked at food sales over two months in two neighboring suburban schools in New York City. They found that when serving "X-ray vision carrots", "Power Punch Broccoli" along with "Tiny Tasty Tree Tops" and "Silly Dilly Green Beans" vegetable purchases went up by 99%! [184]

TIP #4: Give your child a food adventure card! Make tasting new vegetables into a fun game. Create a special card and each time your child tastes a new vegetable, give them a sticker or stamp on their card. When they accumulate ten stamps reward them with a special treat that was agreed upon in advance. Just make sure that treat is not food related; especially not junk food. Instead, reward them with a book, or game, or perhaps a family outing somewhere special.

TIP #5: The kitchen is not a democracy. Remember, at the end of the day, a child eats what *you* feed them. As Buddy Hackett once said, "As a child my family's menu consisted of two choices: take it or leave it." When children are hungry, they will eat what you give them. Be patient, be creative, and be repetitive in the foods you expose them to; do not give up and give in. Help them refine their palates and build an appreciation for *real* food. Let cartoons entertain them on television or in books; not on their plate. Build healthy habits now so they can continue to reap the benefits as they grow.

TIP #6: When all else fails, resort to the covert *hide the veggie* tactic employed by delightfully devious moms and dads across the continent. The idea is that you add veggies in unpredictable places without telling your picky eater so when they least expect it (check out the black bean brownie recipe in chapter 10) they are eating legumes or greens! In general, I am not a huge proponent of this since I want children to enjoy the good stuff knowingly and willingly. That said, when all else fails or as a transitional tactic as you are working on adapting their palate, this is always a foolproof strategy to get both children (and adults) to eat more of the good stuff. In the recipe section in chapter 10, I have included several of my favorite tips for savvy substitutions that make even traditionally unhealthy snack and meals into foods that deliciously adhere to your new manner of eating.

Your *manner of living* is evolving beautifully; your kitchen is now on course to becoming a nutritional safe haven and if you have a child, you are prepared to engage them in your journey! The next chapter will help you to get the most culinary bang out of your buck by revealing how the proper storage and preparation of your foods may be just as important as the food itself.

Chapter 9

Preserve and treat food as you would your body,
remembering that in time food will be your body.
— B.W. Richardson

Food Preparation

Did you know that *how* you prepare a food can make or break its nutritional value? We already discussed how over cooking and processing foods can impact the net caloric intake provided by that food, but food preparation methods can have an even greater impact then just altering a food's digestible calories. In fact, in some cases, poor preparation methods can render a healthful food into a toxic carcinogen while smart preparation methods can elevate a mundane ingredient into super food status. We have often used taste preferences, habits, and convenience to guide the way we store and prepare our food but these preparation and storage methods can actually induce significant changes in the chemical composition of foods. The manner by which we prepare our food is therefore a very important part of maintaining a healthy *manner of living*. It is also one that is most commonly overlooked. It is not enough to just start with healthful ingredients. How you store and prepare them matters.

Consider a tomato, for example. Tomatoes are an abundant source of lycopene; a phytonutrient famous for its anti-carcinogenic effects.

Studies have reported benefits of consuming whole food sources of lycopene particularly with regard to preventing prostate cancer. Lycopene has also been associated with a decreased risk of other chronic diseases including cardiovascular disease.[185] What a wonderful dietary ally! We often default to thinking that raw is better when it comes to fruits and vegetables. However, it is not what you eat but what you *absorb* that matters. When it comes to tomatoes eating them raw appears to short change our culinary *bang for our buck*. A 2007 study conducted at Ohio State University and published in the British Journal of Nutrition found that exposing a tomato to heat and fat during cooking enhanced the absorption of lycopene by a whopping 55%![186] This informs us that to maximize the absorption of lycopene from tomatoes, we are better off passing on the sliced raw ones and instead choose a cooked marinara/tomato sauce made with healthy olive oil.

NOTE: If eating the raw tomatoes, adding a drizzle of extra virgin olive oil or another fat source like a thin slice of mozzarella, can enhance the absorption of lycopene since it is a fat soluble nutrient.

Broccoli is another great example of why preparation matters. As mentioned previously, broccoli has long been celebrated for its sulforophane content, a known potent anti-carcinogenic phytonutrient. A study published in 2000 indicated that exposure to heat reduced the nutritional value of broccoli and suggested that we are better off eating broccoli raw to retain its glucosinolates content (glycosinolate is the precursor to sulforophane).[187]   However, with food we need to balance science and palatability to ensure optimal consumption. While raw broccoli is certainly delicious, not everyone appreciates eating in its raw state. Which begs the question, what if we cook it? Can we still retain broccoli's healthful properties when we turn up the heat?

In 2007, Spanish researchers explored this precise question. They cooked broccoli but used a variety of different types of fats as part of the preparation. Low and behold they found that if you prepare the broccoli with extra virgin olive oil or sunflower oil, it preserves the same sulforophane and vitamin C levels as can be found in broccoli when it is raw.[188]

In 2009, researchers in China looked at the effect of five common cooking methods, including steaming, microwaving, boiling, stir-frying, and stir-frying followed by boiling, on the nutrients and health-promoting compounds of broccoli. However, instead of just looking at vitamin C and glucosinolates, they looked at a variety of nutrients in broccoli including chlorophyll, vitamin C, total carotenoids, total soluble sugars, total soluble proteins, and glucosinolates. They found that in general, steaming led to the lowest loss of nutrients, while stir-frying and stir-frying/boiling lead to the highest loss.[189]

One of the explanations for the findings in the aforementioned studies can be understood through simple nutritional biochemistry. Certain nutrients are fat soluble and others are water soluble. This means that we cannot absorb fat soluble nutrients without fat and water soluble nutrients without water. That is why the researchers found participants absorbed more lycopene when it was prepared with olive oil since lycopene is fat soluble. This also explains why water soluble nutrients are leached out of foods if those foods are prepared submersed in water. That is why boiling decreased the nutrients in broccoli. Therefore, regardless of the nutrients in the food in their raw form, the way we prepare it will impact which nutrients our body can actually access. Remember, *it is not what you buy or eat, but what you absorb that matters.*

Another interesting study illustrates this very nicely. In 2004, researchers gave three groups of participants a salad full of carotenoid rich spinach, carrots, romaine lettuce, and tomatoes. One group had fat-free dressing, the other a low-fat dressing, and the third groups had a full fat dressing. Each group consumed the salad and then researchers measured the subsequent absorption of the carotenoids in eat participant. Guess what? The group with the fat-free dressing had virtually *zero* carotenoid absorption. In the other two groups, the individuals who consumed the full fat dressing saw a greater absorption of carotenoids then those who consumed the low-fat dressing.[190] This makes sense since carotenoids are fat soluble. If there is no fat, there is no absorption. We can learn from this and other similar studies that simply adding a little healthy fat to a salad whether it is in the form of a few seeds, nuts, avocado, or extra virgin olive oil, can actually make or break the nutritional value of that salad.

Consider water soluble nutrients such as the essential vitamins B and C. If we prepare vegetable in a water bath, then chances are we are losing the majority of the nutrients down the drain. Water soluble vitamins have an affinity for water so it goes without saying that if you prepare them in a pot of water; those vitamins are staying in the water. The only time I recommend using boiling as a preparation method for vegetables is if you plan to keep the water. If you retain the water, you retain the vitamins. So use the water for a soup, a stew, or a sauce. Just do not expose this precious water to too much heat. These water soluble vitamins are often also quite heat sensitive.

When Good Oils Go Bad

We all know about the health benefits of extra virgin olive oil. It is a rich source of healthful monounsaturated fatty acids, a strong antioxidant, and offers an abundance of anti-inflammatory compounds. It is also fantastic drizzled on salads (we now know it even helps us enhance the absorption of the nutrients found in our salad!), it adds flavor and heart healthy fats to all sorts of foods and it is wonderful to cook with at low temperatures. That said, what is not commonly discussed about this oil is that while it is a healthy and flavorful addition to food, it is not the most stable oil.

Every type of oil has a **smoke point**. This is the temperature at which oil changes into a gaseous vapor. Cooks intuitively know to toss oil when it accidentally hits this stage of overheating since the delicate flavor will break down at this point. But it is not only the flavor that we are losing. The smoke point is the temperature at which oil will begin to degrade and along with losing its delicate flavor, it also begins to lose some of it vital nutrients. Furthermore, when oils are heated past their smoke point, they produce toxic aldehydes, compounds that are known carcinogens, linked to genetic toxicity and potentially causal agents of various diseases.[191,192] Thus, when olive oil or any oil is heated to temperatures exceeding its smoke point, the oil begins to denature. Its chemistry is altered from being a health promoting food to one that is potentially harmful.

How do you know what is an oil's smoke point? The precise temperature varies depending on the oil and even on how it was manufactured. For example, manufacturers of extra-virgin olive oil list their smoke points as anywhere from "just under 200 degrees" to well over 400 degrees. In general, highly refined oils have higher smoke points. The highest smoke point olive oils are the "light" ones which have been thoroughly refined and are often virtually colorless and tasteless. Unrefined, cold-pressed extra virgin olive oil is the healthiest form of olive oil but also has one of the lowest smoke points of all forms of olive oil. It is the least refined, most nutrient dense, and also the most flavorful. The method of cold-pressing (or cold extraction) is the best way to preserve the delicate flavor and nutrients within an oil, while "virgin" implies that no heat or chemicals were used during the extraction process, and that the oil is pure and unrefined. An extra virgin, cold-pressed olive oil will have a beautiful color varying from a light green to a warm yellow hue, which is a reflection of the fact that it contains the largest concentration of fragile nutritive components. It also has a spectacular flavor.

One study reported the smoke points of three commonly used oils as follows: [193]

Oil	Smoke Point
Coconut oil	175° Celsius or 347° Fahrenheit
Extra virgin olive oil	195° Celsius or 383° Fahrenheit
Canola oil	238° Celsius or 460° Fahrenheit

However, this is not a perfect guide. Different oils, depending on the degree of processing they have undergone, will have different smoke points. These days many manufacturers are noting the smoke point of their oils directly on the package. Generally, some good options for high heat cooking (such as stir frying, searing, or dry heat methods like grilling, roasting and baking) include avocado oil, select olive oils, or rice bran oil. However, keep in mind that it is advisable to keep high heat cooking to a minimum. For low to moderate heat cooking (such as poaching, steaming, braising, or stewing), oils such as extra virgin coconut oil or extra virgin olive oil are often good options.

If your brand of oil does not indicate the smoke point, then the best way to monitor this is while cooking, **if at any time the oil begins to smoke and produce an unpleasant odor and flavor, then discard that oil.** Start again and either use a more heat stable oil if you are using a high heat cooking method or simply prepare your food using less heat.

To get the most out of the fine oils, consider the following five tips:

1. Whenever possible (when preparing food with low or no heat) choose organic, unrefined, cold-pressed oils. These are the highest quality and healthiest oils; they are also the tastiest!

2. Test the temperature of the pan before adding oil. Water boils at 212 degrees Fahrenheit so add a drop of water to the pan before adding the oil; if it at or above this temperature the water drop will sizzle and evaporate within a second or two. This will inform you that oils with a smoke point below 212 degrees should not be used until the heat is reduced.

3. Use high quality oils for preparing sauces at low heat.

4. Add high quality oils to dishes *after* cooking to enjoy their full flavor and nutritional value.

5. Use the high quality oil cold, drizzled over salads.

Storage of Oil

The heat sensitivity of oil expresses itself during storage and not only when cooking. Do not to keep olive oil or any oil, near to a heat source. For convenience, we often place oil beside the stove so it is in arms reach during cooking. Resist the urge to do this. The heat will break the oil down and so will the bright kitchen light.

Delicate oils are not only heat sensitive; they are also light sensitive and even time sensitive. Italian researchers compared oils stored in the light or in the dark for 12 months and found that oils stored in clear bottles under standard supermarket lighting lost at least 30% of their tocopherols (vitamin E) and carotenoids. That is before you even brought the oil home from the store! Another team of Italian researchers wanted to learn about the shelf life of oils so they analyzed a variety of olive oils and found that after 6 months of shelf life almost all of the oils had a 40% reduction in antioxidant activity levels.[194] Spanish researchers looked at virgin olive oil that was storage for 12 months under the best controlled conditions and found Chlorophyll content dropped by as much as 30%, beta-carotene dropped by 40%, and vitamin E dropped (alpha-tocopherol) by 100%! [195]

Here are three useful tips for storing oils that we can learn from the Spanish and Italian researchers:

1. Purchase or store oils in tinted glass, non-reactive dark plastic, or metal containers. These are the best choice for preserving oil's beneficial compounds.

2. Store oils in a cool (less than 67-77°F), dark and dry pantry. You can even keep it in the refrigerator. The cloudy appearance that ensues with refrigeration will subside as it sits at room temperature and will not damage the oil. Most importantly, keep the oil away from any heat source. As mentioned, many people for convenience sake keep the oil below the sink or beside the stove but this sort of placement will expose the oil to excessive heat that will inevitably and prematurely denature that oil and render it potentially harmful.

3. Dispose of any unused oils after six months. High quality oils should not be purchased in bulk quantities. Invest in high quality oils in sizes that you expect you will use within three to six months.

Is Your Cooking Method AGE-ing You?

In recent years, there has been emerging research on the effect of compounds referred to as dietary Advanced Glycation End Products. The acronym AGE, is quite appropriate since it appears that the greater our dietary intake of AGE compounds, the greater the effect these compounds have on aging us. Exposure to AGEs is unavoidable; they are a produced as a *normal* byproduct of our metabolism and all of us have these compounds circulating in our systems. They only appear to become problematic when levels become excessive. In fact, recent studies have implicated high level of AGEs in the pathogenesis of conditions as diverse as poor skeletal muscle strength and sarcopenia, to diabetes, Alzheimer's and cardiovascular disease. [196,197] It appears that if excessively high levels of AGEs accumulate in human tissue, it increases levels of systemic inflammation and in turn, this can precipitate early aging and the onset of disease.

The million dollar question is, if AGEs are produced as a natural byproduct of human metabolism, how on earth can we reduce levels of AGEs and more importantly, what on earth do they have to do with the preparation of food?

The answer is simple: AGEs are formed naturally, but they are also present in food – particularly, uncooked animal-derived foods. Furthermore, depending on the way we prepare these foods, the cooking method can results in the formation of additional AGEs. AGEs are formed in cooking when a sugar molecule hooks onto amino acids of a protein or when a sugar combines with certain fats or other compounds. For all you chefs out there, you may have heard this reaction referred to as the Maillard or browning reaction. Cooking temperatures over 120°C (248°F) greatly accelerate this reaction.[198] Animal-derived foods that are high in fat and protein are generally higher in AGE content and more prone to new AGE formation during cooking. Conversely, foods high in carbohydrates and low in fat such as vegetables, fruits, legumes, and whole grains contain relatively few AGEs, even after cooking.[199]

The next question is, how much is too much? How do we know when our AGE intake is excessive? Unfortunately, the answer to this question is not quite as simple. At this time, a safe and optimal dietary intake of AGEs has not yet been established. The best guide we have is from a study that looked at a group of healthy New Yorkers. The average dietary AGE intake in a group of healthy adults from the New York City area was assessed and found to be roughly 15,000 AGE kU/day.[200] To put this into context, pork bacon, fried for five minutes with no added oil has 91,577 AGE kU. Previously frozen farmed Atlantic salmon steamed in foil for 8 minutes at medium heat has 1,000 AGE kU. A snack of hummus with vegetables has 487 AGE kU, grilled vegetables have 261 AGE kU, red kidney beans cooked for 1 hour have 298 AGE kU; a banana has 9 AGE kU.[201]

As you can see even healthy, whole, real foods contain AGEs. The idea is therefore not to avoid them altogether but rather to simply keep intake to a reasonable level; perhaps under 15,000 AGE kU/day. The good news is that the manner of eating recommended in this book satisfies this recommendation beautifully.

In general, here are some tips to minimize your intake of AGEs:

1. Avoid eating the browned or charred portions of cooked meats.
    o   Food that is "browned" (particularly high-fat, high-protein food) is also likely to be high in AGEs.

2. Limit intake of processed foods.
    o   Many processed foods have been exposed to a high cooking temperature to lengthen their shelf life so as a result, they may also have high content of AGEs.
    o   Additionally, food manufacturers have *added* AGEs to foods as flavor enhancers and colorants to improve appearance.

3. Increase fruit and vegetable intake.
    o   Cooked or raw, fruits, and vegetables are naturally low in AGEs, and contain compounds such as antioxidants that can decrease some of the damage done by AGEs.

Changing the way you prepare your food can also impact AGEs intake dramatically. Here are some cooking tips that decrease the formation of AGEs: [202]

1. Cook foods *slow and low!* Use a low amount of heat (ideally at or below 120°C or 248°F) and a longer cooking time when preparing foods.

2. Maintain the water content in food. Marinate meats and/or cook with moist heat (such as steaming or poaching, etc.)

3. Methods of cooking to reduce AGE intake:

    ✓ steaming
    ✓ boiling
    ✓ poaching
    ✓ stewing
    ✓ stir-frying
    ✓ using a slow cooker

4. Limit the following cooking methods known to accelerate AGE formation:

    - grilling / barbequing
    - baking at high heat
    - broiling
    - roasting
    - searing
    - frying

5. If using one of the above cooking methods, minimize AGE formation and exposure by:

    ✓ Wrapping food in foil before grilling.
    ✓ Using acidic marinades such as lemon juice and vinegar, before cooking and marinate the meat for a few hours prior to exposure to high, dry heat.
    ✓ Adding garlic or herbs and spices like turmeric, ginger, or rosemary to the meat as they contain protective antioxidants. (And they taste great!)
    ✓ Increasing your intake of fruits and vegetable with that meal which as mentioned previously, will help mitigate some of the damage done by excessive intake of AGEs.

Remember, it is not about avoiding AGEs in our food completely, it is simply about minimizing our exposure. Once in a while it is fine to enjoy that grilled grass-fed beef burger or steak, but make it a rule for yourself: for every one serving of grilled (or any dry/high heat prepared) meat, enjoy three servings of delicious vegetables!

Additional Considerations Regarding High Heat Cooking

In addition to AGEs, concerns have also been voiced over three other compounds produced in high heat cooking namely: heterocyclic amines (HCAs), polycyclic aromatic hydrocarbons (PAHs), and acrylamide. HCAs and PAHs are formed in the same way that AGEs are produced in foods. The concern over these compounds stems from the fact that in animal studies HCA and PAH exposure led to cancer in animals.[203] While no study has been able to definitively demonstrate that HCAs and PAHs cause cancer in humans, many experts suggests that HCAs and PAHs may be one of the reasons that an increased risk of certain cancers is seen in people that consume large amounts of red meat and processed meats.[204]   High consumption of well-done, fried, or barbecued meats has been associated with increased risks of colorectal,[205] pancreatic,[206,207] and prostate,[208] cancer. Whether this increase can be attributed to the AGEs, HCAs, PAHs, nitrites, nitrates, the high iron and saturated fats content, or a combination of some or all of these factors, remains to be seen.

Acrylamide is a little different. Unlike HCAs, PAHs, and AGEs, it is not found in abundance in animal proteins exposed to high heat cooking, but rather in baked and starchy foods exposed to high heat. In fact, food plans that are higher in protein and raw foods will be *lower* in acrylamide. It is formed when an amino acid reacts with sugars in high carbohydrate foods. If you eat a lot of commercially processed foods you probably have consumed a lot of acrylamide since it is rampant in foods like French fries, breakfast cereals, crackers, pretzels, pastries, and chips. Regrettably, it is even present in coffee. Many concerns have surrounded consumption of acrylamide, a toxin also found in tobacco smoke, but at this time, we do not have evidence that dietary consumption can cause cancer in humans. It is considered to be "probably carcinogenic in humans"[209] but to date; scientific studies have only shown carcinogenicity in animals and not in humans.[210]   In fact, a 2012 review of all the published literature on the topic of dietary acrylamide intake has failed to demonstrate an increased risk of cancer.[211]

The Bottom Line:
Based on the best available scientific evidence, it is reasonable to limit our intake of dietary sources of HCAs and PAHs, and to use cooking methods that minimize their formation. This means limiting our consumption of meat overall, especially processed meats, and avoiding high heat cooking methods when we do consume meat. The good news is that just as HCAs and PAHs are produced in the same way that AGEs are, our intake can be reduced using the same approach described previously for reducing dietary AGEs.

Concerning acrylamide, lack of evidence of risk is not evidence of safety. Since the foods that contain acrylamide are mostly processed foods, it is sensible for many reasons to choose to eat whole, real foods instead. Regarding coffee, at this time it seems that the benefits of consuming coffee outweighs any theoretical risks so if you enjoy a cup of coffee, continue to enjoy that *cup of Joe* – in moderation.

Pots and Pans

What we cook in can be just as important as what we are cooking. Perfluorooctanoic acid (PFOA) is a chemical used in making of nonstick and stain-resistant material. It is known to be a hormone disrupter in humans, linked to cancer and birth defects in animals,[212] and if you have non-stick Teflon pots and pans at home, you have been exposed to this toxic substance, perhaps at every meal. New research suggests that PFOA may also be linked to obesity. In 2012, researchers in Norway and Denmark found daughters of women exposed to PFOA during pregnancy were up to three times more likely to be overweight.[213] How ironic, considering the major reason most of us invested in non-stick Teflon pans in the first place was to cut fat from our cooking methods to help us stay trim. It is time to reduce your exposure to PFOA by replacing those non-stick Teflon pans.

Here are my favorite options for cookware:

Cast Iron and Enameled Cast Iron
These are by far my favorite pots and pans. I can remember my grandmother cooking using cast iron pots that were beautifully seasoned with love and time. Enameled cast iron cookware are cast iron with a glass enamel coating. They have a naturally nonstick

surface making them one of the best alternatives to non-stick pans; they are also durable and can withstand high heat cooking even in the oven. While costly, they are truly an investment that lasts. And as an added bonus, at a few pounds each every time you lift them they are also providing a great workout for your arms!

Stainless Steel

Stainless steel is another great cooking surface. I use these often for preparing everything from fish to omelets, and for sautéing. Many chefs appreciate that stainless steel can brown food better than nonstick surfaces. Although, keep in mind that while certainly tasty, that browning of proteins reflects the Maillard reaction and hence, the generation of AGEs. So remember to keep the browning of proteins to a minimum if you tend to consume a high intake of animal proteins.

Glass Bakeware

Choose glass for baking, storing, and preparing foods. It is high-heat safe and transfers nicely from oven to table.

Bamboo Steamers

Bamboo is a great material to use for steaming vegetables and fish. It is also remarkably inexpensive.

Food for thought: Concerns exist that cookware made of metals can release nominal amounts of heavy metals like iron and aluminum into our food. Some studies have suggested that this is not a cause for concern.[214] However, in general this is not a robust area of research so it is hard to draw firm conclusions regarding long term safety. As mentioned previously, Tephlon cookware should be avoided. But it is also reasonable to avoid using aluminum cookware due to concerns that overtime, it may leach potentially toxic amounts of aluminum into our food. Copper cookware should also be avoided for everyday use for the same reason. Even cast iron may pose a concern by releasing iron. But do not fret, this does not mean we have to resort to cooking on banana leaves!

When it comes to cast iron, while small amounts of iron may leach from the pan into our food, for many of us this generally does not appear to be a problem. It may even be beneficial for vegans, vegetarians, and others that are at risk of iron deficiencies or that simply have a low iron intake. That said, if you have a condition of iron overload or consume excessive amounts of animal product already high in iron, it is reasonable in such cases to avoid using cast iron cookware altogether.

To minimize concerns, choose *enameled* cast iron which has a non-reactive surface which means it prevents chemicals and metals from leaching into foods. Replace the enameled cookware only if the enamel chips since it may then expose the user to the reactive metals beneath.

NOTE: often the cheaper products are the ones more inclined to chip. High quality enameled cast iron while costly, can last a lifetime. Another tip is that if you use cast iron pans, alternate them with other types of cookware (like enameled or stainless steel) and avoid cooking soups and highly acidic foods (like tomatoes or lemons) in cast iron or stainless steel pots and pans as the acidity will tend to increase the amount of metals leached from the cookware. Personally, I prefer using enameled cookware for this purpose.

Stainless steel is a great option but discard pots and pans with scratches. Stainless steel in the least reactive metal but once scratched, these pans are more likely to release metals like nickel and chromium into our food.

NOTE: Stainless steel products are labeled as 18/10, 18/8, or 18/0 meaning that they contain 18% chromium and 10%, 8% or 0% nickel, respectively. Do not assume that the 18/0 is a safer choice just because it does not contain nickel. In fact, it is quite the opposite. Without nickel, stainless steel is more likely to rust and often is reflective of a poorer quality product. You are better off purchasing 18/10 or 18/8 and again, simply discard if and when scratches occur.

TIP! Does your food seems to have a metallic taste? That may be a sign that it is time to discard old cookware.

NOTE: The internet abounds with articles recommending ceramic dishware which may be a reasonable option as well. However, keep in mind that the glazes used on some ceramic dishware particularly antique ones, may contain lead. When the cookware cracks or chips it

136

can therefore leach lead into our food which eventually may become dangerous to our health. Ceramic coated cookware is generally not recommended since often these coatings are made from synthetic materials and furthermore, overtime they may degrade and expose the user to the reactive metals beneath.

The Bottom Line:

Enameled cast iron and stainless steel cookware appear to be among the safest and most useful cookware. Replace cookware when chips or scratches occur. Glass bakeware and bamboo steamers are also excellent cookware options whenever appropriate.

Presentation Matters

After we select our food, prepare it, and finally serve it, we also need to be mindful of the serving vessel we use. If you are trying to control the quantity of food you consume at each meal, take some advice from Dr. Brian Wansink. His research has revealed that that we consume *more* when our plates are larger and our cups are wider. Simply switching from a 12-inch to a 10-inch dinner plate leads people to serve and eat 22% less![215] Because of visual illusions, people pour 28% more into short wide glasses than into tall ones.[216]

ACTION STEP: To help control portion sizes at each meal, begin with your plate. Ditch the massive, oversized dinner plates and invest in small, but pretty salad size plates to use for meals instead. Also, choose the tall, thin drinking glasses instead of the big gulps to enjoy beverages without overdoing it.

Chapter 10

He showed the words "chocolate cake" to a group of Americans and recorded their word associations. "Guilt" was the top response. If that strikes you as unexceptional, consider the response of French eaters to the same prompt: "celebration."
— Michael Pollan

These Are a Few of My Favorite Things

I love food. I take delight in the pleasure of eating and I want the same for you. Healthful eating should never be about deprivation; it is about celebration! Eating beautiful, whole, real foods nurtures the body, delights the mind, and tantalizes the palate. Remember, there are no good foods or bad foods; just *real* food made with real ingredients to savor. It is the consumption of artificial, overly processed, edible food-like products that deceives the palate. Such artificial "foods" prey on our vulnerability to the taste of fat, sugar, and salt and trick us into an insatiable overindulgence that never truly satisfies. Overtime, these artificial foods hurt us. They impact our health in a detrimental way, which in turn limits our productivity and potential. Real food has the opposite effect and therefore should be celebrated and enjoyed. As you journey towards your new manner of eating, to help you make the most of nature's delightful culinary bounty, I have outlined in this chapter some of my favorite recipes and methods of food preparation that I hope will help make your journey even more delightful.

My Food Philosophy

I have long maintained the mindset that the distinction between breakfast foods, lunch foods, dinner foods, and snack foods is all wrong. There should be no rules! No boundaries! I suggest you feel free to enjoy breakfast foods at dinner and lunch foods as snacks and vice versa. To honor this counter culture approach to dining, I have listed below some of my favorite recipes for you to enjoy as entrees or snacks. Simply decrease the serving size if you choose to enjoy them as a snack and increase your serving size if they are to be enjoyed as a complete meal. Most of these recipes are ones that I came up with over the years, some are my mom's and grandmother's healthy spin on traditional family recipes, and others are ones I adapted from friends or esteemed chefs. As most of these have evolved to include my own personal touch to them, I encourage you to do the same. Treat these recipes as guidelines, not gospel! Feel free to get creative; add spices and herbs that taste good to *you*, experiment with ones you are not familiar with, but most of all, have fun and enjoy! Play music in the background as you prepare each meal, smile as you add each ingredient, and take that extra few seconds to make the presentation of the dish look appealing since we eat with our eyes as well as our mouth. Last but not least, every great chef knows that the one indispensable, secret ingredient that transforms every dish into a masterpiece is… *love.* Find the joy in each meal you prepare and…

Bon Appetit!

Recipes and Creative Combinations

Green Bean French Fries

Warning, these are addictive! French fries never stood a chance next to these.

Place green beans in a large bowl. Add olive oil, salt, and pepper, to taste. Toss to ensure green beans are lightly coated. Optional: add any herbs and spices you enjoy; get creative, try cayenne pepper for a kick!

Layer beans onto a flat pan. Preheat oven to 375 F and roast green beans for about 30-45 minutes until they have a slightly shriveled look and brown color. Their crunch and taste will delight!

140

TIP! This also works great with carrots. Toss thin long French fries-like slices in salt, pepper, and olive oil and roast for at 450 F for approximately 15 minutes.

Sweet Potato French Fries[217]

For a more traditional French fry without the saturated or trans fat but with added phytonutrients and fiber; this is sure to please even the pickiest eater.

- o 2 medium sweet potatoes
- o 1 ½ tablespoons olive oil
- o Salt and pepper to taste
- o Optional: add paprika, cayenne pepper, and a pinch of cinnamon to taste

Preheat oven to 450 F. Cover flat pan with parchment paper. Half the sweet potatoes lengthwise. Place on flat slide and slice 5-6 spears (thick and long strips) of sweet potato. Place them on the pan and toss with olive oil and your favorite herbs and spices. Spread them in one layer. It is important that they have space around them and are not piled up on each other. Bake for 15 minutes and turn with tongs or a spatula. Bake for another 5 to 10 minutes, until lightly browned. Add salt and pepper to taste. Serve hot, room temperature, or cold.

"This Will Make You Like Any Vegetable" Roasted Vegetables

Use this recipe for cauliflower, carrots, Brussels sprouts or… any vegetable!

Cut up vegetable into bite sized pieces. If using Brussel sprouts, cut in half or quarters, and then blanch first in boiling water; this will help them retain their bright green color while roasting. Drizzle vegetable with olive oil. Add a pinch of salt and fresh ground pepper to taste.

Preheat oven to 375 degrees and roast vegetables for about 30-40 minutes until they have a golden brown hue. The browner they turn (without burning), the more the caramelization, and thus, the sweeter they taste. Keep an eye on the veggies to prevent them from burning. Serve immediately.

TIP! Spice up the veggies with cayenne pepper for a kick! Or get creative and add onion powder, garlic, cumin, paprika or turmeric or any other herbs and spice you enjoy!

Freedom Frittata

This delightful egg dish is called a freedom frittata because you are free to add any vegetables, herbs, and spices you have on hand!

Over low heat, sauté your choice of vegetables. I love spinach and kale with mushrooms and peppers but any combination of vegetables are great. Seriously! Green peppers are delicious so is zucchini, onions, asparagus; anything goes. Add two or three eggs and mix it up to coat all the veggies.

Now it's time to spice it up! I like to add everything from chia seeds for their crunch and boost of omega 3 fats, to sun dried tomatoes and fresh dill. Add salt and pepper to taste. Cover, and then cook eggs over low heat for about 3-5 minutes. Turn off heat and keep covered to continue to cook in its own steam for an additional 5 minutes. Et voila! Enjoy.

Convenience tip!

Prep and Freeze: Preparing foods in advance is a simple way that you can have healthful recipes that are grab and go each day of the week. I encourage you to prepare recipes in advance and freeze them in portion controlled amounts so you can easily reheat them as needed throughout the week.

Make sure you label it with the date and content so it does not end up lost in the frozen abyss of your freezer.

<u>Serendipitously Sumptuous Smoothie</u>

A serendipitously sumptuous smoothie since as you use your imagination and any vegetables, fruits, and spices you choose, each time you make this smoothie it becomes a surprisingly new and delightfully delicious concoction.

- o Select any fruits you enjoy (I like berries, try frozen ones; cheaper and available any time of the year)
- o Select any vegetable you enjoy (I like kale and spinach)
- o NOTE: use 2 servings of fruit to each serving of vegetable so the vegetable do not overpower the other ingredients
- o Add ¾ cup of water or almond milk
- o Add 1 tbsp almond (or other nut) butter
- o Add (to taste) flavor and nutritional enhancers like cinnamon, nutmeg, vanilla extract or ginger
- o Add a splash of nutritional enhancers like chia seeds or ground flax seed

Blend over ice, and enjoy!

<u>Almond Didn't Realize There Was Kale in This Shake!</u>[218]

This sweet smoothie is sure to please any palate and is a great way to sneak nearly a cup of kale into even a picky eater's food plan!

- o 1 small frozen banana sliced
- o ¾ cup kale (stems removed)
- o ¾ cup almond milk
- o 1/8 tsp each of cinnamon, nutmeg and ground ginger
- o Add a drop of vanilla extract to taste
- o 1 scoop of protein powder

Blend with ice and enjoy!

TIP! Want to add caffeine *and* an antioxidant kick? Add ½ cup of unsweetened iced coffee!

Savory Spinach Cupcakes

A fun way to get a whopping serving of protein and phytonutrients all in one delicious and portable package!

Makes about 12 cupcakes

- 1 package, 12 oz of fresh spinach (can also use frozen chopped spinach, thawed, drained and squeezed well)
- 4 large eggs
- 2 minced cloves of garlic (can substitute or add any other fresh herbs you enjoy)
- Salt and fresh ground pepper to taste
- ¼ cup shredded Romano or parmesan cheese
- ½ cup part-skim ricotta cheese or low-fat cottage cheese

Preheat oven to 400 degrees. In a food processor, chop the spinach and place in a separate bowl. Add the rest of the ingredients and mix by hand until they are all combined. Then, spoon the mixture into a cupcake tin using approximately one large scoop per cupcake. (Spray the cupcake tin or paper slightly with a high smoke point olive oil to prevent sticking) Bake for approximate 20 minutes. Before it is done, sprinkle a little extra parmesan or Romano over top and allow to brown for an extra moment under the broiler. Enjoy!

TIP! Make these in a mini cupcake tin (recipe can make about 24) for delightful hors d'ouvres when entertaining. (Just watch the cooking time; you may only need about 10-15 minutes if making the mini version)

Fresh Bean and Avocado Salad[219]

High in fiber, phytonutrients, healthy fats, protein, anti-inflammatory herbs and spices, with a low glycemic load, and at under $2.00 per serving this salad proves that the healthy food can taste great, be inexpensive, and be filing too!

- 2 cloves garlic, minced
- 3 tbsp fresh lime juice
- 1 tbsp extra virgin olive oil
- 1 tsp cumin

- o Pinch crushed red pepper flakes
- o ½ teaspoon salt
- o 15 oz can black beans, rinsed and drained
- o 1 cup canned chickpeas, rinsed and drained
- o 1 cup cherry tomatoes, halved
- o 1/4 cup minced red onion, finely diced
- o 1/4 cup cilantro, chopped
- o 1 medium avocado, diced
- o Can of tuna (optional)

In a large bowl, combine the garlic, lime juice, oil, cumin, crushed red pepper, and salt. Add the black beans, chickpeas, tomato, onion, and cilantro; mix well. Gently mix in avocado. Enjoy!

Southwestern Medley Salad[220]

Another perfect meal! This salad is not only big on flavor it is also easy and inexpensive to prepare, high in fiber, phytonutrients, healthy fats, protein, anti-inflammatory herbs and spices, and has a low glycemic load.

- o 15-ounce can black beans, no salt added, rinsed and drained
- o 1 cup cooked quinoa (according to package directions)
- o 1 small red bell pepper, chopped
- o 1 cup chopped fresh mango
- o 1/4 cup finely chopped red onion
- o ½ cup chopped fresh cilantro
- o 1 small jalapeño pepper, seeded and finely diced
- o Juice from 1 medium lemon or lime
- o 1 ½ tbsp extra virgin olive oil
- o 2 garlic cloves, minced
- o ½ tsp ground cumin
- o ½ tsp chili powder
- o 1/4 tsp ground turmeric
- o Can of tuna (optional)

Whisk together the lemon juice, olive oil, garlic, cumin, chili powder, and turmeric in a large bowl. Add the beans, quinoa, bell pepper, mango, onion, cilantro, and jalapeño; mix well. Enjoy!

Chopped Salad

Traditionally an Israeli side dish, this salad is the perfect addition to any meal and also serves as a deliciously bite-sized way to enjoy fresh vegetables.

- o 1 cucumber (English or seedless)
- o 2 tomatoes (firm but ripe)
- o ½ red onion
- o ½ red pepper (optional)
- o 3 or 4 sprigs of parsley, to taste
- o 1 lemon
- o Extra virgin olive oil

Chop up the cucumber, red pepper, and tomato finely to about the same small size. Chop up the red onion very small, slightly smaller than the other vegetables. Chop the parsley.

The dressing is simple: a 50/50 olive oil and lemon juice mix, and salt and pepper added to taste. Mix it all together in a bowl and enjoy.

TIPS! Try adding 1 ½ teaspoons of sumac powder, also known as zataar, it is a delicious spice blend! You can also get creative and add crumbled feta cheese, or chickpeas, or 1 to 2 tablespoons finely minced mint or dill. Enjoy this salad with anything: Add to wraps and sandwiches, enjoy as a side dish, add any protein or enjoy on its own!

Kale, Quinoa, and Avocado Salad

High in fiber, phytonutrients, vitamins, minerals, and protein this flavorful salad is sure to make kale into a new dietary staple in your home!

- o 1 bunch kale, washed and de-stemmed
- o (Use Lacinato Kale, sometimes called Dinosaur Kale or Tuscan Kale)
- o 1 cup cooked quinoa (prepare the quinoa using chicken or vegetable broth instead of just water to enhance the flavor)
- o 2 avocados, diced
- o Juice of 2 oranges (lemons work well too but I like the added sweetness from the oranges)
- o 2 tablespoons extra virgin olive oil

146

o   Salt to taste
o   Optional: Add diced tomatoes and cucumbers

De-rib the kale: remove the tough stems of the kale by running down the center of the leaves with your hand or fold the kale along the rib and run a sharp knife down the side. Stack the de-ribbed kale leaves and chop them into small bites or for a fancier presentation, *chiffonade* the kale by stacking the leaves, rolling them tightly, and then slicing them perpendicularly to the roll to create long, thin strips.

Tenderize the kale: this step brings out the sweetness in the kale and minimizes the bitterness. Place the cut kale into a bowl and add the oil, salt and citrus. Knead and squeeze ("massage") the kale with your hands using a sterile glove or very clean hands. Add the other ingredients, mix together and enjoy!

TIP! This salad often tastes better after it has sat for a few hours to allow the kale to tenderize further. It is even great the next day!

Almond Crusted Baked "Fried" Chicken

This is a delicious alternative to fried chicken but trust me…
you will not miss the 'fried'.

o   2 boneless-skinless chicken breasts
o   Salt and pepper to taste
o   Pinch of cayenne
o   ¼ cup unsalted almonds
o   1 small garlic clove
o   4 tsp olive oil

Preheat oven to 425°F. Season chicken breasts with salt, pepper and cayenne. (Can substitute other spices like cumin in place of the cayenne) Place on aluminum foil or parchment paper lined sheet pan. In a food processor, or blender make a coarse paste of the almonds, garlic and oil. Top each chicken breast with half mixture pressing down slightly to adhere. Roast for 15 to 18 minutes until cooked through.

TIP! Cut chicken into strips for healthy chicken fingers for the kids!

Almond Crusted Baked "Fried" Fish

Here is a slight variation on the previous recipe using fish instead chicken. Please note: the proteins and spices are interchangeable in each recipe.

- o 1lb white fish fillets – about 4 medium sized fillets
- o ½ Cup almond meal
- o ¼ cup parmesan cheese, grated
- o Salt, pepper, garlic powder (add any additional spices you like)
- o 2 egg whites

In a shallow bowl beat egg whites, and add salt, pepper, grated parmesan cheese, and garlic powder. Place almonds in another shallow bowl. Dip filet in egg mixture, then coat with almonds. Place on aluminum foil or parchment paper lined sheet pan. Bake at 450° for 10-15 minutes or until fish flakes easily with a fork. Enjoy!

Sautéed Red Cabbage

This is a healthy, low calorie spin on a traditional eastern European dish. It is rich in phytonutrients and anti-inflammatory compounds and makes a tasty accompaniment to any protein dish or is enjoyable just on its own.

- o 1 medium head of red cabbage, shredded
- o 1 medium red onion, chopped
- o 1 tsp olive oil
- o 2 – 3 tbsp apple cider vinegar
- o Salt and fresh ground pepper to taste
- o Optional: ½ to 1 tsp caraway seeds and/or 1 apple cubed

On a stove top over medium heat, sauté the olive oil and onions until the onions turn a golden brown. Lower the heat, and then add the cabbage and vinegar. Add salt and pepper to taste. Cover and allow cabbage to soften over the heat, stirring periodically to prevent burning. Allow to cook for approximately 15 – 20 minutes until cabbage is soft. If adding apple, allow the dish to cook a few minutes longer until apple is softened, then enjoy!

Super Power Veggie Purée Soup

I make this all the time. Consider it like a warm smoothie! A simple and delicious way to enjoy a wealth of vegetables in one satisfying warm cup.

o   Sauté ½ cup of chopped onions in olive oil over low heat until golden brown
o   Add ½ cup each of chopped celery and carrots
o   Add 4 cups of chicken or vegetable broth
o   Add 4 cups of ANY vegetable (My favorite is broccoli) allow it to soften in the soup by simmering soup over a low heat and then blend!
o   Add salt and pepper to taste

Puree the soup until all the ingredients are blended into a smooth consistency. If using butternut squash instead of the broccoli, use 1 can pureed, no sugar added season with cinnamon to taste. If using broccoli, use 1 whole head and try adding a tablespoon of pesto for a special flavor.

Salmon Veggie Scramble

Another dietary staple in my household.
This is a quick, easy meal that everyone enjoys.

o   1 tsp olive oil
o   2 – 3 large eggs
o   1 small red onion, diced
o   ½ cup mushrooms, chopped
o   ½ cup fresh spinach, chopped
o   1 medium tomato, chopped
o   ½ can wild salmon

Heat olive oil in skillet over medium heat. Whisk eggs in small bowl and set aside. Add onions and mushrooms to the skillet and sauté until soft. Add the eggs and stir gently with a spatula for 2-3 minutes. Add spinach, tomato, and salmon and heat for another 2-3 minutes. Season with any spices you enjoy.

TIP! For a portable meal, place in a whole grain tortilla or collard green leaf, roll it and go!

Curried Tuna (or Salmon) Salad

This is a great way to spice up boring tuna or salmon salad using anti-inflammatory curry powder and turmeric, and blood sugar balancing cinnamon. Do not forget to add the pepper! Pepper contains a compound called piperine which helps support the absorption of turmeric. I love eating this salad with green apple slices or in a hollowed out tomato or green pepper.

- o 1 can water packed tuna or salmon
- o 1 tsp plain, unsweetened Greek yogurt
- o ½ tsp Dijon mustard
- o 1 tsp lemon juice
- o ¾ tsp ground cinnamon
- o ½ tsp curry powder
- o ½ tsp black pepper
- o Add fresh cilantro
- o Salt to taste
- o ½ tsp sweet pickle relish (optional, look for ones without or with minimal added sugar)

Mix ingredient together well (add tuna or salmon last once other ingredients are blended) and serve over top red or green peppers, or apple slices.

Fresh Sardine Spread

Did you know that one can of sardines packed in spring water contain 17g of protein, 1,300 mg of omega 3 fatty acids, and significant amounts of vitamin D, vitamin B12, and calcium? Low cost, high flavor, and a nutritional powerhouse! While sardines are great just lightly grilled or drenched in lemon juice, this recipe is a good way to introduce sardines to unfamiliar palates.

- o 1 (3 3/4-oz) can sardines, drained
- o 1/8 cup plain, unsweetened Greek yogurt
- o 1 tablespoon finely chopped fresh flat-leaf parsley
- o 1 teaspoons drained bottled capers, chopped

- o ½ teaspoon finely grated fresh lemon zest
- o 1-2 teaspoons fresh lemon juice
- o Black pepper and salt to taste
- o Splash of extra virgin olive oil (if the sardine were packed in water)

Mash together all ingredients in a bowl with a fork until combined well. Enjoy with veggies, on crackers or a tortilla, or on top of a fresh salad!

Quick Curry

This is not only low calorie, immune enhancing, and anti-inflammatory, it is also deliciously satisfying. Feel free to add any protein or vegetables you enjoy.

- o Sauté ½ a small chopped onion in 1 tsp coconut oil until golden brown
- o Add ½ cup chopped carrots and ½ cup chopped celery
- o Add at least ½ cup mushrooms (any kind you like and the more the better!) and any other veggies you enjoy
- o Add ½ to 1 cup of coconut milk or almond milk (add more or less to achieve desired consistency)
- o Add 1 package of Shirataki noodles
- o 2 tbsp curry powder
- o 1 tbsp turmeric
- o ½ tsp black pepper
- o Fresh ginger root and fresh cilantro to taste
- o Pinch of salt to taste
- o Add a protein over top (chicken, salmon, shrimp, etc.)

Enjoy!

Avocado and Lime Soup[221]

For a taste of Mexico, this soup is sure to delight. It is also a great way to enjoy a satisfying meal rich in protein and anti-inflammatory herbs and spices.

- o 2 ripe avocados, cubed
- o 2/3 cup chopped red onions
- o 2 large cloves of garlic, chopped

151

- o 2 tsp chopped canned chipotle chile in adobe sauce (may substitute ½ tsp of smoked paprika and a dash or more, of cayenne to taste)
- o ¾ tsp salt
- o ½ tsp ground cumin
- o 2 ½ cup nonfat plain Greek yogurt
- o ¼ cup chopped fresh cilantro
- o 3 tbsp fresh lime juice
- o Optional Garnish:4 tortilla chips (try the tofu chip or almond chip recipes!) or ¼ cup store bought (or fresh made) salsa

Puree then stir in ½ cup ice water and lime juice (can add more water to thin if desired) Chill until cold for 1 hour.

TIP! Garnish with chips and salsa before serving.

Dressings and Sauces

Customize Your Own Oil and Vinegar Dressing

- o 3 to 4 parts oil (extra virgin olive oil)
- o 1 part acid (red wine vinegar)
- o Add seasonings: salt and pepper (freshly ground), Dijon mustard and/or garlic or chopped fresh herbs, or minced shallots

May use less oil and instead of the red wine vinegar, add one of the following: Rice vinegar; white wine vinegar; raspberry or other fruit vinegar; champagne vinegar; or lemon, lime or orange juice.

Simple Dijon Salad Dressing

Mix Greek yogurt with Dijon mustard (to taste) and cilantro or chives.

Simple Avocado Salad Dressing

Mash 1 ripe avocado with crushed garlic (to taste), lemon juice, and a pitch of sea salt. Mix until smooth.

Simple Creamy Dill Salad Dressing

Combine ½ cup of cottage cheese and a bunch of freshly chopped dill. Mix until smooth. Add salt and pepper to taste.

Fresh Lime and Garlic Dressing

- o   1 tbsp extra virgin olive oil
- o   Juice of ½ a lime
- o   ½ clove of garlic, crushed

Wisk all ingredient together.

Avo-Yogurt Dressing

- o   1 ripe avocado
- o   ¼ cup plain, unsweetened Greek yogurt
- o   ½ shallot, roughly chopped
- o   1 tbsp apple cider vinegar
- o   Juice of 1 lime
- o   Salt and pepper to taste

Combine in a food processor.

Peanut Sauce[222]

Tastes great as a dipping sauce, dressing, or a marinade.

- o   ¼ cup peanut flour
- o   1 tbsp rice vinegar
- o   1 tbsp sesame oil
- o   2 tbsp liquid aminos, coconut aminos or soy sauce
- o   3 tbsp water

Wisk all ingredient together.

Coconut aminos: a soy free and gluten free replacement for soy sauce. It is also generally lower in sodium, raw, and organic.

Japanese Restaurant Ginger Miso Salad Dressing[223]

- o 1 large carrot, peeled and roughly chopped
- o 1 large shallot, peeled and roughly chopped
- o 2 tablespoons roughly chopped ginger
- o 1 tablespoon white miso
- o 2 tablespoons rice wine vinegar
- o ¼ cup sesame oil
- o 2 tablespoons water

Combine in a food processor.

Party Foods and Entertaining

While all the recipes listed thus far can work for a sit down dinner party, below are a few tasty treats that work well as passed hors d'oeuvres. Whether entertaining for one or one hundred, these foods are great options that are not only portable for the partygoer but also visually delightful and easy to prepare.

Hummus Deviled Eggs

This is a favorite at my home. We serve it all the time as an appetizer when entertaining and there are never any leftovers.

- o 6 large eggs
- o 3-4 tbsp of your favorite hummus

Place eggs in enough cold water to cover. Bring water to a boil over high heat and then turn off the heat, cover and cook for 12 minutes. Promptly chill eggs under cold water so yolks stay bright yellow. Remove shells and halve eggs lengthwise. Remove the yolks and place in a medium bowl. Mash yolks with a fork and add your favorite hummus. Very carefully spoon mixture back into the egg white halves and then garnish with a light sprinkling of paprika.

<u>Options</u>:
Instead of hummus, add guacamole. Seriously! Just mash the guacamole and the yolks together, and then spoon the mixture into the egg white halves. Garnish with fresh cilantro.

To experiment with different and delightful flavors, instead of the hummus, use Greek yogurt and then...

Curry Devilled Eggs: For an anti-inflammatory boost, add ½ teaspoon of curry powder, 1 tsp of Dijon mustard, pepper to taste, and a drop of tabasco or hot pepper flakes to the mixture.

Smoked Herring or Trout Deviled Eggs: For a delicious boost of protein and a whopping serving of omega 3 fatty acids, blend the Greek yogurt with 1 tsp of Dijon mustard and mix with canned, smoked trout or smoked herring. Really! Add in fresh herbs like dill and 1 tsp of lemon juice and pepper.

Crostini with Pea Purée

This is another favorite! My mom came up with this recipe and it has become a staple and a consistent crowd pleaser every time I entertain.

<u>For Pea Puree</u>

- o   1 red onion, chopped
- o   1 pound of frozen green peas (allow to defrost prior to cooking)
- o   Sea salt and fresh ground pepper to taste
- o   1 tbsp olive oil

On a stove top over medium heat, sauté the onions in olive oil until the onions turn a golden brown. Lower the heat, and then add the peas. Add salt and pepper to taste. Mash the ingredients together using a hand mixer or fork.

For "Crostini"

Slice a whole wheat baguette into small ½ inch slices. Lightly brush each slice with olive oil then place in the oven on low heat until slightly toasted. Watch the bread carefully to avoid burning; this only takes a few minutes in a hot oven.

For gluten free or low carbohydrate diners: the pea puree also tastes great on top of my almond or tofu chips.

Scoop a tablespoon of pea puree over top "crostini" of your choice, place on a serving platter and enjoy!

Custom Meatballs

This is a deliciously versatile meatball recipe. I adapted it from a recipe I found in Men's Health magazine and it is always a favorite.[224]
The best part? You can use any type of protein and seasoning you enjoy!

1. <u>Choose your protein:</u> For four servings, start with 1 and ½ pounds of meat or fish. Nearly any ground protein works, try chicken, turkey, lamb or even tuna, salmon or shrimp! For fish, remove the skin and bones, and pulse in a food processor until ground up.

2. <u>Add your binder:</u> 2 large eggs and ¾ cup plain dry whole grain bread crumbs. You can also use almond meal instead of the bread crumbs or use half and half. Quick cooking oats are also a great replacement for the bread crumbs.

3. <u>Season it.</u> Add 1 teaspoon of salt and ½ teaspoon of fresh ground pepper and then get creative! Here are some suggestions:

>   1 tbsp minced ginger
>   ½ cup minced onion
>   1 tbsp minced garlic
>   ½ cup grated Parmesan or Romano
>   1 tbsp minced jalapeno
>   1 tsp ground cumin

¼ tsp ground cinnamon
¼ tsp cayenne pepper
¼ cup chopped fresh herbs (or 1 tsp dried) try parsley, mint, dill or any you enjoy!

4. <u>Form it.</u> Form the protein mixture into 1-inch-diameter balls and arrange them on a baking tray. NOTE: Forming the balls should be messy; if the mix isn't sticky, then the meatballs will be dry. Eggs, ricotta cheese or milk-soaked whole grain bread crumbs all can add moisture.

5. <u>Cook it.</u> Bake at 450°F until they're browned and caramelized, about 12 minutes.

6. <u>Enjoy it!</u> Try using one of the dressing recipes in the preceding pages as a delicious dipping sauce.

Turnip and Parsnip Martini

Pureed roasted root vegetables make a delicious alternative to traditional mashed potatoes.

o 1 onion, chopped
o 2 cups turnips, chopped
o 3 cups parsnips, chopped
o 3 tbsp extra virgin olive oil
o 1 tsp salt and 1 tsp black pepper

Preheat oven to roast at 400°F. Rinse and chop turnips, parsnips, and onion. Toss with olive oil, salt, and pepper. Spread out evenly on a roasting pan. Roast at 400°F for 45 minutes. Puree vegetables in high-speed blender or food processor until smooth then serve.

TIP! Try topping with freshly grated parmesan cheese. Serve the mash in a martini glass for that added touch of class!

Cauliflower Mash

For thanksgiving and other festive meals, this makes a great alternative to the boring, bland, and heavy mash potatoes.

- o 1 medium head cauliflower, trimmed and cut into small florets (about 6 to 7 cups)
- o 1 tablespoon extra-virgin olive oil
- o ¼ cup of low sodium chicken or vegetable broth
- o Sea salt and ground black pepper, to taste

Steam cauliflower until very tender, about 10 minutes. Next, transfer cauliflower to a food processor. Add ¼ cup of broth and oil 1 tablespoon at a time, and puree until smooth. (You can also mash cauliflower with a potato masher). Season with salt and pepper and serve.

TIPS! Just like above, can add garlic or top with grated cheese or chives. To increase the richness can add ½-3/4 cup plain Greek yogurt or 1-2 tablespoons nutritional yeast for a cheese free, cheesy flavor!

Cauliflower Pizza Crust

This is my own spin on a popular gluten-free and low calorie alternative to pizza crust. Consider the recipe a base; feel free to make it your own by adding your favorite herbs and spices and topping it with your favorite pizza toppings or anything else you enjoy: there are no rules!

- o 1 head of cauliflower
- o 1/3 cup grated/shredded parmesan cheese (if you don't have parmesan cheese try using ¼ cup soft goat cheese or ¼ cup grated mozzarella instead. A combination of ¼ cup mozzarella and parmesan works well too!)
- o 1 large egg
- o ½ tsp dried oregano
- o ½ tsp dried basil
- o ½ tsp garlic powder
- o ¼ tsp salt & ¼ tsp pepper
- o A pinch of dried chili flakes
- o 1 tsp almond meal (optional)

Preheat oven to 400°F. In a food processor, blend the cauliflower into small flakes resembling grains of rice. If you don't have a food processor you can also grate the cauliflower using a box grater. Steam the "cauliflower rice" for 5 minutes (preferred) or microwave for 5 minutes. Allow to cool. Dry the cooled cauliflower very well using a cheese cloth. Wring out as much water as you can. Do not skip this step! If the cauliflower is too wet it will make the final crust fall apart. The dried cauliflower should yield about 3 cups but will vary slightly depending on the size of the cauliflower used.

In a large bowl, mix the oregano, basil, garlic, salt, pepper, chili flakes, and cheese with at least 3 cups of the cauliflower. In a separate small bowl, whisk or beat the egg, then add the egg to the cauliflower mixture and mix it all together into a dough-like consistency. NOTE: If it seems too wet you can add a little almond flour to the mix.

Cover a large cookie sheet with parchment paper. On the paper, shape the "dough" into 3 or 4 small or one large pizza. Feel free to get creative with the shape: try squares, rectangles or the traditional circle. I like to keep the outer edges a little thicker to resemble the outer crust on traditional pizza.

TIP! Instead of a cookie sheet, you can prepare the pizza on the parchment paper and then transfer the paper to a pizza stone.

Bake the pizza crusts for about 25 to 30 minutes at 400°F. You will need a slightly longer cooking time for a thicker deep dish style crust and a shorter cooking time for a thin crust. Keep an eye on the crust so it does not burn. When it turns golden brown the crust is ready. Remove crust from oven and top with your favorite pizza toppings!

TIP! Since we used dry herbs for the crust, brighten up the flavors by using fresh herbs like basil leaves as toppings.

Return to oven for 5 to 10 minutes until toppings are ready. Enjoy!

TIP: Seal up well in tin foil and freeze any leftover pizza to enjoy your very own homemade frozen pizza for lunch another day.

Snack Ideas

Baked Tofu Chips

These are easy and fun. The simultaneously chewy and crunchy texture is a great alternative to chips and also makes a fantastic protein packed snack on the go. These are also great added to sandwiches, over salads or of course, on their own!

o   2 blocks firm organic tofu
o   For the seasoning: 2 teaspoons salt, ½ teaspoon paprika, 1 teaspoon onion powder, 1/8 teaspoon black pepper, pinch of cayenne powder or anything you like! These versatile chips can support sweet flavors (such as vanilla, cinnamon, and nutmeg) or savory spices (such as turmeric, cayenne pepper, lemon pepper, rosemary etc.)

Preheat oven to 250 degrees. Slice tofu into very thin pieces, approximately 1/8 inch thick. (Thicker pieces will allow for a chewier texture; thin pieces will lead to a crunchier chip like texture) Place a sheet of parchment paper on a baking sheet. Spray lightly with oil. Lay tofu flat on baking sheet. Bake for about 25 minutes or until golden brown and crisp. Add the seasoning mix and enjoy!

Almond Chips (Or Almond Crackers, or Almond Tortilla Wraps, or Almond Pizza Crust)

This is a versatile recipe that by modifying the thickness and shape of your dough, you can make it into chips, a soft tortilla, or a pizza crust. This is a great one for all of you who are sensitive or allergic to gluten.

o   2 cups of almond flour (almond meal)
o   2 large eggs
o   1 tsp olive oil
o   ½ tsp salt
o   Add seasonings to taste: For a savory flavor try dill, rosemary, cumin, paprika, garlic powder, cayenne pepper, fresh ground pepper or any combination of them. For a sweet delight, add a touch of vanilla extract, cinnamon, nutmeg or cloves.

Preheat oven to 350 degrees. Combine all the ingredients and knead into dough. Place on parchment paper and roll out into desired thinness.

For chips: Get as thin as possible without breaking. Use a knife to cut the chips into little triangles (or any shape you like)
If you are making chips: wait until they are slightly golden brown. Turn them once after about 7 minutes to allow them to brown slightly on both sides. Use savory chips with any dips or add the sweet chips as a side with any dessert dish or just enjoy them on their own!

For tortillas: Keep the dough a little thicker (cut into desired shape and size) and for pizza crust, keep the dough even thicker! (Shape by hand into a large circle or rectangle and into desired size).

Bake for about 8-10 minutes. (Bake for less time if you want it to be flexible for a tortilla wrap; bake a little longer for a pizza crust.)

If you are making pizza crust: remove from oven and add your choice of toppings (tomato sauce, veggies and cheese or anything you like!) then, continue baking as needed to warm up the toppings. If you are making tortilla wraps: remove, add your choice of filling (pre-cooked chicken breast or canned salmon with guacamole and veggies) then roll it up and enjoy!

Cauliflower Popcorn

This is a great snack; Bet you can't have just one!

- o 1 head cauliflower
- o 4 tbsp olive oil
- o 1 tsp salt, to taste

Preheat oven to 425 degrees. Cut cauliflower florets into bite-size pieces. In a large bowl, combine the olive oil and salt, whisk, then add the cauliflower pieces and toss thoroughly. Line a baking sheet with parchment for easy cleanup, then spread the cauliflower pieces on the sheet. Roast for 1 hour, turning 3 or 4 times, until most pieces have turned golden brown. The browner they turn (without burning), the more the caramelization and thus, the sweeter they taste. Serve immediately!

TIP! Spice it up with cayenne, onion powder, garlic, cumin, paprika or turmeric or any other spice you like. Turn on a movie and enjoy!

Desserts

Easy Homemade Date Paste

While not a dessert on its own this is great as a sugar substitute to sweeten any desert recipes. This is great in baked goods or anytime you need a touch of sweetness!

o   Use any type of date (Medjool dates tend to be the sweetest)

Remove the pits from the dates. Soak a cup of dates in enough water to cover them for approximately an hour. Remove the dates from the water but do not discard the water (pour the water into a separate cup). Put dates in a blender or food processor and gradually add the water back to the dates until you achieve your desired consistency. (Imagine the consistency of honey) You may or may not need to add all the water back depending on how thick you would like the paste to be.

TIP! You can store the date paste for up to one week in the refrigerator in a sealed container.

Dark Chocolate covered Strawberries, Blackberries etc.

This could not be easier and is an elegant and healthy dessert. Feel free to get creative; use any fruit you enjoy!

o   6 ounces semisweet chocolate, chopped (Choose a chocolate with 72% cocoa content or higher)
o   20 strawberries with stems (You may also use any other fruits or berries. Be sure fruit are washed and dried *very well* prior to dipping them in the chocolate. Make sure no water gets into the melted chocolate.)

Put the chocolate into a heatproof medium sized bowl. Fill a medium saucepan with a couple inches of water and bring to a simmer over medium heat. Turn off the heat; place the bowl of chocolate into the saucepan over the water to melt. Stir continuously until smooth. (You can also melt the chocolates in a microwave at half power, for 1 minute, stir and then heat for another minute or until melted.) Once the chocolate is melted, remove from the heat. Line a sheet pan with parchment paper.

Hold the strawberry by the stem, and dip it half way into the chocolate. Hold above chocolate for a moment allowing any excess to drip off, then gently place on its side on the parchment paper. Repeat with the rest of your berries or fruit. Allow to set for about 30 minutes and then, enjoy!

Optional: add a pinch of cayenne pepper or even curry powder to the melted chocolate for a delightfully nutritious kick! Or sprinkle the dipped berries with a pinch of sea salt or ground almonds or walnuts before the chocolate sets.

Ricotta Cheese and Berry Delight!

A simple recipe, but a delightful and healthy dose of phytonutrients and protein! Presentation is key; serve in a martini glass for added flair.

- o   6 oz low fat ricotta cheese
- o   ¼ tsp pure vanilla extract (avoid "imitation" extracts)
- o   1/8 tsp almond extract (avoid "imitation" extracts)
- o   1 tsp sugar to taste (Use any dry sweetener you enjoy such as raw cane sugar)

Mix ricotta, vanilla, and almond extract, with the dry sugar. Place a scoop of the ricotta cheese mixture at the bottom of each glass. Top with fresh berries. Optional: For extra sweetness, drizzle with date paste, raw honey or maple sugar.

Chocolate Cranberry Biscotti[225]

This is one of my favorites to serve with coffee or tea at the end of a great meal. I adapted it from a recipe I saw years ago on a television cooking show and at only about 70 calories per serving it makes a delightful treat!

Makes about 1 ½ dozen

- ¾ cup white whole wheat flour (if desiring a gluten free option try quinoa flour)
- ¼ cup finely ground almonds
- 3 tablespoons unsweetened cocoa powder
- ¾ teaspoon baking powder
- ¼ teaspoon salt
- 1 large egg
- 1/3 cup raw cane sugar or date sugar
- 2 teaspoons pure vanilla extract (avoid "imitation" extracts)
- ½ teaspoon pure almond extract (avoid "imitation" extracts)
- ¼ cup dried cranberries (look for ones without added sugar)
- Optional: melted dark chocolate for drizzling

Preheat oven to 350 degrees and arrange a rack in the center of the oven. Line a baking sheet with parchment paper. Whisk together flour, ground almonds, cocoa powder, baking powder and salt in a medium bowl. Beat egg and sugar with a handheld or standing mixer on medium-high speed until pale and thick, about 5 minutes. Beat in vanilla and almond extracts. Reduce speed to low, and gradually add flour mixture. Beat until no traces of flour remain. Stir in cranberries. The dough will be very wet and sticky. Scrape the dough onto the prepared baking sheet, forming a thick line in the center. Wet your hands and pat dough into a 9-x-3-inch rectangle.

Bake until puffed and dry to the touch, about 25 minutes. Cool on pan for 15 minutes; keep oven on. Peel off parchment and carefully transfer rectangle to a cutting board. Cut crosswise into 1/3-inch-thick slices. Lay slices flat on unlined baking sheet, and bake until dry, about 10 minutes. Flip slices and bake for 10 minutes more. Let cool completely. Biscotti will crisp as they cool. Drizzle with melted chocolate if desired. Enjoy!

Cha Cha Chia Pudding

This will surprise you! It is the easiest pudding you have ever made and most likely the healthiest as well. Customize the flavors to whatever you enjoy!

- o ¼ cup chia seeds
- o 1 cup of coconut or almond milk
- o For extra sweetness, add about 1 tbsp of honey or the sweetener of your choice (add more or less to taste)

> **Chia seeds:** These little seeds can be added to anything from soup to omelets. They add a subtle nutty crunch along with a punch of protein, omega 3 fatty acids, and fiber.

Now the fun part, mix in any flavor boosts! Some suggestions include: cocoa powder, instant coffee powder, vanilla or other extracts, cinnamon – anything you like! There are no rules!

Stir chia seeds into milk using a fork to get them fully coated with the liquid. Cover and refrigerate overnight and voila… delicious, healthy pudding. Try it for breakfast with berries and nuts on top!

Baked Banana Bites (B^3)!

The simple preparation of these cookie-esque snacks makes it a great way to get children of all ages into the kitchen! This was inspired by a recipe I came across online[226] that I have adapted into a great base that you can get creative with to make it your own. For example, I love adding chia seeds and almond butter for added protein, added omega 3 fatty acids and added flavor.

Makes approximately 18 – 20 small bites

- o 2 bananas (ripe)
- o 1 cup steel cut oats, quick cook
- o 1 tsp pure vanilla extract (avoid "imitation" extracts)
- o 1 tsp cinnamon
- o Optional: 1/3 cup unsweetened cocoa powder (optional but recommended! Add more for a deeper chocolaty taste and include a pinch of salt if using chocolate to bring out the flavor
- o Optional: 1 tsp pure almond extract (avoid "imitation" extracts)

For added sweetness: add dark chocolate chips, raisins or dry berries

For added crunch: add chopped walnuts, chia seeds or almonds

For added texture and flavor: add peanut or almond butter (or any nut butter)

For a special fall flavor boost: use pumpkin pie spices instead of the almond extract and cocoa powder

For my favorite combination: use only the bananas, oats, 1 tbsp of chia seeds, 1 tsp of pumpkin pie spices and cocoa powder. Yum!

Mash bananas and oats together with a fork (avoid blending it into a complete mush; keep little banana pieces slightly visible) Add other ingredients and mix well. If it looks too moist add more oats; too dry, add more bananas. The final product will become moister if you allow this mixture to sit for at least 10 – 15 minutes before baking. Use a silpat or parchment paper and cover it with a thin layer of coconut oil to avoid sticking. Bake for 10-15 minutes at 350 degrees (longer cooking time for crunchier, shorter for chewier, softer treats – watch so as not to burn). Enjoy!

Deliciously Raw Brownie[227]

I came across this recipe from a blog called My New Roots. It is the easiest and most nutritious and delicious brownie recipe and is always a crowd pleaser. Be prepared to have guests ask you: "are you sure this is healthy?" With no refined sugar and only raw, whole food ingredients you can feel comfortable responding that it is certainly the healthiest brownie they will ever eat!

- o 2 cups whole walnuts
- o 2 ½ cups Medjool dates, pitted
- o 1 cup raw cacao powder (may substitute unsweetened cocoa powder)
- o 1 cup raw unsalted almonds, roughly chopped
- o ¼ tsp. sea salt

Use a mortar and pestle or a food processor (blend on high) to crush the walnuts until finely ground. Pulse in the cacao and salt. Add the dates one at a time while blending. Should look like cake crumbs but, when pressed together will end up sticking together. If it is not sticking then add more dates.

Chop the almonds (do not grind them into a flour, keep them in rough pieces to add texture the brownie). In a large bowl (or the brownies pan), combine the walnut-cacao mix with the chopped almonds. Press into a lined cake pan or mold. Place in freezer of fridge until ready to serve (easier to cut when they are cold). Store in an airtight container. Chill and enjoy!

Raw Pie Crust

This easy pie crust makes the perfect base for any pie filling. Using only dates and nutrient rich nuts, this delicious and nutritious crust will give that "je ne sais quoi" flair to any pie you make.

- o 2 cups of any raw nut flour/meal (almonds, cashew, walnuts etc.) (I like mixing one part almond meal with one part cashew meal)
- o 1 cup Medjool dates, pitted
- o 1/4 tsp sea salt
- o Optional: Add a splash or vanilla extract and/or spices like cinnamon

Mix all ingredients by hand or blender. Blend until dough-like. You can use a mortar and pestle to crush the dates if you don't have a blender. If the mixture is not sticking together then add a couple teaspoons of warm water. Line a pie crust lightly with oil (I like using an organic coconut oil). NOTE: may also use a muffin tin instead of one large pie tin if making mini tartlets

Spread the crust mixture into a pie/tart pan, using your fingers to press it down around the edges. Put the pie crust in the freezer for about 15 minutes. This helps it become more firm and solid.

Add ANY filling you like!

Raw Apple Pie[228]

Easy, nutritious and delicious; give the traditional apple pie a modern upgrade.

For Crust

- o Use *Raw Pie Crust* recipe described previously and add:
- o 1 tsp vanilla extract (avoid "imitation" extracts)

For Filling[229]

- o 8 medium apples (divide into 5 and 3) Peeled, cored and chopped into chunk (For convenience, may use 2 ¼ cups of organic, unsweetened apple sauce to replace 3 of the apples)
- o 5 Medjool dates, pitted (or more for added sweetness)
- o 1 tsp cinnamon (to taste)
- o 1 tsp pumpkin pie spice
- o 1/4 tsp ginger powder
- o ½ tsp vanilla extract (avoid "imitation" extracts)
- o Add juice from ½ an orange or blend ½ orange with apple mixture

Process 5 of the chopped apples into small, chunky pieces. Remove and place in a large bowl. Process the remaining 3 chopped apples with the dates and spices until it forms the consistency of an apple sauce. Mix the apple sauce with the chopped apples.

Spread the crust mixture into a pie/tart pan, using your fingers to press it down around the edges. Spoon the pie filling onto the crust and flatten with the back of a spoon or spatula. Decorate the pie with a few more nuts, apple slices. Chill and enjoy!

TIP! Wait to add the filling until prior to serving to prevent the crust from getting soggy. Also, feel free to prepare the night before. The flavors seem to get better as the merry together overnight.

Raw Blueberry Pie

A phytonutrient rich dessert that is easy and fun to prepare.
Works well with any berry that is in season.

For Crust:

- o   Use Raw Pie Crust recipe described previously and add:
- o   1 tsp vanilla extract (avoid "imitation" extracts)
- o   Sprinkle of cinnamon
- o   2 tsp lemon juice
- o   1 tsp lemon zest

For Filling:

- o   2–3 ripe bananas
- o   2 cups blueberries
- o   1/2 cup Medjool dates, pitted (or more for added sweetness)

Using a food processor, blend half the blueberries with one banana and all the dates. Slice the remaining bananas into small rounds and cover the bottom of the pie with a layer of banana slices. Gently mix in the remaining whole blueberries into the batter. Pour the batter over the sliced bananas that are covering the crust.
Chill and enjoy!

Sweet Potato Pie

Make this healthy and delicious pie a new Thanksgiving staple.

For Crust:

- o   Use *Raw Pie Crust* recipe described above and add:
- o   1 tsp vanilla extract (avoid "imitation" extracts)
- o   2 tsp lemon juice
- o   1 tsp lemon zest

For Filling:

- o   3 large sweet potatoes (enough to fill 1 ½ cups)
- o   1 cup organic almond milk (or coconut milk)
- o   1 tsp vanilla extract (avoid "imitation" extracts)
- o   1 to 2 tsp pumpkin pie spices (or more to taste)

> **Important tip:** When you are cutting the fat in recipes they may bake quicker and at lower temperatures then the original recipes. Often it is a good idea to decrease the temperature by approximately 25 degrees and check on the baked goods frequently to prevent over baking it.

Pierce each sweet potato several times with the tines of a fork. Bake sweet potato for 45 minutes in oven at 350 F. Allow to cool then remove peels. In a large bowl purée sweet potato with almond milk (add more milk if mixture is too thick). Add pumpkin pie spice blend. Spoon filling into pie crust. Chill and enjoy!

TIPS! For a special flavor add freshly grated nutmeg over top. Also, wait to add the filling until prior to serving to prevent the crust from getting soggy. Feel free to prepare the night before. The flavors seem to get better as the merry together overnight.

Vanilla Cupcakes with Yummy Lemony Icing and (shhh....Zucchini!)[230]

This delicious recipe is another one that I adapted from one I saw on a television cooking show. The recipe makes 12 cupcakes and each cupcake tastes like a decadent indulgence but contains only about 200 calories. The phytonutrient infused recipe will leave your guests guessing what your secret ingredient is!

For the frosting

- o   3 large egg whites
- o   1 cup sugar (try coconut palm sugar, raw cane sugar/sucanat or muscovado)
- o   Pinch of salt
- o   ¾ teaspoon vanilla extract (avoid "imitation" extracts)
- o   Finely grated zest of ½ lemon
- o   1 tbsp of water

o ¼ tsp cream of tartar as a binding agent (this will help keep the icing together so it is not too liquid)

For the cupcakes

o 1 ¼ cup white whole wheat flour (if desiring a gluten free option try quinoa flour)
o ½ cup finely ground almonds
o 1 ½ teaspoon baking powder
o ¼ tsp salt
o 2 eggs
o ¾ cup sugar (Try coconut palm sugar, sucanat or, muscovado)
o 2 tsp pure vanilla extract (avoid "imitation" extracts)
o 1 ¼ cups peeled zucchini, finely grated

Preheat the oven to 350 degrees.

To make the frosting:

Combine the egg whites, sugar, salt and vanilla extract in a heatproof bowl set over (not in) a pan of simmering water. Stir continuously over heat until the mixture is warm and the sugar is completely dissolved, 1 to 2 minutes. Remove the bowl from the heat. Using a handheld electric or standing mixer set on high, beat until the mixture is entirely cooled, glossy and stiff, about 7 minutes. Blend in the lemon zest until smooth — once smooth, take care not to overbeat or the mixture will get lumpy. Let frosting set and cool in the refrigerator (at least 30 minutes), while making the cupcakes.

To make the cupcakes:

Arrange a rack in the center of the oven. Line a 12-muffin pan with cupcake liners. In a bowl, whisk together the flour, almonds and baking powder; set aside. In another bowl, beat the eggs, sugar, salt and vanilla with a handheld or standing mixer until thick and light-colored. Beat in the zucchini on low speed until fully incorporated. Add the dry ingredients and beat on low speed until fully incorporated, scraping down the bowl once with a spatula during beating. Spoon the mixture into the muffin cups. Bake until a toothpick inserted into the center comes out clean, about 20 to 25 minutes, turning the pan midway through baking. Transfer cupcakes out onto a wire rack and cool completely before icing. Enjoy!

Chocolate Raw-Vocado Pudding

Avocados infuse this decadent pudding with heart healthy unsaturated fats, potassium, and a special "je ne sais quoi" flavor.

o 2 ripe avocados
o ½ cup cacao powder (or unsweetened cocoa powder)
o 6 large Medjool dates, pitted (add more or less until desired sweetness achieved) (no dates? Add honey to taste, instead)
o 2 tsp vanilla extract (avoid "imitation" extracts)
o ½ tsp sea salt
o ½ cup water or organic almond milk (add more or less depending on desired consistency)
o 2 tbsp plain unsweetened Greek yogurt

To soften dried dates, soak in the 1/2 cup of warm water for 5 -10 minutes (do not dispose of this water, use the same water for the pudding). Pit and peel the avocado. Combine all the ingredients using a blender or food processor until smooth. Spoon into serving dishes. Chill in refrigerator or enjoy it immediately.

TIP! To enhance the flavor, add a splash of strong coffee or espresso. Serve with apple slices or berries.

Black Bean Brownies [231]

This is a great way to enjoy a decadent treat with a secret bit of black beans for added fiber, protein, and phytonutrients!

o 1 15-oz can black beans, rinsed and drained very well
o 3 eggs
o 3 tbsp organic canola oil (Can also use coconut oil or a light, mild-flavor olive oil that is a light golden color – do not use an extra virgin olive oil as it will impart a too strong flavor)
o ½ cup unsweetened cocoa powder
o Pinch of salt
o ½ tsp baking powder

- o   1 tsp pure vanilla extract (avoid "imitation" extracts)
- o   2/3 cup muscovado or date sugar
- o   ½ cup semi-sweet chocolate chips, divided

Preheat oven to 350 degrees. Spray an 8" x 8" baking pan with cooking spray. In food processor, process black beans until smooth. Add the eggs, oil, cocoa powder, salt, baking powder, vanilla extract, and sugar, and process until smooth. Add ½ of the chocolate chips, and pulse a few times or stir, so that the chips are mixed in. Transfer the batter to the baking pan, and sprinkle the remaining chips on top of the brownies. Bake for 30-35 minutes, or until a toothpick inserted at the center comes out clean. Enjoy!

TIP! Experiment with adding different spices or walnuts for an anti-inflammatory and omega 3 fatty acid boost!

Avocado Frozen Yogurt[232]

This recipe will surprise you! A delightfully rich recipe abundant in heart healthy fats, potassium, and satisfying protein. Prepares 2-3 servings.

- o   1 ½ ripe avocados
- o   2 tbsp lemon juice
- o   2 tbsp sweetener or more or less to taste (try maple sugar, date sugar, or raw honey)
- o   8 oz containers Greek yogurt
- o   ½ cup almond milk
- o   1 tbsp lemon zest
- o   1 tsp pure vanilla extract (avoid "imitation" extracts)

Set aside the lemon zest, and place the rest of the ingredients in a food processor or blender, and blend until smooth. Transfer to a bowl or ice cream maker and stir in the lemon zest. If not using an ice cream maker, freeze in an airtight container for at least 2 hours. When ready to use, let it thaw slightly, giving it another stir.

Easiest Ice Cream Ever!

The name says it all.

Cut 1 banana per serving into small ¼ inch slices. Place in the freezer in a sealed container until completely frozen. Remove from freezer and puree the frozen banana until smooth.

TIP! For an extra creamy texture, add in a scoop of plain Greek yogurt while blending.

Add any toping you enjoy! Try cocoa powder, cinnamon or vanilla extract or coconut flakes. Use your imagination with toppings and get the kids involved!

You can also puree the banana with any ingredient you enjoy. Here are some of my favorite combinations:

Strawberry Chocolate Chip: Puree the banana with 1 cup frozen chopped strawberries and blend in 1 tbsp of dark chocolate chips

Mint Chocolate Chip: Puree the banana with a ½ tsp mint extract and 1 tbsp dark chocolate chips

Banana and Peanut Butter: Puree the banana with 2 tbsp of peanut butter

Raspberry Almond: Puree the banana with 1 cup frozen raspberries and 1/2 cup chopped almonds

Banana or Grape Sorbet

If you thought the recipe above was easy then try this!

Simply slice up a banana (thin slices freeze quicker) or if using grapes, remove grapes from the vine. Place into a freezer protected in a sealed container until completely frozen. Then, enjoy! These make a delicious and healthy frozen snack.

TIP! Want a little extra indulgence? Dip the frozen banana slices in almond butter. Yum!

Baked Apple

This is an old favorite that is simple to make, but always satisfying. My grandmother used to make a variation of this and I still remember how intoxicatingly delicious it made the kitchen smell while it was baking.

Preheat oven to 350 degrees. Core apple. Use any type of apple you enjoy – can also use pears. Sprinkle with cinnamon and drizzle with 1 tsp of date paste or any other sweetener of your choice. Bake for 20 minutes until tender. Enjoy!

Savvy Substitutes

With some clever culinary switches you can decrease the calorie load and amp up the nutritional value of everything from Thanksgiving dinner to decadent desserts without sacrificing taste.

Here are a few of my secrets…

Try:	Instead of or to cut back on:	Why and When:
Cauliflower	Potato	Perfect substitute for a mash! (See my cauliflower mash recipe) Cauliflower resembles the taste and texture of potatoes and check this out: ½ cup of potatoes= 67 kcal ½ cup of cauliflower =14 kcals Cauliflower is also an excellent source of vitamin C and contains a variety of important phytonutrients, vitamins, and minerals. 'nuff sad.
Doubling the vegetables	Grain or pasta	Cut out half the grain or pasta in a recipe and instead add double the vegetables: try sautéed onions, tomato and peppers in warm dishes or shredded jicama and raw coleslaw in cool dishes.
Cooked zucchini purée	Butter	In savory recipes, this makes a great substitute to cut the saturated fat without cutting moisture and is also a great way to increase the vegetable power of meals for picky children!

Cooked lentil purée	Flour	In recipes such as muffins or breads replace ¼ cup of the flour the recipe calls for with ¼ cup of pureed cooked lentils. This will add a boost of protein, fiber and nutrients and with a very subtle hint, will even make the recipe taste better!
Arrowroot or Cornstarch	Cream or butter	Can be used as a thickening agent in soups and salad dressings that would normally require a lot of saturated fat.
Greek yogurt	Cream, butter, or mayonnaise	It's thick, rich, and creamy texture can replace other fats in most recipes from dips to dressings. (replaces equal amounts)
Dijon mustard or avocado	Mayonnaise	Serves as creamy and rich add on to sandwiches and dips.
Fresh herbs like chives, dill, garlic and cilantro	Salt	To enhance flavor, without missing the salt.
Lemon	Salt	Brings out the flavor of any dish!
Beets, yes beets!	Sugar	Try using in chocolate cakes or cupcakes to reduce sugar without compromising sweetness.
Ground almond (almond meal)	All-purpose flour	Can be used in baked goods. (replaces equal amounts)

Unsweetened fresh banana purée or apple sauce	Fats (butter or cream) and sugar	In sweet baked good, use to cut back on the amount of fat and sugar recipes call for without compromising sweetness and moisture!
Any fruit purée!	Fats (butter or cream)	Use ½ as much puree (apple, pear, dates etc) as the recipe call for in fat and if the batter looks dry just use a little more puree to moisten it up.
Vegetable purée such as zucchini, butternut squash or sweet potato	Fats (butter or cream)	Up the nutrients and cut the calories in baked good recipes. Can replace all or at least ½ the fat in everything from cupcakes to cookies! Remember, Use ½ as much puree as fat called for in the recipe and if the batter looks dry, simply add a little more of the puree.
Dried fruits such as plums, raisins, apples, pears, peaches, apricots, cherries, and cranberries	Added sugars	Cutting these dried fruits into very small pieces helps distribute their flavor and sweetness evenly and leads to burst of sweet flavors to each bite. Also adds a plethora of nutrients to each bite!
Mini morsels of chocolate	Chocolate chips	Instead of using big chocolate chips use tiny morsels. They will distribute throughout the baked good providing chocolaty goodness and antioxidants in each bite with less overall sugar and calories.

Flavor Enhancers

Flavor enhancers can be used in sweet and savory dishes to enhance other flavors, to add a special signature taste, or to help cut back on other less healthful ingredients a recipe may call for like sugar. The best part is that most of these tantalizing flavors have few or zero calories yet offer exceptional nutritional benefits from antioxidants and phytonutrients to natural anti-inflammatory compounds!

Flavor Enhancer	Suggested Use and Benefit
Orange or lemon zest	Brings out the fruitiness in a dish and heightens the flavors of the ingredients used. Also adds a pinch of nutrients!
Pure vanilla extract and nut flavorings	Produce an aroma of rich, sweetness without added fat and sugar. Avoid "imitation" extracts; choose only "pure" extracts.
Cinnamon, cloves, allspice, ginger, and nutmeg	These sweet-enhancing spices intensify flavors in a dish. Combine more than one for an exotic, depth of flavor and natural anti-inflammatory benefits!
Cold strong coffee	Use this in chocolate recipes as a substitute for the liquid the recipe calls for. The coffee brings out the deep chocolate flavors and adds an antioxidant punch!
Top baked goods with fruit, fruit spread, or a generous amount of cinnamon or a small sprinkle of sugar	Toping baked goods with the main flavors allows the flavors to be on top and tasted immediately and allows us to use less within the baked good itself – creates the taste and appearance of sugar and sweetness while using less!

The Art of Cooking and the Science of Baking

While cooking and eating is an art, baking is no doubt a science. When we cook, we can easily manipulate the ingredients and amount of ingredients to suit our preferences and out palate. Baking on the other hand, does not always lend itself to such flexibility in amateur hands. Consider sugar for example. Sugar performs many important roles in baking. It provides moisture and tenderness to baked goods, caramelizes at high temperatures, and, of course, it adds sweetness. Refined sugar help cookies spread during baking, allowing their crisp texture. These critical functions make it challenging for the unseasoned baker to replace sugar with a different sweetener. So when you are experimenting with the substitutions described above, for savory dishes almost anything goes! When baking sweet dishes, some trial and error may be required.

Another tip when baking is to simply *decrease* the amount of sugar the recipe calls for. In most recipes, you can decrease the amount of sugar by one third without affecting the quality or even the taste of the final product! Also, keep in mind that some natural sweeteners such as honey taste sweeter than granulated sugar. You can therefore use less honey to sweeten a batch of muffins or a cake than you would sugar. In fact, baked goods made with honey are moist and dense and tend to brown faster than those made with granulated sugar.

Chapter 11

*The search for truth is in one way hard and in another way easy, for it is evident
that no one can master it fully or miss it wholly. But each adds a little to our
knowledge of nature, and from all the facts assembled
there arises a certain grandeur.*
— Aristotle

Fine Tuning Your Manner of Eating:
The Business of Food

Food is big business. It is remarkable that our culture has allowed the
most basic human need to go corporate; and has it ever. Our food
selections these days are often determined more by the genius of food
chemists and savvy marketing teams then by wholesome seasonal
harvests and primitive instincts. Since the early 1950's, as agriculture
and food manufacturing processes became more and more
industrialized, we have progressively seen a movement away from the
consumption of whole, real foods and instead, we made a shift towards
eating more fabricated foods. Driven by a desire to appease the hunger
for convenience of modern society, we have allowed this trend to
continue as we were blissfully unaware or perhaps intentionally
ignorant of the depth of sacrifice we were making in the process.

In the fifties we prized TV dinners. Convenience ruled! We reveled in
the innovation of a burger and French fries at the local diner hot spot.
The diner food trend took us right through the sixties. In the seventies

we wanted more and we wanted it faster! The fast food industry rapidly evolved and gained in popularity, and took us straight into the eighties. In the eighties, we thought the more processed the food, the better. Artificial flavors and sweeteners meant we could avoid fat and calories. Along came the nineties and the early two thousands and we loved our refined sugars and fast food meals so much, that we began to demand more and more. We became insatiable. The industrialized food producers heard our cries and responded in spades. Enter the *super-size me* generation, but bigger was not enough. We looked for more creative ways to play Mother Nature so we genetically altered our foods to give us bigger and brighter fruits, we found ways to industrialize our cattle and poultry to give us the perfectly shaped egg and satisfy our need for cheap meat. Our bellies became fat and full but yet we did not feel satisfied. Something went terribly wrong.

Does it Matter what your Dinner Had for Dinner?

The problem that has emerged with the over-industrialization of our food supply is that we have moved away from whole, natural ingredients and the ritual of food preparation. Much of the food we eat today comes cheap, but there is a huge hidden cost. To keep costs low and supply high, methods of food production have been implemented that defy nature. Take cattle for example. Americans love a good burger. Yet, when we explore what goes into making the cheap meat commonly found in most fast food burgers, we quickly lose our appetite.

Did you know that cows are vegetarians? In fact, as natural herbivores they are the strictest kind of vegetarian! Cows are designed to digest grass and leaves and other plant based foods. When left to their own devices, they roam freely in pastures, dining on bountiful blades of grass that have been infused with the energy of the sunshine. They have a four compartment stomach that allows for otherwise indigestible foods to be digested by virtue of repeated regurgitation and re-chewing. They therefore are able to digest grass and convert it into the proteins and fats their body needs to survive and thrive.

This pastoral life is not one that is known to most modern feedlot cattle. This ideal existence costs money and time. It requires huge lots of land for the cattle to live on and time for the grass they eat to grow and be replenished. As we all know, time is money and in order to produce that burger and sell it for 99 cents, fast food companies do not have the luxury of rearing their cattle in such a pastoral existence. Instead, from birth to slaughter, the cattle are frequently reared in a contained environment and in close quarters. Instead of grass, it is cheaper to feed the cattle grains. Since cattle are not designed for such a diet, it leads to digestive complications and infections. When cattle are fed grain, they grow faster but, at the cost of disrupting their normal physiological mechanisms. A grain based diet in cattle has been shown to cause ulcers and even sudden death in feedlot cattle.[233] To ward off infections, antibiotics are added to the feed which can counteract such ailments. The antibiotics also help prevent cross infection that can result due to enclosed and overcrowded living quarters. The tradeoff is that the antibiotics further alter the digestive health and physiologic functions of the cattle.

Now, the normal development of cattle takes time. But alas, time is money, so instead of waiting on the natural development, recombinant bovine growth hormone (rBGH) is injected into the cattle to stimulate abnormally rapid and super-sized development and abundant milk production. However, cows treated with rBGH tend to develop more udder infections so, they also require more antibiotics. In the end, manufacturers are able to produce more meat and milk; quicker and cheaper to feed our super-sized appetites.

My mention of this is by no means an attempt to brainwash you to become a vegetarian. On the contrary, cattle grazing in their natural surroundings, feeding on grass, and roaming wild to build up muscle and mass naturally are a wonderful and healthful source of Omega 3 fatty acids and an excellent source of lean protein. If you enjoy meat, then your meat should come from animals that are reared in the manner that nature designed. It is the meat from cattle that are growing up in the industrialized cattle hotels I described above that we need to worry about. Here are a few reasons why:

1. It is estimated that livestock now consume 70% of the antibiotics in the United States which undoubtedly contributes to the rise of antibiotic-resistant bacteria.

2. There are many concerns of the effect of consumption of growth hormones and the impact on human health. (more on this below)

3. Grain fed cattle produce meat that is high in unhealthy, pro-inflammatory fats. Conversely, meat from free range, grass-fed cattle has higher levels of healthful conjugated linoleic acid (CLA) and the omega-3 fatty acids ALA, EPA, and DHA.[234]

The title of this section asks whether it matters what your food consumed before it made it to your plate. To appropriately address this question, let us look further at a few of the ingredients that may show up on your dinners' dinner plate.

Recombinant bovine growth hormone (rBGH)

Recombinant bovine growth hormone is a synthetic hormone made through genetic technology that is FDA approved in the United States and used by dairy farmers to increase milk production in cows. Its use is not permitted in the European Union, Canada, and some other countries. [235] While rBGH does not appear to have a harmful direct effect on human health, it does have a negative effect on cows. Use of this hormone causes mastitis in the cows so to combat this condition, farmers give the cows antibiotics. This produces insulin growth factors (IGF) in the cows which then, is also present in the milk that we drink or yogurt we eat. There is concern that IGF may have a link to cancer and may also have other harmful effects on human health. While at this time, the evidence for potential harm to humans remains inconclusive, there is sufficient concern to avoid consumption until we know more.

The Verdict? Avoid. If you eat meat or dairy, look for labels that indicate the food is rBGH free.

Hormones and antibiotics in poultry and pork

To clarify, hormones are provided to cows but hormone use in poultry and pork production even conventional production, has been banned since 1959. In fact, The USDA does not permit the use of hormones in chickens, hogs, turkeys (and other fowl), or in venison. However, this does not mean they are not exposed to antibiotics. Buying USDA-certified *organic* poultry and pork *does* ensure that the animals were not given antibiotics.

184

The Verdict? Avoid unnecessary exposure to antibiotics. Organic standards prohibit the use of all hormones and antibiotics. Choose poultry and pork (and *all* meats) that are certified organic.

Grain-fed versus grass-fed meat

Grass-fed animals eat only their mother's milk and fresh grass throughout their lifespan. Simply put, when a cow eats a grass based diet it produces healthier meat that is higher in omega-3 fatty acids and conjugated linoleic acid (CLA) than those animals raised on grains.

The Verdict? Choose meats that have been grass-fed. Grass-fed meats do cost more so if cost is an issue, simply eat meat less often and when you eat it; enjoy the good stuff. Keep in mind that not all grass-fed beef is organic, and organic doesn't necessarily mean grass-fed. The term "grass-fed" alone still does not have a strict definition or regulation. Thus, the best option is to select certified organic, grass-fed meat which ensures the meat is grass-fed *and* free of all hormones and antibiotics.

Depleted soil

Plants eat too. They dine on the soil they reside in and it takes time for soil to replenish its natural nutrient profile for each subsequent generation. While organic farming methods and alternating fields between seasons provide time for the soil to restore itself, most conventional farming practices are selling us short. As a result, keeping up with the demands of modern agricultural practices have left many regions over-farmed. Each subsequent generation of plants grown on these soil are therefore progressively more and more deplete of essential vitamins and minerals that would have been abundant in their counterparts just a few growth cycles back. In fact, a study of British nutrient data from 1930 to 1980, found that in 20 vegetables, over the course of 50 years the average calcium content declined 19%, iron 22%, and potassium declined 14%.[236] Another study of U.S. Department of Agriculture nutritional data from 1950 and 1999 found "reliable declines" over 50 years in the amount of protein, calcium, phosphorus, iron, vitamin B2 and vitamin C for *43 different* vegetables and fruits. [237]

The Verdict? It is best to purchase seasonal produce from local, certified organic farmers. However, the sad reality is that even if you do eat the good stuff and consume a diet rich in whole, real foods, soil depletion may be a reason to consider dietary supplementation to fill in the nutritional gaps. I will elaborate on this issue further in chapter 13.

Wild versus farmed salmon

The debate between wild sources of salmon versus farmed sources does not have a simple answer. While many experts maintain that farmed salmon is safe, emerging evidence suggests that regardless of the omega 3 fatty acid content of the salmon, farm raised varieties may have excessively high levels of environmental contaminants like persistent organic pollutants (POPs), which may negate the beneficial effects of fish consumption.[238,239]   POPs are chemicals such as herbicides, pesticides, coolants, and flame retardants that do not break down in nature and instead, accumulate in the environment. POPs are abundant in the marine based feed of farmed salmon and thus, in the farmed salmon themselves. While nominal exposure may not pose a risk, chronic exposure to POPs has been linked to the development of type 2 diabetes in humans[240] and insulin resistance and obesity in mice.[241] The World Health Organization cautions the public and manufacturers that *excess* exposure to these toxic POPs from food may be damaging to the immune system, alter hormonal levels, cause reproductive and developmental problems, and may be carcinogenic.[242]

In the name of sustainability, more and more farmed salmon are being fed a diet of soybean oil instead of a diet from a marine origin. The good news is that this diet may reduce the amount of POPs in the fish; the bad news is that it also reduces the content of anti-inflammatory omega 3 fatty acids and increases the pro-inflammatory omega 6 fatty acid content.[243]

Yet, not all farmed fish are raised in this manner. Responsible farming of fish may actually produce healthy varieties. According to experts from Harvard School of Public Health and Environmental Defense Fund, the quality of the fish ultimately depends on the fish itself and where it is reared. These two agencies collaborated to disseminate a list of the best fish farmed or wild which can be found by Google-ing "SeafoodWatch".[244] They also offer a "SeafoodWatch" app that is available through the same website. National Geographic also has a new user friendly online tool called the "Seafood Decision Guide"[245] that offers information regarding the omega-3 fatty acid content of fish, the mercury content, and sustainability.

Verdict? While online guides can help you determine the quality of fish in your community, when in doubt choose wild sources. When it comes to salmon, whenever possible, chose wild Alaskan salmon, select small filets that will have less accumulation of pollutants, and periodically, opt for canned salmon as a cost effective way to enjoy wild salmon (most canned salmon are wild). If you eat farmed salmon, limit your intake to no more than a few servings per month.

A Word on Mercury Contamination in Fish

Many types of fish can be described as nearly a perfect food. They are packed with essential nutrients such as omega 3 fatty acids, vitamins D and B, and lean protein. However, the sad reality is that due to ever increasing global pollution trends, nearly all fish and shellfish these days, even wild sources, contain at least trace amounts of persistent environmental pollutants including methylmercury. The concerns with consumption of methylmercury centers primarily on its potential to effect brain development and to cause harm to the nervous system. Some studies suggest that even low levels of this mercury can be potentially harmful to the health of children and the developing fetus in a pregnant woman.[246] Nevertheless, the Environmental Protection Agency (EPA) informs us that the risk from methylmercury by eating *reasonable* amounts of fish and shellfish is not a significant health concern.[247] This notion is echoed by many experts and to a certain extent, I happen to be one of them. Based on the best available scientific evidence at this time, it appears that the benefits of reasonable fish consumption (generally *at least* 3 servings per week not to exceed an average of one or two daily servings per week) far outweigh the risks.[248] That said it is important to be smart about your choices.

Minimize your intake (never more than 1 serving per week *if at all*) of those fish that are known to contain the highest levels of methylmercury including:

- Shark
- Swordfish
- King mackerel
- Tilefish
- Orange roughy
- Ahi tuna (sadly, as this is one of my favorites)

These are all large fish that remain in the water for extended periods of time and consume other fish that contain mercury and therefore, accumulate the highest amounts of the toxin.

Fish and seafood that have the lowest levels of methylmercury are healthful to include in our regular food plan. These generally include:

✓ Shrimp
✓ Canned light tuna (canned albacore tuna contains more mercury than canned light tuna made from skipjack, yellowfin or tongol)
✓ Salmon (Canned or fresh)
✓ Pollock
✓ Scallops
✓ Sea trout
✓ Rainbow trout
✓ Squid (calamari)
✓ Cod
✓ Haddock
✓ Oysters
✓ Mackerel (North Atlantic, Chub)
✓ Herring
✓ Sardines

NOTE: Whenever possible, choose wild sources of these fish and seafood.

If pregnant or planning to become pregnant, consume *only up to* 12 ounces of these low mercury fish each week. High mercury fish and seafood should be avoided completely during pregnancy.

Since methylmercury levels vary by region, if you live in the Unite States, there are local advisories that can inform you about the safety of fish caught in local lakes, rivers, and coastal areas. These advisories can be accessed at: http://fishadvisoryonline.epa.gov/General.aspx and by accessing the other online guides mentioned previously.

The Bottom Line:
Beyond the issue of animal rights or responsible agricultural practices, it *does* matter to your health wholeheartedly, what your dinner eats for dinner. Be sure to choose your food sources wisely.

The good news is that today as I am writing this book, the trend is to go back to traditional farming methods and reign in global pollution. The pollution issue is a bigger challenge but the matter of more widespread organic farming practices is becoming more and more prevalent. Many food producers are hearing the consumers call for quality over quantity and rekindling traditional farming practices that embrace this sensibility. What is even better is that as consumer demand increases, the availability of quality foods increases as well. In turn, the cost will eventually decrease as the supply continues to increase. That said, as with any matters of consumer demand, the buyer needs to beware. Deceptive food labeling practices regarding food production can be misleading. So, in the pages that follow, I have included a primer to help you make informed decision regarding your food.

Standardizing Organic

In the United States (US), Canada, Europe, Australia, and Japan organic standards are formulated and overseen by the government meaning that strict legislation is in place to ensure that only certified producers use the term "organic." In these countries the definition of organic is generally quite similar allowing for trade without the need for recertification. In other countries that do not have government guidelines, certification is generally handled by non-profit organizations and private companies. However, select countries including Israel, Ghana, and Argentina are now certifying organic products according to the same standards used by the US and Canada in an effort to facilitate international trade.

USDA Organic Labeling

In the US, the United States Department of Agriculture (USDA) is in charge of organic certification. If a food is authenticated as being organic it means the following:

Organic crops: The USDA organic seal verifies that irradiation, sewage sludge, synthetic fertilizers, prohibited pesticides, and genetically modified organisms were not used.

Organic livestock: The USDA organic seal verifies that producers met animal health and welfare standards, did not use antibiotics or growth hormones, and used 100% organic feed, and provided animals with access to the outdoors.

Organic multi-ingredient foods: The USDA organic seal verifies that the product has 95% or more certified organic content. If the label claims that it was made with specified organic ingredients, you can be sure that those specific ingredients are certified organic.

The chart that follows lists some common terms seen on food labels and describes what the label means. An unregulated term means that there is no independent third party authenticating the validity of the claim it is therefore generally considered unreliable and often can be misleading."[249]

What the label says	What it means
100% Organic	Products that are completely organic or made of all organic ingredients
Organic	Products that are at least 95% organic. Products that display this USDA organic seal means product is certified to be at least 95% or more organic

190

Made with Organic Ingredients	Products that contain at least 70% organic ingredients with strict restrictions on the remaining 30% including no GMOs (Genetically Modified Organisms)
All-natural	Unregulated term
Free-range	Unregulated term
Hormone-free	Unregulated term

NOTE: Products with less than 70% organic ingredients may list organically produced ingredients on the side panel of the package but may not make any organic claims on the front of the package.

Is Organic Better?

This is the million dollar question. The answer to this question appears to depend what you mean by "better" and depends on who you ask.

One consideration is simply the issue of regulation of organic foods. While this regulation aids the consumer and establishes a common standard and language, it is not without its critics. Independent organic farmers argue that organic farming used to be based on trust between the farmer and the consumer and not regulation. Opponents argue that it is the non-organic producer that should be regulated tighter and not the organic one! Organic should be the standard. Formal regulation increases cost and bureaucratic barriers and therefore puts the small, independent organic farmers at a disadvantage. Opponents also argue that some large food manufacturer apply creative interpretations to organic standards and even worse, corporate lobbyist drive legislation that impacts the organic standards. For example, in 2006, the US agricultural appropriations bill with the Organic Trade Association rider was passed with USDA approval allowing select synthetic additives to be used in organic foods. While these issues are certainly thought provoking and even alarming, proponents of organic food manufacturing generally agree that while the regulation and the bodies governing regulation are imperfect, legislation is important to help control adherence to at least minimally acceptable standards.

The other major issue surrounding organic food is whether they are more nutritious than conventionally produced food. A 2012 study from Stanford University found that in reviewing 240 studies from around the world, the current published literature lacks evidence that organic food is significantly more nutritious than conventional foods. However, the researcher did acknowledge that consumption of organic foods may reduce exposure to pesticide residues and antibiotic-resistant bacteria.[250] For most advocates of choosing organic foods, that is exactly the point. The main reason for advocating an organic manner of eating is not what is in the food, as much as what is *not* in the food; pesticides, synthetic hormones, and genetically modified compounds.

Pesticides used in the manufacturing of conventional food items are not permitted in organically grown foods. But, are pesticides harmful? If you look to the website of the Environmental Protection Agency (EPA), it explains that consuming pesticides in low amounts is considered not to be harmful. The EPA elegantly quotes Paracelsus, the Swiss physician, alchemist and the "father" of modern toxicology (1493-1541) who said, "The dose makes the poison."[251] They explain that since the dose of most pesticides is so minimal, the potential harm is minimal as well.

Yet, studies show an association between pesticides and health problems ranging from cancer, attention-deficit (hyperactivity) disorder, and nervous system disorders and others report that exposure can weaken immune systems.[252,253] Concern exits that children's growing brains are the most vulnerable to pesticides in food. [254,255] Furthermore, The National Cancer Institute reports in its 2011/2012 update that general studies of individuals with high exposures to pesticides such as farmers, have found high rates of blood and lymphatic system cancers; cancers of the lip, stomach, lung, brain, and prostate; as well as melanoma and other skin cancers.[256] Yet, even with these concerns voiced, data from long-term studies are not yet available so many experts argue it is premature to *conclusively* support or refute the use of pesticides.

The Bottom line:

If you do not eat organic foods regularly due either to cost or accessibility, a viable strategy is to at least attempt to minimize your exposure to pesticides until we learn more. Choose organic foods when the food does not have *natural packaging*. For example, for foods with a removable peal (natural packaging!) such as bananas, avocados, or oranges you can save your money and purchase non-organic versions of these foods as the peels may serve as a bit of a barrier to pesticide exposure. However, for foods like strawberries, blueberries, or peaches splurge on organic. Also, since most pesticides are fat soluble, meaning they are stored in fats, for your oils and high fat foods, invest in organic.

A Word on Genetically Modified Foods

Another major consideration surrounding organic food is the issues of genetic modification. There has been much banter lately about whether we should consider genetically modified foods healthy or harmful to humanity. After all, a tomato or apple can be genetically modified. A grain of rice can be too, and this process can actually enhance the quantity of nutrients these foods possess beyond that which is found in nature. Proponents argue that this is good thing that uses the ingenuity of science to elevate natural foods from good to great. Critics challenge that notion by arguing that tampering with the food provided by nature will ultimately harm human health similar if not worse to the concerns seen with consumption of other highly processed, "fake" foods. So, which side is right? To arrive at an informed conclusion, let us explore the facts.

A genetically modified organism (GMO) is an organism (animal, plant, or bacteria) whose genetic structure has been altered by incorporating a gene that will express a desirable trait.[257] The resulting food is described as genetically modified (GM). Genetically modifying foods is theorized to reduce production costs and at the same time, allows for the opportunity of creating plants that will produce food that is more resilient and more nutrient dense. For example, adding beta carotene to rice is theorized to be beneficial for preventing nutritional deficiency in developing nations where food is scarce. The concerns of GMO consumption include potentially unpredictable interactions with other processes of the human body, undesirable interactions with other foods and medications or potential allergic reactions or sensitivities. These concerns inevitably lead us to the question of what effect does the consumption of GM foods have on human health?

The answer is that we simply do not know. At this time, we have far too little valid scientific evidence to definitively say whether GM foods truly have a negative or positive effect on human health (benefits outweigh risk or vice versa). Animal studies have raised concerns of a link between GMOs and cancer and even reduced lifespan.[258] But at this time, no studies exist that demonstrate these same findings occurring in humans when consuming GMOs. Regrettably, this is quite a common challenge that we encounter with many controversial topics related to human nutrition. That said, when issues in nutrition are equivocal regarding safety and/or efficacy, as a healthcare practitioner I have always defaulted to communicating the following stance when advising my patients:

I have no interest in serving as a human guinea pig. Do you?

Unless necessary, do not by choice assume the role of a human guinea pig or test tube. Until we learn more, choose to consume, whenever possible, non-GMO foods.

This may be easier said than done. I do hope this will change by the time this book goes to print but currently, a major challenge in making informed choices about whether we eat GM foods or not is that food manufacturers in the US are simply not required to notify consumers of GM food ingredients on food labels. In response, many manufacturers that do not use GMO ingredients have selected to voluntarily notify consumers that the ingredients in their foods are *non-GMO*. Fortunately, significant efforts are being made to establish new legislation that will mandate labeling of foods that are genetically modified. This labeling is not about making a statement of whether GM foods are good or bad; it simply respects the consumer's right to make informed decisions about what they eat. In the meantime, if you wish to avoid consumption of GMOs, choose USDA certified organic foods (by definition, certified organic food cannot be subject to genetic modification) or look for foods that state "non-GMO" on their package.

The Bottom Line:

In the battle between organic, non-organic, and even local foods; if one winner must emerge; my bet is on local, organic food. In a perfect world, my recommendation is to eat locally produced organic foods. Why local? The less your food has to travel, the more nutrients it retains. I will discuss this further in chapter 13 but in the meantime, the ideal situation is to find a local organic farmer for your produce. This is the culinary Holy Grail! In a more realistic and more budget friendly world, my suggestion is choose local whenever possible and choose organic for meat, dairy, fats/oils, berries and other hard to clean produce. Save money by opting for non-organic when purchasing foods with their own natural packaging like bananas and avocados.

Chapter 12

Gluttony is an emotional escape, a sign something is eating us.
— Peter De Vries

Emotional Eating

Anyone that has ever struggled with an inner dialogue prior to, or following eating has an emotional influence over what they eat. In fact, anytime we consume food when we are not hungry we are responding to an emotional influence over what we eat. Food *is* emotional. Cake is inextricably linked to the happiness that imbues birthdays and weddings, we associate desserts and culinary decadence with the joy of holiday celebrations; many holidays like Thanksgiving, are centered on the meal itself. In religious traditions foods hold special significance and meaning such as salt water consumed at the Jewish Passover meal to represent the tears of slaves or the bread consumed in Catholic traditions to represent the body of Christ. Even at death, mourners are comforted with gifts of food and the life well-lived is often toasted with fine drink.

For better or worse, food and emotions are inextricable linked. This is one of the reasons food is such a beautiful part of life. It has the remarkable ability to conjure up memories of family traditions, a taste can trigger a feeling of a mother's hug, and a smell can bring you right back to a special memory or event of childhood. It can connect you to the past and soothe you in the present. Whoever claims that food is just about filling an empty belly is either lying or missing out.

We often program our likes and dislikes of many foods based on memories that food item conjures up and not just the flavor the food triggers on our taste buds. As adults, the memory and the emotion evoked by a food is often more influential than anything else to determine our food plan. The term *comfort food* encapsulates this sentiment as it is a food item or taste that evokes a satisfying and soothing feeling from the past. While some comfort foods can be universal to a culture or region such as mac and cheese or meatloaf in North America, comfort foods can also be very personal. For my dad it was barley soup; for you it may be French toast.

Interestingly, there is also a physiologic reason we lean towards comfort foods. They are generally high in carbohydrates and carbohydrates trigger the release of serotonin, the "feel good" chemical. It therefore makes sense how a food that can release this feel good chemical and trigger a great memory makes cravings for that food so nurturing.

When that *food hug* feeling is desired, do not deny yourself that pleasure. There are times when such foods offer a value to us beyond the nutrients in the food alone. Interestingly, studies have explored that our mood when eating and the pleasure we get from food may actually enhance our ability to absorb essential nutrients from food. In his highly acclaimed book *The Gospel of Food: Everything You Think You Know about Food is Wrong*, Barry Glassner references a study from the 1970's that looked at two groups of women, one Swedish and one Thai, that were both fed a spicy Thai meal. The Thai women — who presumably liked the meal more than the Swedish women did —absorbed almost 50% more iron than the Swedish women. However, when the meal was served as a mushy paste, the Thai women absorbed 70% less iron than they had before — from the same food! Next, both groups were served a traditional Swedish meal. This time, the Swedes absorbed more iron! The researchers concluded that food that is unfamiliar (Thai food to Swedish women) or unappetizing (mush rather than solid food) becomes less nutritious than food that looks, smells, and tastes good to

198

the individual.[259]   It seems that the anticipation of eating something one enjoys appears to stimulate the digestive system and increase its efficiency at absorbing nutrients.   So, never deny the emotional pleasure that joyful eating provides.

The connection between emotions and eating does thread a fine line. While at times emotions are a beautiful complement to our dining experience if misdirected or misunderstood, the link between eating and emotion can also become out of control and destructive. When we rely too much on food to help us cope and as a source of comfort, this connection becomes dangerous.   This can result in excessive food intake leading to fat gain and obesity, not to mention the masking of the underlying emotion that is being blunted by the food.   If you can recognize this behavior in yourself, rest assured that you can move past it.   The key is to get reacquainted with what your body is telling you and to regain control of your eating behaviors and emotional needs.

Getting Reacquainted with Yourself and Regaining Mindful Control

It is common for us to progress to a point when we no longer are able to hear the authentic hunger cues from our body.   Our eating habits become so wrapped up in responding to patterns of behavioral and emotional triggers that the feeling of hunger, the voice from our belly telling us that we are genuinely hungry becomes foreign to us.   Or, that voice is silenced by the distracting sound of our emotions.   One of the best strategies for becoming reacquainted with your hunger and satiety signals is to learn to listen to your gut.

First, before you reach for that next snack or meal, ask yourself:

Am I hungry above the neck or below it?
True hunger is below the neck.   It is a hunger pang felt in your gut.   It is satisfied when you eat.   Emotional hunger is above the neck.   It is often signaled by boredom, sadness, anger, pain, or frustration.   Food is an attempt to quiet the voice of this emotional hunger but at its best it simply dulls the emotion temporarily.   At times, emotional eating may become the product of habit.   Consider activities such as coming home after work or school, sitting down to watch television and instinctively reaching for a snack, even if you are not hungry.

Emotional hunger may seem to call for food, but it is never satiated by food. In fact, in some cases eating especially over-eating, will make you feel worse. Emotional hunger requires connection, communication, support; not food. It requires recognition of the emotion, the cause of the emotion, and then reaching out for help and support. Understanding and treating the cause of such emotions reaches beyond the scope of this book but the recognition of it is a pivotal first step. Becoming reacquainted with yourself begins with recognizing the distinction between gut hunger and emotional hunger so you can learn to listen for what your body truly needs. If you determine a hunger is above the neck, then, seek help and support by a friend or doctor to find a way to satiate the emotional hunger pangs.

In Brian Wansink's book *Mindless Eating*,[260] Dr. Wansink does an excellent job at illustrating the differences between physical hunger (below the neck, gut hunger) and emotional hunger (above the neck, emotional hunger). I have summarized some of these differences in the chart that follows:

Physical Hunger	Emotional Hunger
Builds gradually	Develops suddenly
Occurs several hours after a meal	Unrelated to time
Goes away when full	Persists despite fullness
Eating leads to feeling of satisfaction	Eating leads to guilt and shame

Now that you recognize true hunger, gauge it.
The difference between being 'not hungry/satisfied' and being 'full' can be several hundred calories so pay careful attention to the signals of hunger and satiety that your body is sending you. One trick that I like to use is to visualize a hunger gauge with a dial that moves from zero to ten. When the dial is at zero you are starving; when the dial reaches ten you are holiday dinner full, undo the top button on your pants full, I can't believe I had the third helping full! The idea is that you want to avoid both of these extremes. You never want to be excessively hungry or excessively full. So, when you identify that feeling of hunger, and you verify that it is below the neck genuine gut hunger, ask yourself, how hungry am I? Where does my hunger fall on my hunger

gauge? If the dial is at 3 or 4; eat. Never go below 3 on your hunger gauge, when you are starving you will be more likely to overeat and make poor food choices. Once you reach 7 or 8; stop eating. If you eat more than this you will feel uncomfortably full leading to the increased likelihood of skipping future meals and the consequent undesirable spikes and crashes in blood sugar levels.

Establish a mantra to eat until you are satisfied.
My father could have a feast fit for a king set before him but his food choices were always guided by his gut and not his eyes. Part of his routine at mealtime was the often inclusion of what in hindsight, can be considered a mantra. Whenever my dad was dining and he reached the point of satiety (achieving a level 7 or 8 on his hunger gauge), he would often boldly state: "I eat until I am comfortable" and then promptly stopped eating. Why should you learn this habit from my dad? He maintained the same weight, brilliance, energy, and vibrant passionate existence throughout his lifespan. Furthermore, my dad was not alone in proclaiming a mantra at the close of each meal. In the Japanese Island of Okinawa, portion control is deeply rooted into the culture with the statement *Hara Hachi Bu* meaning *eat until belly is 80% full*. This mantra has assumed a prominent role in the culinary vernacular of Okinawans and serves as a guiding principle of dietary practices. Why should you listen to the people of Okinawa? Okinawans are among the global leaders in adults living to be 100 year of age or older, and their longevity has often been attributed to their remarkable *manner of living* including their dietary habits. If that does not convince you, a Japanese proverb cleverly warns of what happens if you do not follow this mantra: *eight parts of a full stomach sustain the man; the other two sustain the doctor.*[261]

Establish a mantra for yourself to mark your point of satiety when you eat. Make it your brand and say it out loud and proud, or just keep it to yourself; either is fine as long as you say it. Make it your special symbolic closing to your meal; a statement to acknowledge to yourself that you are now hearing, paying attention and responding to what your gut is telling you.

Taste your food.
This may seem obvious, but I encourage you to challenge that notion. Often mindless eating means eating for energy or to feed an emotion

rather than eating for pleasure. Food is pleasure; it is joy! Enjoy the food. Savor it. Smell it. Taste the flavors. Detect the nuances of each flavor within your food. Think about tasting a wine. You first look at the color and how it captures the light. You then smell it and savor each layer of its aroma permeating the air. The last thing you do is taste it. But you do not merely consume it, you savor it. You allow it to swirl around your mouth to pick up all the flavors and the nuances that make it unique. I challenge you to do this with everything you eat.

Consider eating a blueberry. Pause to appreciate its deep blue pigment, smell it to appreciate its gentle sweetness, and then finally taste it but allow it to melt in your mouth so you can revel in the flavors and textures from the sweetness of its juices to the texture of the little seeds, the skin, the meat - is it bitter, sweet, sour, salty? Now *that* is eating mindfully.

TIP! Select to enjoy one meal this week alone, just you and the food. Turn off the television, put away the book and the crossword, shut down that smartphone and tablet, and even avoid conversation. Sit at a table just you and the food and with each bite, using all of your senses, taste it; use the advice described above to *really* taste it.

Slow down.
It can take twenty to thirty minutes for our brain to get that signal of satiety when we eat,[262] so do not rush your meal. To slow things down, plan to chew each bite at least ten to twenty times and put the fork or spoon down between each bite. Taking the time to taste your food will also help slow you down *and* draw more pleasure from each meal.

Sit down at a table while eating.
Do you find yourself standing while you eat? Lying on a couch, reclining like a Greek god or goddess? Are you eating while walking? Sitting at your desk at work, multitasking? Avoid engaging in other activities while eating. Activities such as watching TV, driving, working, checking email all shift focus away from food and lead to mindless eating which leads to overeating. The only activity that you should participate in while eating is socializing. Focus on your food while you eat.

Share.

Everything taste better when you share it! Discuss the flavors, compare the taste experiences. Derive pleasure, savor, and interpret flavors. Ask your dining partner about their experience with the food. They may even offer insight that allows you to take even more pleasure in the food.

Respect your food.

Buddhism teaches us to consider the past of our food; to mindfully respect each stage of our food's journey prior to its presentation upon our plate. The seed that allowed for its growth, the farmer that turned the soil, nurtured the land, the worker that harvested it and the grocer that selected it and placed it upon the shelf; the cook who purchased it and spent time preparing it for you to enjoy. When we consider the many hands that contributed to the possibility that this food would be here to nourish us, it gives us an enhanced respect for the profound value of that food.

Eat to satisfy your needs.

Do not eat because someone tells you too, because it is healthy, or because you do not want to insult the chef. Respectfully thank them for their efforts but communicate your preferences and needs. Do not impose your preferences on others but do surround yourself with those that respect your needs.

Interpret your cravings.

Our cravings can be a window to our needs. But do not give into them mindlessly. Consider them thoughtfully. Below is a strategy to help you assume control over your cravings.

Ask Yourself:	Example:
What do I need/ what am I craving?	French fries
Why am I craving that food?	The flavor, the texture and taste
What is it about the flavor that I like?	Filling and salty
What does that flavor make me feel like?	Comforting, satisfying
Where else can I get that feeling from?	Call my mom, take a bath

This simple self-reflective activity can offer insight into your subconscious needs and help you gain control over your cravings. It can help you determine if your craving is really for food or something else. Are you getting sweetness and comfort from food instead of from life? Are your cravings for cake or a donut really a craving for joy, pleasure, and happiness from life? Consider what you can do to achieve sweetness and comfort in your life that does not require a donut.

Chapter 13

Men occasionally stumble over the truth, but most of them pick themselves up and hurry off as if nothing ever happened.
— Winston Churchill

To Supplement or Not to Supplement?

Linus Pauling, PhD was a brilliant Nobel Prize winning scientist who can be credited with putting dietary supplements on the contemporary, mainstream map. He maintained a position that the amount of vitamin C the body needs to thrive and heal cannot be attained through diet alone. He therefore advocated the use of high dose dietary supplementation with vitamin C pills to treat and prevent a variety of health conditions. While this brought new attention and understanding (and criticism) to dietary supplementation, supplements have long been an integral part of the culture of health and wellness worldwide. For centuries, cultures across the globe have used vitamin, mineral, and herbal dietary supplementation to enhance everything from beauty to virility, and to treat diseases as diverse as tooth decay and cancer. How can we forget the fabled stories of how to the disgust of children from the late 1800's to the 1950's Cod liver oil was seen as a non-negotiable essential for supporting healthy childhood development? (Cod liver oil has high levels of omega-3 fatty acids and vitamin D so no wonder it was thought to be so good!)

Over the past few decades, dietary supplementation has become synonymous with a healthy lifestyle. Just like carrying a water bottle, taking daily dietary supplements became a marker of a healthy lifestyle. Supplementation even emerged into the mainstream of conventional medicine with recommendation of calcium and vitamin D supplementation becoming nearly as commonplace as the prescribing of antibiotics. Supplements of essential, naturally occurring nutrients simply made sense. But over the years, as more and more people were taking dietary supplements, research studies slowly came out that challenged the notion that simply because it was natural, it was beneficial or even safe.

In general, the benefits of appropriate dietary supplementation appear to outweigh any risk. However, dietary supplementation is not without risk and does not always provide benefits, so it is important that you do not take supplements with reckless abandon but rather, make informed choices when it comes to supplementing your manner of eating.

First of all, there are generally three reasons to consider taking a dietary supplement:

1. To correct a deficiency
2. To benefit a specific health condition
3. To optimize health, prevent disease, and promote longevity

Supplementing a Deficiency

Historically, in the context of public health, nutritional supplementation was most often recommended purely on the basis of preventing clinical deficiencies. Even today the Recommended Daily Intake (RDI) for vitamins and minerals reflect the amount of nutrients our body needs to prevent a deficiency that is significant enough to lead to overt signs and symptoms. This is different than the amount of nutrients that may be required to *optimize* health.

At a time when obesity is emerging as a principal public health concern, it is hard to believe that we would still need to worry about nutritional deficiencies. However, as I mentioned early in this book, many Americans are overfed yet they are also undernourished. People can have an excess of energy (calories) leading to fat gain, but if the sources of energy they consume are deplete of nutrients (as are most foods that make up the Standard American Diet[263]), these same people can suffer from nutritional deficiencies. The reality is that if we are not getting nutrients from our food, supplements may be the next best thing.

The greatest risk of deficiency is among those of us that eat mostly packaged and processed foods, and those that adhere to a restrictive manner of eating. Vegetarians, those who limit or restrict intake of gluten, grains, dairy, and/or other foods or food components may also be at risk of deficiencies. Vegans for example, often do not get adequate amounts of iron and vitamin B12 in their diet which can lead to the onset of anemia. To prevent this, it is often advisable for vegans to increase their intake of these nutrients by taking supplements.

Another well-established need for supplementation is during pregnancy. Globally, it is recognized that supplementation with folic acid is important during pregnancy to avoid the possibility of a deficiency which can lead to neural tube defects in neonates. Interestingly, new research suggests that the use of prenatal folic acid supplements around the time of conception is also associated with a lower risk of autistic disorder.[264]

Finally, certain medications can lead to the depletion or inadequate absorption of nutrients leading to deficiency. Anytime you begin a new medication, talk to your doctor to find out if that medication can lead to a nutrient deficiency.

A very common nutrient deficiency is vitamin D.[265] The sun can help support our needs for this nutrient since our body is able to produce vitamin D when ultraviolet rays from sunlight strikes the skin and triggers vitamin D synthesis. However, this means of synthesis can be inefficient in some adults and may be inadequate for those among us living in cool climates where access to sunlight may be limited most of the year. Vitamin D can be found in foods including fatty fish such as salmon, tuna, and mackerel and small amounts are found in beef liver, cheese, and egg yolks.[266] However, we often do not consume adequate amounts of these foods to meet our vitamin D needs. It is therefore no surprise that recently, it has been recognized that many adults are deficient in this vitamin. This is a problem since vitamin D is essential to support a variety of our basic needs. You may be familiar with the importance of vitamin D in supporting bone health, specifically in helping promote the absorption of calcium. But an adequate vitamin D level is also essential to support neuromuscular and immune function, reduction of inflammation, and has been shown to play a role in the prevention and management of type 1 and type 2 diabetes, hypertension, and even multiple sclerosis, congestive heart failure, and certain types of cancer.[267,268,269,270,271,272,273,274] There is some uncertainty as to whether it is a low vitamin D level that causes or contributes to such diseases, or if poor health is what causes vitamin D levels to drop in the first place. Either way, if your levels are low it is prudent to take supplemental vitamin D until your levels are restored and maintained within normal ranges.

You can determine your levels of vitamin D by asking your doctor to order a blood test for **25-hydroxyvitamin D** [25(OH) D]. This blood test is the best indicator of one's vitamin D status.[275] If your levels are below the normal recommended healthy ranges, or even if they are in the low end of normal then supplementation is likely warranted.

NOTE: Recent studies suggest that the optimal levels of vitamin D may be slightly higher than once thought with many practitioners now recommending patients achieve and maintain slightly higher serum levels of 25(OH) D in order to *optimize* health. For example, while some references suggest that a 25(OH) D level of 30 ng/ml (75 nmol/L) is within the normal acceptable range, studies on vitamin D and breast, colorectal, and prostate cancer prevention only reported benefits at 25(OH) D values between 40 to 60 ng/mL (100-150 nmol/L).[276] Work with your doctor to determine what is best for you.

Another important note: if you are deficient in vitamin D and supplementation is not resulting in an increase in 25(OH) D, the main issue may not be the vitamin D after all. Instead, the problem might be low levels of magnesium. Magnesium is a mineral involved in the synthesis and metabolism of vitamin D. When magnesium levels are inadequate as is common in many adults, this may contribute to low 25(OH) D as well. Therefore, supplementing magnesium alongside the vitamin D may help increase levels of 25(OH) D in those who are not responding to vitamin D supplementation alone.[277]

208

In general, there are certain people that are at the greatest risk of nutrient deficiency. If you or any of your loved ones fall into one of the categories below, then talk to your doctor about nutritional supplementation.

Are You at a Risk for a Nutrient Deficiency?

1. If you qualify as a person that until now has been overfed and undernourished (adhering to the S.A.D. aka. the Standard American Diet) then you are at risk.

2. Vegans and others with restrictive dietary patterns including those who limit intake of gluten, grains, dairy, and/or other foods or food components may also be at risk.

3. Those among us with dangerous lifestyles habits such as smoking or drinking alcohol to excess are at risk.

4. High-performance athletes and those with high stress occupations are also at risk of nutrient deficiency. While increasing intake of vegetables and other whole foods can often satisfy needs, at times supplementation may be appropriate.

5. If you are a woman of child-bearing age, you may be at risk for a deficiency as well; not necessarily for you but for your unborn child. Basic nutritional needs increase during pregnancy to meet the developmental needs of the fetus. With so many unplanned, or surprise pregnancies, it is advisable for all sexually active young women to talk to their doctor about ensuring they maintain the proper nutritional foundation in the event of pregnancy. During pregnancy, our demand for adequate levels of certain nutrients like folate/folic acid is essential to support the needs of the developing fetus and to reduce the risk of neural tube defects. Keep in mind that most pregnancies are only discovered several weeks after conception so it is important that you have the proper nutritional foundation in place beforehand so as not to compromise nutritional status during the vulnerable first few weeks of development.

6. If you are taking medications you are also at risk for nutritional deficiency. Many medications can deplete or inhibit the absorption of certain nutrients leading to dangerous deficiencies. Common culprits include oral contraceptives, cholesterol-lowering statins, and antibiotics. For example, diuretics medications used to treat high blood pressure are known to deplete minerals such as magnesium, potassium, and zinc[278,279] while statin drugs commonly used to treat high cholesterol have been shown to deplete coenzyme Q10,[280] which is an essential nutrient used for energy production. If you are taking any medication talk to your doctor about drug induced nutrient deficiencies.

7. If you have been diagnosed with a specific health conditions such as heart disease, osteoporosis, digestive problems, diabetes, arthritis, or high blood pressure, than you may also be at risk.

8. Finally, if you are over the age of 55 your age alone may put you at risk. The natural production of certain nutrients often becomes less efficient as we age making targeted supplementation essential to avoid deficiency.

The Bottom Line:
Through an assessment of your dietary intake and through targeted blood work, your healthcare provider can determine if you are deficient in important nutrients. If so, supplementation is not only beneficial, it is essential. Talk to your doctors about disease, medication, lifestyle, and/or age induced nutrient deficiencies and make certain these are managed with appropriate supplementation. Also, be aware that nutrient deficiencies rarely present in isolation. When a sign or symptom of one nutrient deficiency appears, it is highly likely that you are also lacking in other key nutrients; they simply have not yet presented with overt clinical signs or symptoms. Therefore, while supplementing that individual nutrient, you should also be vigilant to ensure that your manner of eating is supplying adequate amounts of other essential nutrients as well.

Supplementing Disease

The other common reason to take dietary supplements is to help support the management of specific health conditions. Inspired by their big pharma counterparts, the nutritional supplement industry coined the term 'nutraceutical' to describe supplemental nutrients that can be used as a means of managing and/or preventing disease. More and more evidence is emerging to substantiate this role of dietary supplements. For example, a 2012 study reviewing all other studies completed to date on the topic of supplements and osteoarthritis concluded that there was evidence to support the use of nutraceuticals to provide symptomatic relief to patients with osteoarthritis. The researchers reported that there were benefits to using these supplements as adjunct therapy for osteoarthritis management.[281] Other studies have found that Vitamin C, E, β-carotene, and zinc may help treat and prevent age-related macular degeneration.[282] Omega-3 fatty acid supplementation has been shown to help treat mood disorders[283] and improve the symptoms of rheumatoid arthritis.[284]

Countless studies inform us of the safety and benefit of using nutraceuticals to help manage the symptoms of a diverse array of diseases. However, just like with medications, there is no one size fits all approach. While generally safer than pharmaceuticals, the quality, form, and dose of the nutrient can have profound implications on the safety and effectiveness of supplements. Also, many times nutrients can interact in potentially harmful ways with other nutrients, foods, and/or medications so it is important that you discuss these matters with your healthcare provider before taking any nutraceutical.

The Bottom Line:

Strong evidence is emerging in support of the value of dietary supplements to help manage many types of disease. However, before beginning to take any nutraceutical it is essential to respect the fact that *just because something is natural does not mean it is safe*. Ask your healthcare provider about nutrients that may benefit any specific health condition that you have been diagnosed with. Inquire about safety, effectiveness, and potential for side-effects or interactions with other foods, drugs, or nutrients. Be sure to also inquire about proper dosing and about how long you should take the supplement before you can expect to see a benefit. If your medical doctor has not been sufficiently trained in nutraceutical use, ask them to refer you to a healthcare provider such as a chiropractor, nutritionist, or naturopathic doctor that can offer informed guidance on the smart and safe use of nutraceuticals. By the way, you should be asking your doctor the same questions about any prescription or over the counter medication you take as well.

Supplementing Health

The third common reason to take a dietary supplement is to optimize health, prevent disease, and promote longevity. For years I have maintained a healthy *manner of living*. I rarely have been ill. My blood work has always been optimal, I have no existing disease and my risk factors for chronic disease are minimal. My manner of eating is impeccable. I engage in activity frequently, but not excessively. Over the years I have taken a low dose vitamin D3 supplement on and off, and periodically I take omega 3 fatty acid supplements from fish oil, and a probiotic. As a teen and young adult I was known to take vitamin C supplements, but admittedly it was primarily because I enjoyed the orange flavor of the chewable pills. Truth be told, if I had to swallow them as flavorless capsules, I rarely would have taken them! As far as a multivitamin goes, in the past I have tended to vacillate between periods of time when I would take a multivitamin regularly and then for just as long, I would go through periods when I avoided multivitamins altogether. The reason for my inconsistency was that I was not convinced that as a healthy adult there was an added benefit derived from taking a multivitamin. Furthermore, I was not convinced that synthetic nutrients could offer me the same benefit as consuming whole, real food sources of these same nutrients. I therefore always chose whole, real food instead. However, as a doctor and professor it was not good enough for me to simply rely on my instincts; I had to look to the evidence. I therefore sought out to answer the following question:

If I adhere to a healthy manner of living should I still take a multivitamin?

In doing my research I found that to respond to this question, there are two important considerations one must keep in mind:

1. We cannot always depend on food alone for essential nutrients
2. Natural does not always equate to safe

Is Eating Whole, Real Food Enough?

As mentioned, I adhere to an impeccable manner of eating. I have a predominantly plant based food plan, eat mostly whole, real organic foods and choose wild and organic sources of protein. My manner of eating is precisely the one I describe in this book. I practice what I preach. The question is therefore not whether I am choosing to eat the right foods but rather, can I depend on food alone for all the essential nutrients that I need? Sadly, the answer in some cases appears to be no. Even when we choose to eat the best types of food there are certain factors that may compromise the quality of that food by the time it reaches our dinner plate.

1. **Soil depletion**

   As mentioned in chapter 11, the mass-production that characterizes modern agricultural practices leads to the depletion of nutrients from the soil without sufficient time to replenish them. When the soil is deplete of essential minerals and other nutrients, so is the byproduct of that soil, namely the vegetable or fruit that grow upon it. Each time that soil is planted and harvested, less and less nutrients remain. The foods may look the same as their predecessors but may possess a very different nutrient profile compared to the same produce farmed of that land a decade earlier. This issue can apply to organic and nonorganic foods.

2. **Food storage and transportation**

   Time is of the essence. All foods deteriorate as they age. Many foods are shipped over great distances these days before they are stocked in our local grocery stores. Overtime, many of the nutrients have therefore been lost before you even had opportunity to take that food home. Eating locally grown food is a smart way to help minimize the effect of time and transport on our food.

3. **Commercial food processing**
   Processing may expose food to light, heat, oxygen, or dramatic fluctuations in temperature or humidity. These exposures can destroy vital but fragile nutrients.

4. **Food irradiation**
   Food irradiation is a means of extending the shelf life of food by destroying microorganisms, inhibiting sprouting, and delaying ripening. The problem is this process may also destroy vital nutrients, especially antioxidants and fat-soluble vitamins. Note that certified organic foods cannot be subject to irradiation.

5. **Preparation and cooking of foods**
   As discussed in chapter 9, the way we prepare our foods can make or break its nutrient value. Cooking certain foods, especially overcooking, can in some cases diminish or even destroy vital nutrients.

The Bottom Line:
Even if one adheres to a healthful manner of eating, a low dose (less than 100% of the Recommended Daily Intake) and ideally, a whole food based multivitamin (more on this in a moment) is smart insurance to help fill in the nutritional gaps caused by some avoidable and other unavoidable compromises to our food supply. NOTE: Take multivitamins with food to enhance the absorption of the nutrients.

Natural Does Not Always Equate to Safe

When we look to the published research, at this time the scientific evidence remains rather equivocal in showing whether dietary supplementation with a multi vitamin/multi mineral formula can help optimize our health, prolong our life, and/or prevent chronic disease. There are certainly studies out there that have discovered meaningful benefits to taking multivitamins for optimizing health and even prolonging our lifespan. For example, a 2009 study found that multivitamin use is associated with longer DNA telomere length among women.[285] Shorter telomeres have been associated with increased mortality[286] and increased risk of select chronic diseases including cancer, dementia, and cardiovascular disease.[287,288,289,290] To put it simply, the longer your telomeres, the longer your lifespan is likely to be. Therefore, this study suggests that taking a multivitamin may be a promising ally to support living a healthy and long life.

Another study published in 2012 in the esteemed Journal of the American Medical Association, looked at over 14 000 US male physicians aged 50 years or older and gave them either a placebo or a multivitamin and then monitored them for almost 15 years. The study found that those taking the daily multivitamin supplement had a significantly reduced total cancer risk.[291] Interestingly, the same study found that taking a daily multivitamin did *not* reduce their risk of heart attack, stroke, or cardiovascular disease mortality even after more than a decade of treatment and follow-up.[292] Researchers studying adults in California and Hawaii came to a similar, although even bolder conclusion stating that there was no clear decrease or increase in mortality from *all* causes, cardiovascular disease, or cancer and in morbidity from overall or major cancers among multivitamin supplement users. Another study found there was no association between multivitamin supplement use and breast cancer risk in women.[293] Yet another study found that in older women, several commonly used dietary vitamin and mineral supplements may even be associated with *increased* total mortality risk; particularly when it comes to supplemental iron.[294]

In fact, when it comes to isolated nutrients, the research has really challenged the value of *preventive* supplementation (supplementation in the absence of a clinical deficiency). One study reported that in patients with vascular disease or diabetes mellitus, long-term vitamin E supplementation did not prevent cancer or major cardiovascular events and may even increase the risk for heart failure.[295] Another study found that calcium supplements might raise myocardial infarction risk.[296] Yet another study found omega-3 fatty acid supplementation was not associated with a lower risk of all-cause mortality, cardiac death, sudden death, myocardial infarction, or stroke.[297] One study called the "Alpha Tocopherol, Beta Carotene Cancer Prevention Study", found that smokers who took beta carotene had a *higher* chance of dying from lung cancer than those taking the placebo.[298] Another study called the "Beta Carotene and Retinol (Vitamin A) Efficacy Trial" (CARET) found that after an average of 4 years of taking the pills, there were 28% *more* cases of lung cancer diagnosed in smokers taking the supplements.[299] It is important to note that these findings were not replicated in smokers that consumed beta carotene from food sources as part of their food plan. In fact, a recent study found that participants eating (not supplementing) higher intakes of the micronutrients vitamin C, vitamin E, and Selenium and were 67% *less* likely to develop pancreatic cancer than those eating lower amounts.[300]

While I realize it may appear that I am not making a very strong case in favor of supplementation for the purpose of optimizing heath, prolonging life, and chronic disease prevention, it is essential to note that many of these studies are not without significant limitations that we must consider before drawing conclusions. In fact, there are four critical limitations to many of these and other similar nutrient studies that we must keep in mind:

1. Correlation does not imply causation
2. Nutritional supplement research is challenging
3. Not all supplements are created equal; product quality matters
4. A synthetic nutrient may act very different that one derived from whole food

Correlation Does Not Imply Causation

When it comes to dietary supplement research, many of the studies that make headlines are observational studies. What this means is that researchers are observing individuals who have chosen to take a dietary supplement. While these studies at times can reveal interesting and novel correlations between two seemingly distinct variables, it is important to understand that *correlation* is not the same as *causation*.

Consider a headline making study in 2013 that linked high blood levels of omega 3 fatty acids to prostate cancer.[301] This observational study had reporters chomping at the bits with breaking news claiming that omega 3 fatty acids *caused* prostate cancer! Yet, if these reporters would have read past their own headlines, they would have seen that the while the study showed a statistical relationship between high blood levels of omega 3 fatty acids and prostate cancer, it did not show that omega 3 fatty acids *caused* prostate cancer. There is a huge difference.

Correlation means that a connection or association between two variables was made. But just because two things occur together does not mean one *causes* the other; the connection may be completely arbitrary. For example, I can say that whenever I wake up at 9:00 AM the sun is up in the sky. The time that I wake is one variable; the sun in the sky is another. I therefore can claim that I observed a correlation between the time I wake up and the sun being up in the sky as they occurred at the same moment. However, it would be absurd to say that I can now draw the conclusion that my waking up at 9:00 AM *caused* the sun to be up in the sky!

In the omega 3 fatty acid and prostate cancer study as in other observational studies, a correlation was described but no mechanistic relationship was identified, and no intervention was done to prove that any cause and effect association exists. Once a connection between two variables is identified, other studies are required to determine whether the connection was purely by chance or if a relationship between the two really exists. Otherwise, this type of study is interesting... but without more evidence, that is *all* it is.

The Challenges of Nutritional Research

Investigating the efficacy of a nutrient or dietary supplement is not like studying a drug. When we study a drug, we can compare a group of people that are taking the drug with those that are not taking the drug and then monitor the difference between these two groups. This is challenging to do with a dietary supplement. You can have one group take the supplement and one group not, but there is an inherent problem. The group not taking the supplement may not be taking that nutrient during the study but it is highly likely that they were exposed to it previously (or even during the study) from food sources. It is not like a drug that they were never exposed to. They are not a clean slate.

Therefore, when we attempt to draw a comparison between two arms of a nutritional supplement study, it may not be a fair comparison. This is one of the major criticisms of many nutrient studies. Critics argue that the conclusions are skewed perhaps even invalid since participants in the non-intervention arm of the study may have had a history of consumption of the nutrient under investigation prior to their participation in the study as a part of their normal dietary intake.

Additional challenges with studying nutrients is that it is not always clear if certain combinations of nutrients works better than other combinations, if synthetic forms of nutrients impact health in the same way as whole food based ones, or if an isolated nutrient will have the same effect on health as it does when it is consumed as part of a whole food. Remember, most studies look at one nutrient at a time, but vegetables for example, present numerous compounds at once. The benefit may therefore come from simultaneous expose to many nutrients. To add more confusion to the picture, the microbes that reside in our gut ferment select phytonutrients found in fruits, grains, and vegetables which may contribute to their benefits and which may also be yet another variable that makes nutrient research challenging. In other words, one's gut microbial composition can potentially impact their response to select nutrients.

While studies are attempting to seek answers to these questions and assess each of these variables, these challenges also bring to light the issue of whether the reductionist approach of isolating a single compound, which is how randomized controlled trials (RCTs) for drugs are typically designed, is the best way to study nutrients. Researchers are exploring ways to devise a better framework for studying the impact of nutrients/dietary supplements on our health. In the meantime, we simply must be mindful of these potentially confounding factors when we interpret the conclusions of research articles related to isolated nutrients and dietary supplements.

Product Quality Matters

One important factor that is often neglected in interpreting and applying the findings of research involving dietary supplements is that there is very little regulation controlling the quality standards of supplements. Simply put, not all supplements are created equal; products made by different companies can actually be very different and react in the body very differently. As a result, the findings from observational studies can at times be questionable, as it is unclear what type and form of the supplement the participants were taking. To really understand this issue, let us first consider the matter of quality and then, we will explore the topic of nutrient form; synthetic versus natural.

When it comes to product quality, for better or for worse (and there are two sides that argue vehemently for and against this issue) under DSHA (the Dietary Supplement Health & Education Act of 1994) there are minimal regulations by the Food and Drug Administration (FDA) defining a standard of practice for manufacturing supplements in the United States. As of June 2010, all manufacturers must adhere to the US FDA published Current Good Manufacturing Practices (cGMPs). These new standards were seen as a major milestone. However, many feel these standards are still inadequate and poorly regulated. Each manufacturer (not the FDA) ultimately remains responsible for monitoring the identity, purity, strength, composition, and safety of their products. In other words, the FDA generally leaves it up to supplement manufacturers to control the total quality of their product. The advantage to this is that supplements are not as strictly regulated as a medication so there is no need to have a prescription in order to purchase them; consumers can access supplements directly. The disadvantage is that we are putting trust in manufacturers to produce quality products. This is potentially problematic since for some manufacturers, maximizing profits may be a greater priority then maximizing quality. As a consumer you therefore must be certain that you buy your supplements for a reputable manufacturer.

Here are a few fundamental things to look for when buying a supplement:

1. **Independent, third party certified manufacturing**
   Since supplements are not strictly regulated by the FDA, nutraceutical manufacturers can authenticate the quality, stability, purity as well as the absorption, dissolution, and bioavailability of their products by receiving certification by an independent third party. Many reputable, independent groups have emerged that offer third-party testing and certification. These groups include: National Sanitation Foundation (NSF) which is an international designation[302], the Natural Products Association (NPA GMP)[303], Therapeutic Goods Administration (TGA) from Australia[304], ConsumberLab.com[305], and the United States Pharmacopeia (USP).[306]

How do you know a supplement manufacturer is third party certified? Ask! When a manufacturer is certified by a third party, they are awarded the distinction of using the group's "mark" or "seal" on their product in hope of increasing consumer confidence in their brand. Typically, most manufacturers will post their badge of certifications directly on their product packaging. Some may only list it in product catalogs or on their website. Either way, manufacturers are proud of this certification so if you do not see it on their product, contact the manufacturer and ask. If they are reluctant to share this information, if they give you excuses such as a claim they cannot tell you since it is proprietary information, or if they tell you they "adhere" to good manufacturing practices they just do not bother with the certification due to cost, then in my opinion, they should lose our business. If manufacturers want to retain control of their industry, the burden is upon them to demonstrate product quality to us, the consumer.

2. **Comprehensive scientific evaluation to verify quality and efficacy**

Naturally, the priority is to ensure the product is safe and high quality; that it includes exactly what it says it should on the label, nothing more and nothing less. Once quality is authenticated by third party certification then, when using supplement formulas that combine multiple nutrients, the next thing to look for is whether the manufacturer has pursued testing of their proprietary products. A common practice among even high quality supplement manufacturers is to take findings from studies on each individual nutrient a product contains, and use these studies to demonstrate the efficacy of their overall product blend. The issue with this practice is that sometimes when we combine more than one nutrient it is plausible that the effect of the combination of nutrients may be very different than if the nutrient is taken alone and the effect is not always better. This begs the question of whether a finding from a study of an individual nutrient remains the same when that nutrient is combined with others. Does combining it with other nutrients enhance its effectiveness? Negate it? Change it? This is generally not known unless the blended formula itself has been studied. For this reason, more and more high quality dietary supplement manufacturers are doing their own product research and clinical trials. Such companies offer comprehensive safety reviews on their proprietary product blends along with human clinical evaluations to assess safety and efficacy of their products.

Referring back to the studies I cited earlier in this chapter, with few exceptions, in many cases there is little control over the quality of the brand of dietary supplement that is used in the studies. This fact challenges the validity of the study findings, calling into question the reliability of the researcher's conclusions.

Synthetic vs. Whole Food Nutrition

The other consideration brought to light by these studies is that a synthetic nutrient may act very differently than one derived from a whole food source. When we attempt to replicate a healthy dietary pattern with nutritional supplements we make one tragic flaw: fruits and vegetables do not only contain isolated vitamins or minerals. They also contain hundreds of other phytochemical compounds whose functions are not yet well understood. To take an isolated nutrient and think we are replicating the benefits of consuming that nutrient in it whole food form is naïve. At this time, there is no substitute to whole real foods. Therefore, when manufacturers create supplements, multivitamins specifically, the specific nutrient they include, the quantity of these nutrients, the form of that nutrient (natural or synthetic), and the combination of nutrients are all important considerations often neglected in multivitamin research studies.

Select synthetic nutrients like folic acid are better absorbed then their naturally occurring counterpart, which in the case of folic acid, is folate. Conversely, many experts argue the synthetic form of vitamin E is not an appropriate substitute for the natural occurring forms of the vitamin. Synthetic vitamin E is known as dl-alpha-tocopherol. However, naturally occurring vitamin E exists in eight chemical forms (alpha-, beta-, gamma-, and delta-tocopherol and alpha-, beta-, gamma-, and delta-tocotrienol). Therefore many experts argue that clinical trials involving the supplementation of only the isolated synthetic form of vitamin E are deceptive and unreliable. It is suspect whether synthetic vitamin E reacts even remotely similar in the body to the naturally occurring forms of this nutrient. In fact, there are concerns that synthetic vitamin E is rejected by the body and may even lead to imbalances in other nutrients which can perhaps explain some of the negative findings attributed to it in some of the studies I cited earlier.

Another similar issue is with vitamin A. When supplemented as its synthetic form retinyl acetate or retinyl palmitate, study findings have not always been positive. In fact, studies have shown that too much retinyl acetate or retinyl palmitate has been linked to birth defects in premenopausal women and increased risk of bone fractures and decreased bone density on postmenopausal women. However, when consuming vitamin A from naturally occurring beta carotene source, the effects are different. Beta carotene must be metabolized within our cells into to retinal and retinoic acid, the active forms of vitamin A. When we consume too much retinyl acetate or retinyl palmitate, it accumulates in the body's tissue and can become toxic. This however, is not the same with beta carotene. When we consume beta carotene, the body only converts as much as it needs to retinoic acid; whatever excess remains is safely excreted. The source of vitamin A in your multivitamin should therefore primarily come from beta carotene.

The final issue is the combination of nutrients. Certain nutrients can compete for absorption with one another, while others can facilitate each other's absorption. For example, if we consume iron with vitamin C, the vitamin C will facilitate the uptake of iron. This is good if we have an iron deficiency but not so good if we already have adequate iron levels. Excessive intake of iron can then lead to toxicity. While vitamin C supports the absorption of iron it inhibits the absorption of copper. But, if you take in too much copper it can lead to a vitamin C deficiency! Then consider zinc. Consume too much and you now inhibit the absorption of both iron and copper! Whew! It can be challenging to keep track of this. Unfortunately, this fact is not considered either in many of the clinical trials conducted on multivitamins, which once again raises questions regarding the reliability of their conclusions.

The Bottom Line:
Although multivitamin supplements are commonly used to optimize health, promote longevity, and prevent chronic disease, their efficacy in this regard remains unclear, partly because of the inherent challenges

we face when we study them. That said, there appears to be sufficient evidence of safety and potential benefit to support taking a *high quality*, daily, *low dose*, and *whole food based* multivitamin. However, if you choose to take a multivitamin do not take just any product. If you are looking to supplement your diet then choose a low dose multivitamin (less than 100% of the RDI of each nutrient) made from whole food sources. Ideally, it is important to find a multivitamin that replicates whole food as much as possible. Your multivitamin should list the majority of each of its nutrients as derived from whole food sources. This way you are getting the natural form of the nutrient as well as the additional phytonutrients found in the host plant.

Furthermore, avoid mega dose supplements. Not only do you risk consuming toxic levels of specific nutrients, you also run the risk of increasing or inhibiting the absorption of other key nutrients. A good multivitamin should have between 70-100% of your daily need of each vitamin. Also, choose reliable manufacturers that have undergone third party testing (with current certification) and that do their own product formula testing and clinical trials. This will help ensure that each nutrient is well placed in the product to avoid undesired interactions and to optimize their benefits. When in doubt, talk to your healthcare practitioner. Often they have done the work for you and can recommend reliable products and brands that can meet your personal needs. In the resource section of this book, I have included links to the websites of some of my favorite nutritional supplement manufacturers.

Chapter 14

Lack of activity destroys the good condition of every human being while movement and methodical physical exercise save it and preserve it.
— *Plato*

Move It!

Did you know there is an amazing thing that can cut your risk of heart disease in half? Recently, studies have found that this same thing can also cuts the risk of breast cancer and colon cancer. It has also been shown to work as well as medications to reduce depression and acts as a natural anti-aging agent by increasing endogenous growth hormone production without any side effects. The good news is that it is available worldwide and without a prescription. The best part? It is completely free! The bad news? It does not come in a pill.

This amazing thing is... activity.

The above paragraph describes the impact of activity on our health and is inspired by a similar account offered by the esteemed physician, Tierona Low Dog, MD at a conference on integrative medicine I attended several years ago. Her words had such an impact on me that I had to do my best to paraphrase and share them with you in hopes that you too will find them impactful.

The effect of activity on our heath is truly remarkable. If we bottled it we would have our first great anti-aging panacea! Think about it, if you engage in physical activity each day for just 30 minutes without even changing a darn thing about your food intake, you will lose ten pounds of fat in one year and drastically reduce your risk of chronic and degenerative disease. It will help stimulate circulation, promote the removal of waste products from the body, and at the same time encourage the delivery of essential nutrients throughout the body. It is the ultimate anti-aging, anti-depressant, anti-disability, and anti-disease agent that exists; it is an evidence-based intervention with countless reliable, scientific studies to corroborate its exceptional benefits so why on earth are we not all actively pursuing it?

It really is amazing when you think about it; if we could encapsulate the benefits of physical activity into a pill, everyone and their baby would be taking it. Just because the delivery mechanism is a little more advanced than swallowing a pill, even though it is at our disposal any time of day, so many of us still opt out. This of course begs the questions, why? Why are we not all regularly participating in activity and reaping the benefits?

It is either funny or sad (or perhaps a little of both) that the proliferation of the fitness industry - with gyms on every corner, fitness video empires, countless television programs about fitness, and endless amounts of books on everything from yoga to running for dummies - has paralleled the increase in rates of obesity. The fitness industry is clearly offering us solutions to the obesity epidemic, so why is it not working?

There is no simple answer to that question. Many experts agree that one of the greatest obstacles to our fitness and health these days is our *obesogenic environment*. What this means is that our environment, the modern world we have created for ourselves, promotes weight gain.[307] This is not only about the excessive quantity of poor quality foods we eat. Our modern world has made it increasingly less necessary to integrate activity into our daily routine. Blame it on what some describe as *the curse of modern man*; our advances in technology have made our life so effortless that for most of us, strenuous physical activity is virtually unnecessary. For many cultures, gone are the days that entire afternoons are spent walking on uneven roads to a market to purchase food for the week and then carried home so every meal can be prepared by hand from scratch. Gone are the days of entire afternoons spent walking to a friend's home to discuss current events. Today's modern conveniences have made us so efficient and productive without ever leaving the comfort of our computer or car that we can actually go days at a time with little more movement than the trip it takes to get to and from our vehicle or desk top.

We get in our car, drive to work, take the elevator, and get seated at our desk. Send e-mails and text messages instead of visiting co-workers or friends, order lunch to be delivered straight to our desk or meeting, go to the drive-through on the way home to pick-up dinner, then sit with (or without) the family and consume the meal before retiring to the computer or TV for the rest of the evening. Repeat.

Strap a pedometer (or step counter) onto the person I just described and maybe, if he or she is lucky, he or she would have taken only about 400 steps and even that depends on whether he or she got the far parking spot or the close one. To offer you some context, it is suggested that the ideal daily step goal should be closer to 7,000 to 10,000 steps, not 400. Let's face it; modern convenience has made the basic function of movement more of an option then a necessity. If we want, most of us have access to every convenience these days. While these luxuries are groundbreaking and practical they can also help make us fat and lazy – if we let them.

But alas, it seems we *are* letting them. And the consequences of this sedentary lifestyle are far greater than just weight gain.

An article in Harvard Business Review described sitting as "the smoking of our generation".[308] A study of 9,000 adults reported that with each additional hour of television a person sat and watched per day, their risk of dying rose by 11%.[309] A 2012 study, of over 6,000 adults reported that prolonged sitting-time was positively associated with all-cause mortality.[310] That's right; the more time you spend sitting, the greater your risk of death by *any* cause. Yet another study, this time looking at over 100,000 adult men and women in the U.S. found that the amount of time spent sitting was *independently* associated with total mortality, regardless of physical activity level.[311] This means that regardless of whether an individual participates in some consistent form of daily activity (such as going to the gym to work out for an hour, going for a morning walk or running, attending an aerobics class, etc.) their risk of death is *still* increased if they also happen to sit too much during the day. This echoes the results of a Canadian study that found a *dose-response association* between sitting and risk of death and heart disease.[312] This means that as the time we spend sitting increases, so does our risk of dying and of developing heart disease. Once again, this association was present regardless of the amount of leisurely physical activity engaged in by the study participants.

The reason for this relationship between increased risk of mortality and sitting still needs to be elucidated, but it is clear that the body needs consistent daily movement to thrive. A remarkable study shed some light on this issue by exploring the connection between our muscles and genes. The researchers identified a key gene (called lipid phosphate phosphatase-1 or LPP1) expressed by muscle tissue that helps prevent blood clotting and inflammation. They found that this gene is significantly suppressed when sitting for hours, thereby increasing the risk of blood clots and inflammation. Amazingly, they also found that LPP1 is not impacted by movement and activity if the muscles have been inactive most of the day.[313] At a genetic level, this study helps us begin to understand why sitting too much appears to be so deadly.

Now do not get me wrong, I am not preaching that the solution is for us to leave all our modern conveniences behind, work the land, and live as our ancestors did; I too am guilty of being lost for hours at a time seated and working on my computer, playing mindlessly with a new apps on my iPhone, or driving my car one block up the road to buy coffee instead of taking the 5 minute walk to the cafe. It is not necessarily about giving all that up. Rather, it is about finding a balance, and learning ways to reintroduce activity as part of our *daily* routine. After all, our body is designed for movement and it clearly requires it for longevity and good health.

In Dan Buettner's bestselling book *The Blue Zones*,[314] he uncovers the common threads that are interwoven into the lives of individuals worldwide who are living to 100 years of age and beyond. One common thread he found among these centenarians is frequent activity integrated into their daily life. In most cases, in the original Blue Zone communities including Okinawa, Japan, Nicoya, Costa Rica, and Ikaria,

Greece this daily activity is not necessarily by choice, but rather out of necessity. There are no fast food restaurant drive-throughs. No fast food. If you want food; you make it. But you do not make it just by nuking it in the microwave, to prepare lunch you must bike or walk to the market, gather the bounty, grind the seeds, and mix it by hand. And there is a real joy in this. When one has to work a little harder for their food, when one sees where our food comes from, there is a greater sense of value and appreciation for the food we eat. We are less likely to overindulge unnecessarily. From an activity stand point we also learn a great lesson. That fitness leading to the ultimate goal of longevity is not only found in a gym. It is found in the way we live our life and in how we choose to participate actively in our daily existence. Since our contemporary lifestyle often allows us the luxury of being sedentary, we have to make a conscious decision to value our ability to move, and then, choose to exercise that ability.

So, Where Do You Begin?

To infuse more movement into your daily routine, you can start by just creating conditions that necessitate additional activity. Ask yourself:

What can I do to be less sedentary in my daily routine?

A 2013 study of 6,000 American adults found that just having an active daily routine appears to be as effective as structured activity for offering health benefits including preventing high blood pressure, high cholesterol, and metabolic syndrome.[315] So from today on, start celebrating when you find the furthest parking spot! Take the stairs not the elevator. Want to use almond meal in a recipe? Use a mortar and pestle to grind the almonds yourself! Walk the long way home and enjoy the journey. Invite a friend to meet you for a walk rather than for drinks. Instead of staying home and sitting in front of the television, go to the mall or market or museum or art gallery and walk around enjoying the view or even to window shop. Save money on the gardener and do the gardening yourself. Commit to standing and walking around every time you are speaking on the phone or inviting a co-worker for a walking meeting instead of sitting around a boardroom table. Stand at the back of class instead of sitting for hours on end. Do jumping jacks during the commercial breaks. When all else fails, even just fidgeting is better than just sitting there motionless!

ACTION STEP: Become less sedentary. As described in the previous paragraph, there are innumerable ways to seamlessly incorporate more movement into our daily routine. Pick one today and do it.

As you are becoming less sedentary, your next step to further reap the benefits of physical activity is to find an activity you enjoy, and participate in it. If you are not sure where to begin, then start by simply asking yourself:

Which activities did I enjoy participating in as a child?

Did you enjoy dancing? Swimming? Tennis? Maybe bicycling or flying a kite? Ballet? Perhaps going to the beach or tobogganing? Skiing? Playing catch with your dog? Whichever activities you enjoyed as a child can also bring you joy as an adult. Remember, movement should be fun! It is a privilege. Just ask anyone that is immobilized due to injury or disease. Celebrate your ability to move each day. Keep in mind that physical activity does not only occur in a gym. The world is your gym and opportunities for movement are endless!

ACTION STEP: Select one of your favorite childhood activities and do it! You will be surprised how much fun you have and the wonderful side effect will be the development of your fitness.

Ultimately, the goal is to include activities on most days of each week that develop your sense of balance, strength, and that get your heart racing. Start by choosing a fun; get your heart racing, aerobic activity as described in the action step above. As far as strength and balance training goes, if you are not sure where to begin, then I have the perfect plan to offer you! To make things easy, I have provided in the pages that follow a resistance game you can add to your daily routine without ever leaving the comfort of your own home. After that, you will see some easy and convenient steps for improving your balance and stability.

> **IMPORTANT:**
> When performing any of the following activities, muscles should feel fatigued, but not painful. Stop any movement that causes pain. Attempt to adjust your posture and body alignment to ensure you are performing the activity properly and as described. Then, attempt that movement again slowly and safely. If the pain persists, stop the activity completely and contact your healthcare provider.
>
> If you experience pain, dizziness, loss of balance, or similar symptoms with any of the following activities STOP the movement immediately and contact your healthcare practitioner for further advice.

The Equipment Free, Full Body, No Cost, Do Anywhere, Resistance Game!

These five movements are the most basic, tried and tested movements to engage your full body in a resistance routine. They will help you to maintain or even increase your muscle mass. These movements can be performed anywhere, whether at home or while travelling and the whole series can be completed in only 10 minutes (I do not care how busy you are; we *all* can find 10 minutes) and this resistance game can accommodate any level of fitness so, no excuses! I have included modifications if you are a beginner and additional challenges for the expert. I have also included notes on variations for each movement if you have an injury and pain that may limit your activity.

NOTE: If your goal is to *maintain* your current muscle mass, perform the series at least 2 to 3 times every week. If your goal is to *increase* your muscle mass, perform the series at least 3 to 4 times every week, if not daily.

TIP! To add an extra cardiovascular boost to this routine, between each movement either a) run in place, b) alternate lifting one knee at a time up towards your chest or c) do jumping jacks. Perform for 60 seconds and then take a 20 second break before moving on to the next movement.

ACTION STEP: Incorporate this 5 step activity game into your daily routine. Before brushing your teeth in the morning, take 10 minutes to run through these movements. That little routine will pay off in exponential dividends in terms of increasing bone density and muscle mass, not to mention all the other wonderful benefits that come along with the improvement in your body composition.

One more thing: take note of the SUCCESS TIPS and MIND GAMES I have listed with select movements described below. The "success tips" are strategies to improve the quality of each movement and to prevent common errors when performing each motion. The "mind games" are little tricks you can play with your mind to help you challenge yourself and get the most value from each movement.

Let the game begin!

1. PUSH-UP

This movement engages your chest, shoulders, triceps, back, and abdominal muscles.

Beginner or if you have shoulder or lower extremity pain, begin with the wall push-up:

➤ Feet on the floor positioned parallel to one another and placed approximately 2 feet from the wall. NOTE: The further your feet are from the wall the more challenging this will become - as it gets easier, step further away from the wall.
➤ Place your hands parallel to each other on the wall. The further apart they are, the more it will engage your pectoral muscles. The closer together they are, the more you will feel this in your triceps muscles.
➤ Using your arms, lower your torso towards the wall and then, push yourself away.
➤ Repeat!
➤ Perform up to 12 repetitions or until you feel like your muscles have fatigued; and then, *do just one more*!

Intermediate and advanced: Using the same steps described above, but instead of leaning against the wall, get down on the floor. Place your hands on the floor and for intermediate, start with body weight on your thighs just above your knees (not on your knee caps) with bent knees. For advanced, progress to having your lower body weight on your toes.

SUCCESS TIPS! Keep your core engaged throughout this activity by imagining that you are pulling your belly button in towards your spine and then up into your lower rib cage – this will help to protect your lower back. Also, squeeze your buttocks to keep your lower body strong and stable throughout. Challenge yourself by changing your arm position from a wider to a narrower placement on the wall to engage different muscles in the upper body.

MIND GAMES! As you straighten your arms, imagine that you are pushing the wall (or the floor) away from you!

2. LUNGE

This movement engages most of the muscles in your legs including your quadriceps, hamstrings, calves, and gluteal muscles.

➤ Focus on a point ahead of you so that you keep your chin up and your body upright (not leaning forward). Keep your shoulders down and away from your ears (resist the urge to contract them, visualized pulling your shoulders down and back through the entire activity). Pull your belly button in towards your spine and up your rib cage – this will help to engage your core and protect your lower back.
➤ Take a large step forward with one leg.
➤ Lower your hips down as you bend both knees to up to a 90 degree angle but never past that point. Your back knee should lower to a point where it is almost parallel to the floor but not to the point that it touches the floor. Your back foot will be on its toes.
➤ Look down and check to ensure that your front knee is directly above your ankle and not past your toes.
➤ As you rise back up, put your weight into your front heel to push yourself up.
➤ Repeat!
➤ Perform up to 12 repetitions on each side (right and left) or until you feel like your muscles have fatigued; and then, *do just one more*!

SUCCESS TIPS! Begin by doing these stationary, alternating sets with the right foot forward first and then the left. If you feel wobbly, pull your belly button in tighter and squeeze your buttocks; the more you engage your core muscles the more stable and steady you will be. If you still feel unbalanced, support yourself lightly by holding onto a chair or the wall. When you feel ready, progress by alternating between sides and moving forward with each step as you lunge. If you feel discomfort in your knees, start by taking a smaller step. As you progress and gain strength it will become easier; you may then be able to then increase the size of your step without the discomfort.

3. SQUAT

This movement engages your gluteus maximus, quadriceps, hamstrings, and calves.

➢ Begin by positioning your feet facing forward on the floor slightly wider than shoulder width apart. Keep your knees above your ankles and your belly button in towards your spine. Focus on a point ahead of you to help keep your chin up and your body upright.
➢ Slowly bend your knees then hips then ankles until your knees are at a 90 degree angle.
➢ Then rise up by pushing your heels into the ground to return to your starting position.
➢ Repeat!
➢ Perform up to 12 repetitions or until you feel like your muscles have fatigued; and then, *do just one more*!

Beginner: Practice by using a chair and sitting down towards the chair just until the point that you butt skims the top of the chair then, using your legs push yourself up by pushing your heels into the ground. Wall squats are a great way to progress from working with the chair; they are also a great way to ensure you have good form while doing the squat. Start with your feet about 2 feet ahead of you, lean against the wall with your back being sure to still keep your belly button pulled in towards your spine. Bend down at your knees and hips until they reach 90 degrees but not past that point. Then rise up and repeat.

SUCCESS TIP! Watch the position of your knees; they should always stay behind your toes. Look down as you squat; if you can no longer see your toes then step further out or lean further back.

4. BASIC CRUNCH

This movement engages the abdominal muscles.

Beginner and Intermediate:
- ➤ Lay on your back, bend your knees with your feet flat on the floor (you may also have your toes up and heels on the floor which will engage more of your lower abdominal muscles), place your hands on the sides of your head.
- ➤ Start by crunching up to approximate your pelvic bone towards the tip of your chest bone or sternum; lifting your shoulder blades up off the floor about 1 or 2 inches. At the same time pull you belly button down towards the floor flattening your lower back and keep it there throughout the crunch. To protect your lower back, avoid allowing your lower back to arch at all during this activity.
- ➤ Keep your head in line with your back throughout the crunch to protect your neck.
- ➤ Hold the crunch for a few seconds but *do not* hold your breath.
- ➤ Slowly lower yourself down.
- ➤ Repeat!
- ➤ Perform up to 12 repetitions or until you feel like your muscles have fatigued; and then, *do just one more*!

MIND GAME! Imagine a rod through your neck and back so it is moving as one unit - the movement should be coming entirely from the belly; not from the neck. If this is still hard to do, try pushing the back of your head into your hands as you lift up to prevent you from jutting your chin forward and straining your neck.

Advanced: According to a study at San Diego State University,[316] the Bicycle Crunch was found to be one of the most effective movements for engaging the abdominal muscles. Here's how to do it:

➢ Begin laying on the floor in the same position as you would for the crunch. Engage your core muscles and keep them engaged throughout the activity.

➢ With your hands lightly resting at the back of your head, raise your knees up to a 45 degree angle, with your hips bent to about 90 degrees.

➢ Slowly at first and then moving quicker, move your legs as if you were pedaling a bicycle.

➢ Alternate bringing your sternum up towards the left knee, then twist to bring it up towards the right knee.

➢ Repeat! Repeat! Repeat!

➢ Perform up to 12 repetitions on each side or until you feel like your muscles have fatigued; and then, *do just one more*!

SUCCESS TIP! Keep your belly pulled in towards your spine throughout the activity and remember not to hold your breath; keep breathing!

5. PLANK

This movement engages the muscles in your abdomen, back, arms, and legs.

➢ Lie face down resting on your forearms, with your palms flat on the floor.

➢ Push off the floor, raising up onto your toes and resting on your forearms.

➢ Keep your body in a straight line from the top of your head to bottom of your heels.

➢ Hold this position for as long as you can; up to 60 seconds.

BEGINNER: If the above seems too difficult, begin by resting your weight on your knees instead of on your toes. All the other steps described above will remain the same but you will find the degree of difficulty a little more manageable. As this becomes too easy, progress to moving from your knees to your toes.

SUCCESS TIPS! Keep your gaze directed towards to floor to prevent yourself from hyper-extending your neck. Pull your belly in towards your spine to keep your lower back flat. Actively squeeze/tighten the muscles in your buttocks to offer additional support. Do not let your rear end stick up into the air or to sag down in the middle.

BALANCE TRAINING

This is one of the most overlooked forms of training that is just as important for the 80 year old sedentary grandma as it is for the 25 year old professional athlete. Therefore, regardless of your age or current level of activity, the following movements will help you improve your sense of balance to help improve your stability and prevent falls as you age.

To improve your balance and stability, progress through the following 3 stages:

Stage 1: Stand with both feet on a pillow (an unstable surface). Hold position for 60 seconds.

Stage 2: *When stage 1 becomes too easy,* stand on one foot at a time on the floor. Hold position for 60 seconds.

Stage 3: *When stage 2 becomes too easy,* stand one foot at a time on a pillow. Hold position for 60 seconds.

SUCCESS TIP! Be sure to have a wall or sturdy piece of furniture nearby to gently lean on as you perform the following activities just in case you feel unstable or lose your balance.

ACTION STEP: Every time the phone rings, stand up and while talking on the phone stand on one foot at a time to integrate balance training into your everyday routine! Again, when first beginning be sure to have a wall or sturdy piece of furniture nearby to support you in case you lose balance.

NOTE: Activities like tai chi and yoga are excellent ways to help further develop your sense of balance and prevent falls. If you are an older adult and new to fitness I encourage you to attend a tai chi class. It is fun and safe for all levels of fitness and can benefit you in improving balance, muscle flexibility, and joint mobility.

Breaking the Plateau

When you first begin a new fitness routine and a new manner of eating you start to see significant changes in your body for the better. However, it is not uncommon that overtime you may notice you begin to hit a plateau. The same activities and manner of eating that once supported your body composition change, now no longer seem to be working. If you encounter this, there is a simple explanation and a simple fix.

The body is always striving towards efficiency. It wants to get the most benefit by using the least amount of its valuable resources. Another way to consider this is that our body is fighting to maintain balance. This is typically a good thing except when we are trying to shed body fat or build muscle. The body initially may respond beautifully to our imposed request to shed fat in the early stages of change, but as the body gets accustomed to our new activities and our new food supply, it starts to accommodate and reestablish a new normal, a new balance. Therefore, as we continue to try to shed fat or build muscle we need to keep the body from getting too comfortable. To do this, you need to mix up your routine once in a while.

There are three keys to breaking through the plateau. Try one or all three!

1. Challenge your body by participating in a new *type* of activity
2. Alternate between a relatively higher and lower intensity of effort *during* activity (interval training)
3. Alternate between a relatively higher and lower energy intake on different days

To help break through the plateau, challenge yourself! Participate in new activities, engage different muscles with new movements, or modify the amount of resistance you use, the intensity of effort, or even the type of terrain you work-out upon. They key is simply to change things up to challenge your body in a new way.

Your food intake can also help with breaking through the plateau. Avoid sticking too consistently to a set caloric intake each and every day. Instead, mindful of your estimated daily caloric needs, alternate between days when you may eat a little more (for example, an extra 100 or 150 calories above your typical daily intake on the days when you engage in more activity) and other days when you may eat a little less (consume 100 or 150 calories below your typical daily intake on days when you are less active). But whatever you do, make sure you eat! Believe it or not, one of the biggest mistakes we can make that leads us to a plateau in fat loss, is not eating enough.

Often, we reach a plateau since we are not eating adequate amounts of food to support our body's needs. When the body thinks it is in a period of famine (insufficient calories/inadequate energy intake to maintain basic functions) it slows down your metabolism to conserve energy and thus, you will plateau. That is why it is so important to eat enough food *especially* when you are trying to lose fat. If you are unsure about the amount of energy your body requires, or if your energy needs may have recently changed due to an increase in physical activity or fat loss, then turn back to chapter 6 to calculate an estimate of your daily energy needs based on your current level of activity. By modifying our routine and challenging our body in different ways we can prevent our body from settling into a state of efficiency and we can succeed in breaking the plateau.

Interval Training

When it comes to movement, whether you are a novice or expert interval training is a wonderful way to challenge your body in a new way that will also help break the plateau. It may sound complicated, but interval training is actually quite simple to implement. Interval training is a technique that prevents our body from settling into a predictable routine by alternating between bursts of intense activity and periods of lighter activity. Interval training results in increased calorie burning during your activity of choice, and increases your aerobic capacity, endurance, and speed leading to improvement in your overall physical fitness and body composition.[317] The other advantage of interval training is that it helps prevent the onset of boredom with your routine. Here is an example of how to put this into practice.

Interval training while walking: Next time you go for a walk instead of walking at a steady pace, modify your pace and intensity. If you tend to walk at a leisurely pace, then alternate your leisurely pace with

239

periods of faster walking. If you tend to walk at a brisk pace, incorporate short bursts of jogging into your regular walks. You can opt to increase the intensity for 1 minute or even just 30 seconds as you first begin.

For example: warm up by walking at a low intensity for about 5 minutes. Now, choose to walk for 30 seconds to 1 minute at a moderate or high intensity followed by 3-5 minutes of low intensity walking. Repeat alternating between this routine of high and low intensity effort approximately 6 - 8 times throughout the duration of your walk. Finish the walk with a low intensity cool down for at least 5 minutes.

If you walk outdoors, instead of time you can also have fun by picking a landmark as your guide to change intensity. For example, decide that when you reach the blue car up ahead you will begin increasing your intensity and choose to maintain that intensity until you reach the big tree at the end of the block.

If instead of walking you participate in swimming, bicycling, running, or any other similar aerobic activity, then you can apply the same steps to your sport of choice as described above. Remember, the key to interval training is simply to alternate between a low intensity effort and bursts of moderate or high intensity effort. Whether novice or expert you will be amazed at how this manner of movement will transform your body and help you break through the plateau!

Eating Before and After a Workout

Patients repeatedly ask me whether it matters if they eat before or after they workout and if so, whether it matters *what* they eat. The answer to both questions is a resounding yes; it matters. However, this position is not without some controversy.

The question of whether or not one should eat prior to engaging in vigorous physical activity has actually been a rather contentious topic of debate among many sport medicine practitioners. There is a school of thought and some evidence to support the notion that if one is looking to lose body fat, they are better off *not* eating prior to a workout.[318,319,320] One study in 2011, compared the amount of fat burning in athletes participating in endurance training without eating before activity versus those who ate. The researchers found that the athletes who had not eaten prior to training burned more fat.[321] Critics of this approach argue that even if there are short term metabolic advantages with a person burning more fat, the long term impact is negligible. Particularly, since without sufficient energy prior to a workout, the overall quality of the workout may be compromised.

Working out on an empty stomach can lead to low blood sugar during the activity which can lead to fatigue, lightheadedness, dizziness, and even faintness. In turn, this can lead to a less effective workout, compromised form and increased susceptibility to injury. The latter is a major concern. Those among you that have experienced an injury related to activity are all too familiar with the physically and emotionally damaging effect of being sidelined by an injury. Recovery from musculoskeletal injuries can be long and frustrating; the risk is most certainly not worth any negligible potential benefit of working out on empty.

Another concern if one does not eat prior to activity is that it may lead to overeating *after* the activity. In general, it is reasonable that one should adhere to the same practices to maintain normal blood sugar levels throughout the day whether they are working out or not. This approach helps optimize energy, function, and prevent overeating.

So yes; you should eat before a workout. In fact, for optimal function your body demands it.

The next question is: what should you eat?

Time for a little biochemistry! We already know that the type of food we eat has an essential role in keeping our body alive and well. It therefore stands to reason, that when we engage in an activity that challenges our muscles and cardiovascular system even more than usual, the fuel source is going to be critical. When participating in any challenging activity, the body has two fundamental needs:

1) The body needs fuel to support the activity and,
2) The body needs the resources to rebuild and recover afterwards.

Pre-Workout Fuel

So, how do we fuel activity? Remember, carbohydrates are made of sugar or glucose molecules. When we eat a carbohydrate, it is broken down through the digestive process into its smaller glucose components. Whatever glucose we do not use right away we store as glycogen. Glycogen is our energy stockroom. (However, consuming too many carbohydrates will fill up our glycogen stores and force any additional carbohydrates to then be stored as fat.) Glycogen is a chain of glucose molecules that is located primarily in the liver and muscle. When we engage in any activity, particularly for an extended period of time, our body releases the glucose from the glycogen to produce energy. This is what fuels *every* muscle contraction! Our glycogen stores are limited and usually can sustain us for anywhere from 30 to 90 minutes depending on the intensity of the workout. That is why athletes that are engaged in prolonged high level endurance activities will continue fueling with carbohydrates not just before, but during the activity as well.

Complex carbohydrates are the best food source for building up our glycogen stores. That is why small amounts of foods such as oatmeal, nuts, nut butters, vegetables, fruit, or a few whole grain crackers, are great to consume pre-workout. If you eat refined carbohydrates like white bread, sugary cola, or candy before a workout it can lead relatively quickly to a state of hypoglycemia/low blood sugar (remember the vicious cookie cycle?) making you feel tired and weak before the workout is over. Complex carbohydrates raise blood sugar levels at a slower rate so they offer more sustained energy during your day and during your workout.

It is important that we consume enough carbohydrates before we engage in vigorous activity since if the body does not have enough carbohydrates to use for energy, it will turn instead to protein. In the absence of adequate carbohydrates, the protein stores in our body will be broken down to make glucose for energy. This is not a good thing since we never want to use up our protein stores for energy. This is merely a back-up mechanism for times when we are in a state of desperate starvation. Consider protein as a building block, not as a fuel source. Protein builds muscles and other essential body tissues. If you are burning it up for energy then you are also compromising your ability to build and maintain muscle and other tissues. Furthermore,

242

over time the byproducts produced when using protein as energy can be damaging to our kidneys.

Therefore, in addition to a small source of complex carbohydrates it is also a good idea to consume some protein pre-workout so that you can begin to supply the amino acid building blocks your body will need to support your recovery after the workout. As a general rule, if your workout will entail mostly strength training, then eating a little more protein beforehand is a good idea in addition to the complex carbohydrates. On the other hand, if the workout will consist mostly of aerobic activity, then a little less protein during the pre-workout meal or snack is fine.

Fat should not be consumed in substantial amounts immediately prior to your workout. A teaspoon of nut butter on apple slices is fine pre-workout; a big slab of cheese is not. Fat can take over 6-hours to digest so it is not the best source of energy before a workout. It is not accessible for immediate energy and can even make some people feel sluggish if eaten too close to activity. Furthermore, converting stored body fat to energy takes time. One pound of stored fat on your body provides approximately 3,600 calories of energy. However, stored fat needs to be broken down then transported to the muscle; it is not as immediate to access as glycogen. When we perform quick, intense efforts like sprinting or weight lifting we really do not access this fat energy that much. Instead, the stored fat is accessed more during longer, slower lower intensity, and endurance activity such as prolonged cycling, swimming, and walking. However, the more muscle we build even by participating in short duration activities, the greater our metabolism becomes so the more of that stored fat we will burn up, even at rest!

Post-Workout Recovery

After the workout the body needs to recover. It needs to adapt to the training load by building and repairing the muscle tissue. You see, any vigorous activity (such as walking, running, swimming, or dancing) or resistance activity (such as free weights, jump-training, and isometric training), that challenges our muscles is actually tearing our muscle tissue. But this tearing is a good thing! Before a muscle can get stronger, it needs to undergo this microscopic damage. Together with the accumulation of lactic acid that builds up in the muscle, this microscopic damage is what induces that feeling of soreness in your muscles after intense activity. But again, this is a good thing. The breakdown of the muscle fiber is essential to allow for re-growth and development of the muscle tissue. A muscle requires approximately 24 to 48 hours for repairing and rebuilding itself. This recovery process is what allows for us to develop more toned and stronger muscles afterwards.

It is important that we support this rebuilding process appropriately by choosing the right type of food following our workout. You must supply your body with amino acids (found in protein-rich foods) which are the building blocks of muscle tissue. By having a snack that contains approximately 10 to 20 grams of lean protein within thirty minutes following activity, we can support and enhance the repair and rebuilding of muscle tissue post workout. Combining that protein with some healthy carbohydrates is your best bet, as this combination has been shown to result in increased glycogen storage and more efficient muscle repair and development.[322,323] Then, within approximately 2-hours post activity, consuming a balanced meal with carbohydrates, protein, and some healthy fat is ideal. This meal will further replenish protein and glycogen stores and prepare your body for future needs. Remember, the amount of food you consume before and after vigorous activity should still remain within your daily energy needs as outlined in chapter 6. The chart that follows includes some examples to help fine tune your pre- and post-workout food choices.

The Bottom Line:
You would never take road trip without a full tank of gas; do not embark on a workout without a full tank of glycogen. You also would not put low octane gas in a Ferrari or Bentley! Feed your body the right types of foods to optimize performance during activity and recovery afterwards but do not consume more than you need. Eat fewer calories than you use up during your activity, but not less than your body needs to fuel the workout.

The following chart offers some guidelines to help fuel your workout along with some specific food choices. Keep in mind, this is intended to support the energy and recovery needs of those among us that participate in moderate to intense aerobic and/or resistive training activities lasting within 30 to 90 minutes. If you are a beginner and your activity of choice is a short, gentle walk, no need to modify your intake around light activity. Conversely, if you participate in extreme, high level athletics like marathoners, tri-athletes, or competitive weight trainers, your nutritional needs should be customized to your sport. If that is the case, talk to a qualified athletic trainer or healthcare practitioner with a specialty in sports nutrition, to help tailor your intake. For the rest of us, use the chart below to help maximize energy, function and recovery during and after your workout.

Fueling your Activity

If you eat:	Quantity	Choose
2 to 3 hours before activity	Consume a regular, balanced meal	*Any regular meal that contains lean protein, carbohydrates, and vegetables (refer to chapter 6 for suggestions)* NOTE: If eating a regular balanced meal within 2-3 hours before activity, no need to eat again before the workout.
1 to 2 hours before activity	Consume enough calories to equal approximately half those you expect to burn during your workout (200-300 kcals)	*Choose relatively high-carbohydrate, moderate protein, low-fat snack/meal: (avoid high-fat foods or large quantities of any food)* ✓ Fruit and low fat plain Greek yogurt parfait ✓ Almond milk blended with frozen fruit, nut butter, and greens to make a smoothie ✓ A small serving of tuna salad on a whole grain tortilla or cracker ✓ Turkey wrap with vegetables ✓ Steel cut oatmeal topped with blueberries and slivered raw almonds ✓ Grilled chicken breast with brown rice and broccoli ✓ 2-3 hard-boiled egg, half of the yolks removed and replaced with hummus ✓ Hummus and raw veggies

		✓ Half an almond butter or tuna/turkey/chicken sandwich on whole grain, sprouted bread, or gluten free crackers
30 minutes before activity	Consume within 100-200 kcals	*Choose relatively high-carbohydrate, moderate protein, low-fat snack/meal: (avoid high-fat foods or large quantities of any food)* ✓ Any of the food choices above in smaller quantities or: ✓ whole grain crackers with nut butter ✓ ½ banana with 1 tsp almond butter ✓ ½ apple with 1 tsp nut butter
Activity!		
0 to 30 minutes post activity	Consume enough calories to equal about 50% of the calories you burned and include approximately 10-20 grams of protein	*NOTE: modify portion sizes below to suit your desired intake* ✓ 4 ounces turkey, 1 cheese wedge, and 1 apple ✓ 4 ounces turkey, wrap in 1 large collard green leaf with Dijon mustard, avocado and raw sliced veggies ✓ 2 devilled eggs with a sliced green apple ✓ Veggie omelet (2 eggs and 1 cup sautéed seasonal veggies) ✓ 2-3 whole eggs scrambled with a handful of chopped onion, spinach, and bell peppers ✓ Blend 4 cups spinach, ½ cup Greek yogurt, 1 cup almond milk, 1 banana, and 1 tablespoon peanut butter, vanilla extract to taste with ice ✓ turkey or chicken sandwich ✓ vegetable stir-fry with chicken, shrimp, or tofu ✓ whole-wheat tortilla filled with black beans, salsa, and cheese

246

		✓ smoothie with almond milk, yogurt, or added protein powder ✓ smoothie with 2 scoops of whey protein powder combined with water and ½ banana Any light meal that contains lean protein, carbs, and vegetables: ✓ Bowl with tuna, brown rice, avocado, and kidney beans ✓ Nicoise Salad with spinach, tuna, red peppers, green beans, and tomatoes and ½ an egg
0 to 30 minutes post activity		If the workout was intense from a cardiovascular standpoint, be sure to also replenish any lost electrolytes (minerals such as chloride, potassium, and sodium). Unsweetened coconut water (look for one with at least 110 mg of sodium per cup) or a banana with a little salted almond butter are good options (may be incorporated into the post workout snack above)
2 hours post activity	Consume a regular, balanced meal	*NOTE: if workout was in the evening, no need to consume this meal – continue to adhere to guidelines in chapter 6 that recommend not eating within approximately 2 hours prior to bedtime.* Any regular meal that contains lean protein, carbohydrates/vegetables, and healthful fats (refer to chapter 6 for suggestions)

TIP! If you tend to get very hungry after strenuous activity, plan your workouts around your regular meals or snacks times (such as before lunch or prior to dinner) so you do not end up adding an extra meal after your workout.

A Guide for Choosing a Protein Powder

It is smart to have a high quality protein powder on hand to make quick post workout smoothies or even to add to cooked and baked goods to enhance their protein punch! There are many types of protein powders on the market but not all are created equal. The following are the two forms of protein powder that I recommend.

Whey Protein: *Recommended!*

Various studies, including a 2011 double-blind, randomized controlled trial, have found that the consumption of supplemental whey protein can help improve body composition and reduce waist circumference.[324]

NOTE: Whey protein *isolate* is not identical to whey protein. The isolate form does not contain lactose thus making it easier to digest for those with lactose intolerance than whey protein which is generally only 20% whey protein and 80% casein protein. The main advantage of including casein protein is that it takes longer to digest than whey, so it can be beneficial as a meal replacement, but should only be consumed in individuals *without* a dairy allergy or intolerance to lactose.

TIP! Choose organic whey protein powders sourced from grass-fed cows not treated with rBGH just as you would choose other dairy foods.

<u>Vegetarian Protein Powder</u>
Pea Protein and Rice Protein: *Recommended!*

These are excellent options not only for vegetarians, but also for those with allergies to gluten, soy, or dairy, lactose intolerance, and in those just looking to vary their protein source. Both pea and rice protein generally have high digestibility and a low potential for allergic response. Rice protein is commonly mixed with pea protein powder to improve their amino acid profile. Together, they are comparable to dairy or egg protein in terms of their amino acid profile.

NOTE: While I *am* a proponent of consuming whole, organic soy foods such as tofu, tempeh, and edemame as part of an overall healthful dietary pattern, (assuming one does not have an allergy or sensitivity to soy) I do not recommend consuming *isolated* soy protein powders and other processed soy products like soy meats (think fake'n bac'n!) made with *soy protein isolate* or *textured soy protein*. While studies have demonstrated benefits of soy protein supplementation,[325] there is also sufficient concern raised in the scientific literature to advise against the consumption of these *isolated* forms of soy until more research demonstrating its safety is available.[326]

Hydration

Do not forget to stay hydrated throughout activities. As a general rule, on top of your normal daily fluid intake, add at least one 8 ounce glass of water for every 30 minutes of aerobic activity per day. Also, have at least one 8 ounce glass of water prior to activity and at least one 8 ounce glass of water following activity.

If you work out first thing in the morning, your hydration needs may be even greater. We often wake up in a dehydrated state since we have not consumed fluids for hours while sleeping. Therefore, if you like to participate in vigorous activity at the crack of dawn, be sure to consume adequate amounts of water prior to and during the activity.

If you engaged in prolonged (over 60 minutes) of intense, aerobic activity such as long distance running or cycling, you may also want to consider replenishing lost electrolytes both during and following your activity. Instead of reaching for the artificial sports drink, replenish lost electrolytes with unsweetened coconut water (look for one with at least 110 mg of sodium per cup) or choose a banana with a little salted almond butter following the workout. These whole foods are rich in electrolytes without the added sugars or artificial ingredients found in most commercial sports drinks.

Popeye was Right; Spinach Does Build Muscle!

Who knew that an iconic muscle-bound cartoon character was so far ahead of his time? Dietary nitrates are found *naturally* in foods such as spinach, beetroot (beets), kale, and all dark green leafy vegetables. Recently, studies have elucidated how nitrates in these foods have a range of beneficial effects on our health including reducing blood pressure, inhibiting platelet aggregation, (preventing our blood from getting too sticky) preserving or improving the health of our blood vessels, and enhancing exercise performance in both healthy individuals and those with peripheral arterial disease.[327] A 2012 Swedish study done in mice also found that plant sources of nitrates boost the production of two key proteins that help build muscle mass. Please note that nitrate supplements are not required, as the same daily dose of nitrates used in the study can be obtained from consuming a few servings of spinach or from eating two to three beetroots.[328]

As mentioned in chapter 8, there has long been a perception that dietary sources of nitrite and nitrate are harmful, as some studies reveal an association between foods that contain nitrite and nitrate (such as cured and processed meats) and cancer. Yet, this paradigm has recently been challenged in light of the current research demonstrating an undisputed health benefit of food plans that are rich in *plant sources* of nitrites and nitrates.[329] It is important to clarify that the current research suggests potential carcinogenic effects of nitrites and nitrates are linked *only* to cured and processed meats and *not* to dietary intake of nitrates when consumed in fruits and vegetables.[330]

The Bottom Line:

Plant sources of nitrates appear to enhance performance during physical activity and increase muscle mass. To ensure you optimize your dietary intake of nitrates but minimize the potential risk of any side effects from excessive ingestion when used as an additive, choose whole food fruit and vegetable sources such as spinach and beets, minimize intake from cured meats, and *avoid* intake from processed meats and dietary supplements.[331]

By now I trust you are gaining confidence in the steps to take as you proceed in the journey that defines your new *manner of living*. I recognize there are special considerations that for some of us, can serve as obstacles or challenges along our path. For this reason, the next few chapters offer support and empowerment through knowledge and tips that will help you diminish these obstacles and overcome any perceived challenges. My job is to make your journey as seamless and pleasurable as possible, so turn the page to reveal tried and tested ways to enrich your new *manner of living*. First, let us start by conquering stress.

Chapter 15

*The mind is its own place, and in itself can
make a heaven of hell, a hell of heaven.*
— John Milton, Paradise Lost

Stress

Stress is frequently the culprit in our undoing. For many among us, as
we embark upon a path paved with healthful habits and best intentions,
as soon as we are confronted by a stressor we unravel. Furthermore, if
that stressor is ongoing or repeated we often use that to justify our
inability to fully embrace a healthy *manner of living*. If this resonates
with you, then that pattern is now about to change.

The connection between weight and stress has been quite elusive since
in response to chronic stress some people lose body weight; whereas
others gain. Either way, this response can be unhealthy in the long
term. Recent cutting-edge research has revealed clues to help us better
understand the connection between stress and body composition. One
study showed that chronic stress unlocks the body's fat cells by
stimulating a special chemical called neuropeptide Y (NPY). NPY
unlocks certain receptors in fat cells, causing them to grow in both size
and number. Researchers found that stressed mice fed high-fat, high-
sugar foods developed more body fat than unstressed mice fed the

same food.[332]   Another fascinating study used animal models to demonstrate that extreme stress such as war, injury, or traumatic grief typically results in decreased food intake and body weight. However, ongoing every day social stresses such as public speaking, exams, job and relationship pressures, appear to have the opposite effect, leading to overeating and weight gain.[333]

Part of the reason the connection between weight and stress remains so elusive is that stress is personal. There are certainly events that can be thought of as universal stressors such as war or loss of a loved one. However, it is not the event itself that dictates our response to the stress; it is our perception of that event that matters.

Stress is not a bad thing. It triggers a brilliant physiologic mechanism that is essential for human survival. The stress response allows us to think under pressure, cram before that big exam, respond quickly when put on the spot; it can even give us the "superhuman" strength to respond in moments of danger or confrontation.

Think back to the time of Paleolithic man.   A caveman would go about his day hunting and gathering to survive. If he was confronted by a lion the stress response gave him the power to quickly respond to the situation. The stress response allows the body to redirect its efforts so that the body can mobilize its energy more efficiently to respond to a challenging situation. In response to the stress, stress hormones are released. This "fight or flight" response halts unnecessary actions of the body and sends the body into high alert. Heart rate and blood pressure increase, blood sugar levels rise to supply the muscles with energy, blood vessels constrict on the skin to send blood to the muscles, and muscles tense up. Non-essential body systems like the digestive system and the immune system are shut down so the body can focus its energy on responding to the emergency. The caveman is now empowered with the ultimate strength to fight or run as fast as he can from the threat. Then, once the stressful situation has passed, the body restores its normal balance and function. But, what if that stress *never* goes away?

Stress becomes a problem when it is chronic and unremitting. Consider the stress of the modern world. We do not have wild beasts to worry about these days; instead, we have a boss, spouse, kids, tests, bills, deadlines, traffic, or commitments. These stressors do not go away instead, they are chronic and persistent, and so may be our stress response. This means our blood pressure and stress hormones can remain elevated, our digestion can remain inhibited, we can remain constipated and so on. You do not need a doctorate to understand how this state of being eventually leads to chronic disease.

But there is a secret to managing stress and the stressor itself has nothing to do with it. We cannot change always our boss, or our spouse, or our kids, and fortunately, we do not have to! The negative effects of stress are never about the stressor itself, it is about our perception and resilience.

I live in southern California so for me, bumper to bumper traffic is a daily reality. You may drive in the same traffic that I do. We both may travel along the 405 freeway in Los Angeles during rush hour. This is the same road that Angelinos attribute its designation as the 405 to the fact that it takes 4 hours and 5 minutes to get anywhere on it! Needless to say this is one freeway that sees its share of traffic each day. So let us consider that we are driving in separate cars but in the same traffic jam on the 405 freeway in Los Angeles. You may be listening to music, thinking about your day, and just driving along observing your surroundings. You use this time as an opportunity to think about issues that have been on your mind and enjoy a moment of alone time to ponder thoughts and enjoy music. Your blood pressure is stable and your body is calm and relaxed. Someone cuts in front of you and you hit the breaks to accommodate their sudden movement but otherwise, you remain calm and relaxed. You arrive at your destination unfettered and go about your day.

Now imagine that a few cars over, I am sitting in my car in that same traffic jam on the 405 freeway in Los Angeles. Same road, same traffic jam but I am experiencing it in a drastically different manner. I am frustrated that I am stuck in a traffic jam; thinking about all the things I need to do today: the appointment I may run late for, the call I need to make, the projects I need to finish, all the other things I could be doing right now. I curse the drivers ahead of me and blame them for causing me to be stuck here. I am frustrated at the waste of my time this traffic has imposed upon me. My blood pressure is rising and my body is releasing a cavalcade of stress hormones. Someone cuts in front of my car and I curse at them like a sailor for the careless maneuver and my blood pressure continues to rise. I arrive at my destination late, angered, and frazzled.

The above scenario illustrates two identical situations with two drastically different responses. At face value we chock this up to two different personality types; no big deal. But physiologically it is a big deal. How we experience and respond to situations is the major factor influencing whether the situation is seen as a stress or not. In other words, a situation itself is only a stress if we experience it to be so. (For the record, I actually enjoy driving so in reality, I fit more into the first scenario I described and not the second!)

Do not get me wrong, there are certain situations that universally can be perceived as stressful. Take war for example. By definition, it is a horrifically stressful event for anyone that has ever experienced it. Yet, despite the obvious emotional trauma exposure to such a stressful life event can impose upon ones psyche, two people with the same traumatic experience can respond in a drastically different manner.

In the 1997 Italian film *La Vita e Bella* (Life is Beautiful), the lovable Italian actor Roberto Benigni depicts the story of a man attempting to survive with his family in Italy during the Holocaust. While enduring this most horrific chapter in modern history, in an attempt to protect his son he employs his imagination to create beauty and humor within the unimaginable misery of a Nazi death camp.

My father, who was a Holocaust survivor, shared this same remarkable ability to harness strength, optimism, and imagination. However, for my father it was not for the benefit of a film; it was for the benefit of his life and survival. My dad lived through the holocaust as a 17-year old young man. I could never and will never be able to wrap my mind around that reality. When I was 17-years old I was still a child; a pampered teenager dependent on my parents to protect me from the harsh realities of the world. To this day I am pained and halted in my tracks in an inexplicable manner at the mere attempt of thinking about the horrific atrocities that my dad experienced. Right now as I write this I have tears in my eyes and searing pain at the thought.

Yet, my father always told my brother and me stories of that period in his life as if they were adventures. His stories to us about his experiences during the war were heroic, humorous, and amazing tales of adventure and not of misery and sadness. Part of the rationale for this was undoubtedly to protect my brother and me from the horrific realities he witnessed, but a major part of it was just him. Throughout my dad's adult life he would often stop and proclaim *La Vita e Bella!* This was in response to, and in appreciation of the wonderful little moments of daily life. My father had an incredible ability to find and appreciate beauty, strength, and awe in all moments of life, especially the good ones, but even in the most difficult circumstances. This quality is no doubt at least part of the reason for his exceptional resilience throughout his life. I am quite certain this attribute is a critical part of explaining how he could survive and then thrive after enduring the unimaginable horror of the Holocaust and then 50 years later, survive two of the deadliest cancers and talk about those experiences again, as a challenge and adventure. His unrelenting strength, passion, optimism, and awe for life was contagious and inspired many. In fact, it was he that unknowingly inspired me to write this book.

As I write this book my father is always beside me. Originally, as I began to write it in a hospital room by his bedside and now, as he is in my heart and my mind and in my very being. My dad survived two of the deadliest cancers in seemingly inexplicable ways – through his brilliant intellect in discerning innovative approaches to his treatment and through his superhuman reliance and strength of mind and spirit, he defied all odds. His survival mystified oncologists. He served as an advocate for others going through cancer therapies and served as their and forever my, inspiration. He only passed away when the cancer attacked his brain. It was the only way the cancer could hurt him; if it accessed his mind. Until then, his mind could outsmart and overpower anything, including cancer.

For many, the trauma of war has unraveled lives. Cancer has worn down spirits. These are the same experiences that my father endured, but for many people the effect is far different than it was for my father. Not due exclusively to the experience itself, but rather due to their perception of, and response to it. Remember, we cannot always change the experiences in our lives, but we CAN always change how we choose to respond to them.

I began this chapter with a quote from the epic poem *Paradise Lost*, written by the 17th century English poet John Milton, "The mind is its own place, and in itself can make a Heaven of Hell, a Hell of Heaven." This quotation illustrates perfectly how stress is ultimately about perception and response. It is also beautifully empowering. It reveals how we can regain control over our perceptions. You *can* change your mind. In fact, the science of *neuroplasticity* informs us that our brain is constantly going through remodeling that is affected not only by life experiences, genetics, and biological agents but also by our chosen behaviors and thought patterns.[334] Even deeply rooted behavioral patterns can therefore be overcome at any stage of life with conscious intent and repetition. So, there is scientific proof that you *can* teach an old dog new tricks. You can build resiliency and assume control over your response to any of life's stressors. Choose to start doing it today.

Building Resilience

A 2012 study in the Annals of Behavioral Medicine found that how people respond to the daily stressors in their lives is predictive of future chronic health conditions. The researchers found that people who become upset by daily stressors such as an argument with a spouse or an impending deadline, and continued to dwell on the stressor even after it passed were more likely to suffer from chronic health problems especially pain, 10 years later![335] In order to mitigate the negative effects of stress, the key is recognizing that as described before, while we cannot always avoid stress, we can always strengthen our resilience to it.

Resilience is essentially the ability to *bounce back* in the face of adversity. It is about embracing ones self-efficacy and is arguably one of the most important allies we have to help us retain control over our minds and our lives when we are faced with stressors. Some of us may innately possess this ability, but for the rest of us we can develop it. I have listed below twelve tips that will help you hone this critical coping skill. As you read these tips, do not just skim through them, consider them deeply in the context of *your* life and make a conscious effort to put one or more of them into practice each day. Have confidence and trust in your strength and ability to build resilience. Consider the words of Ralph Waldo Emerson: "What lies behind you and what lies in front of you, pales in comparison to what lies inside of you."

1. **Think like an optimist.** Look at life's challenges and setbacks as temporary and changeable. Resist feelings of helplessness and anxiety.

2. **Take action.** Assess the situation: Can you influence the outcome or not? If not, *let it go*. If you can, establish a plan and do something about it! Do not get caught up indefinitely in the stressor and allow it to linger, but do not just ignore it either. Make a decision and take action. NOTE: Choosing to let it go is an action too.

3. **Look ahead.** Often a stressful event locks us in time. It seems insurmountable as we become short sighted and only can see the moment. In such instances, step back and look at the big picture of your life. The big picture lets us see all the possibilities ahead rather than just becoming fixated on the one obstacle that is before our eyes. The further you pull back, the more perspective you can gain and the smaller and more manageable that obstacle will seem.

4. **Accept failure like a success.** Do not give up after failure. Recognize that all people with great success stories have encountered failure at one or more points in their life. Use failure as an opportunity to learn and grow, not to retreat.

5. **Laugh!** Learn to laugh at the unpredictable nature of life. Stop taking things so seriously. Life has good and bad moments; the good only feel good if you have also experienced the bad.

6. **Have a willingness to grow and learn.** When things go wrong, use that as an opportunity to grow. Could you have avoided this? What can you do differently to prevent this from repeating? Can this teach you something about yourself? Who you are, who you are becoming? Friedrich Nietzsche said it best: "That which does not kill us makes us stronger."

7. **Be competent.** Learn what you need to know; read, speak with experts, empower yourself with knowledge and understanding so you can make well informed decisions.

8. **Be confident!** Trust your gut and instinct. Do not give other the power to unravel you; celebrate your uniqueness even if others do not.

9. **Be connected.** Surround yourself with people that make you feel good and support you.

10. **Find calm.** Any type of meditation whether it takes the form of deep breathing, yoga, guided imagery (described later in this chapter) or just repeating a meaningful mantra quietly to yourself, can help you focus your thoughts and calm your mind during moments when you feel overwhelmed.

11. **Accept help.** Reach out to family, friends, books, support group, associations, or professionals. Often novel perspectives can offer comfort and revelations.

12. **Embody Tip #1. Become an optimist.** *Life IS beautiful*; it is up to you to choose to embrace a willingness to find and appreciate the beauty in any situation.

Changing Your Mind

We all talk about heart health, skin health, and bone health but strangely the organ that does the most work for us, seems to get the least amount of respect and attention. It is time we pay more attention to the brilliantly beautiful and complex organ that is the brain. Part of the reason that we may have overlooked the brain, is that we often see it as so complicated and enigmatic that we think there is little we can do to influence its activity. But in reality, the brain while astonishingly complex, may not be as clever as we think. You see, we can easily play tricks on our mind and harness its strength to help us heal and recover.

Imagine there is a lemon in your hand. Picture its bright yellow skin and its firm, cool texture. Imagine slicing the lemon with a sharp knife into four segments. Picture yourself picking up one of those segments and bringing it towards your mouth, smelling its fresh citrus fragrance. Now, imagine biting into it. Imagine the sour taste that sucking on the lemon wedge elicits in your mouth.

Are you salivating? If you visualized the scenario with the lemon that I just described (particularly if you do so with your eyes closed), chances are; you are.

What happened?

You tricked your brain.

The brain, as brilliant and complex as it is, cannot always distinguish between reality and imagination. Just now, simply by imagining the experience of tasting a lemon you did such a compelling job convincing your brain that it was biting into a real lemon that you were able to trigger the same response that biting into an actual sour lemon would trigger. You caused the brain to send a signal to the glands in your mouth to salivate.

Imagine using this same technique to trigger the brain to release hormones and other chemicals that allow us to relax, to heal from disease, to enhance the effectiveness of medications, or even eliminate the need for medications. Imagine convincing our mind to stimulate our immune system to fight off cancer cells or to trigger our body to become calm, decrease our blood pressure, or not feel pain. Sounds like science fiction? Well, it's not.

Research has revealed seemingly unbelievable possibilities of harnessing the power of our mind to make us well. The beneficial effect of the mind-body connection is understood both through epigenetics mechanisms,[336] and through the science of psychoneuroimmunology (the study of the connection between the mind (*psycho*), the nervous system (*neuro*) and the immune system (*immunology*)). This big word helps us understand how the amazing and often misunderstood placebo effect[337,338] can help us heal. We can also harness the power of this connection intentionally, through therapeutic activities such as guided imagery.

Guided imagery is a means of guiding your imagination to support well-being and healing. Compelling evidence is emerging in support of the diverse benefits of guided imagery for everything from helping to decrease pain and anxiety[339,340,341] to improving athletic and professional performance[342,343] and boosting immune health.[344] It can even help build your resilience.[345]   I have long been a proponent of guided imagery and have included some links to books, recordings, and practitioner organizations within the resource section of this book.   In the meantime, to experience a taste of this powerful intervention, try this simple activity: Find a relaxing place and assume a comfortable posture.   Close your eyes and imagine yourself within a tranquil, calm scene. Visualize yourself experiencing vibrant health in that moment; free from any pain or stress you may have been experiencing, free from any disease you may have been diagnosed with. If you feel pain or stress, simply expel it out of your body - picture it leaving your body through the tip of your toes and being replaced with a soothing, healing energy that blankets your mind and body. With each breath you take picture your body healing. With each breath you take, picture your body becoming stronger and more vibrant yet calm and comfortable. Revel in this experience for at least 5 minutes. Then, open your eyes.

Chapter 16

If you want to lift yourself up, lift up someone else.
— Booker T. Washington

No Person is an Island

Throughout this book, I have shared with you the value and benefit of sharing your *manner of living* with all those around you; guests, children, friends, and family. In the previous chapter, one of the tools for enhancing resiliency was developing a sense of connectedness. Seeking help and counsel from others. Regardless of how effective we are on our own or how successful, life is always better when we can share our experiences with others. A healthy *manner of living* is best when it is shared! For this reason I wanted to take a moment to reinforce the value of retaining a sense of connectedness in life as a means of achieving your new *manner of living*.

For many of you this may be a no brainer. You may have a huge extended family, several kids, coworkers, and a huge sphere of influence. (By the way, Facebook friends do not count!) If you do not have this strong sense of human connection around you then this chapter is for you. Perhaps you have lost a loved one or have many acquaintances but few true friends. Perhaps you have a big family around you but still feel alone. Perhaps you feel sad and empty. If any of these scenarios relate to you, consider volunteering.

Volunteering

The last thing that tends to come to mind when considering volunteer work is that it is self-serving but in reality, the value and benefit to you the volunteer is priceless.

One of the best things you can do when feeling sad, dealing with depression, or feelings of loneliness or worthlessness, is to give back. It seems counterintuitive, if you feel worthless how and what can you give? But the truth is, as cliché as it sounds-there is always someone worse off than you. Beyond that cliché, there is always someone for whom what you have to give, even if it is just your smile and time, is of exceptional worth and value. When times are tough, one of the best ways to gain perspective and resilience is to find a cause you value and give nothing else but your time and compassion. This act of stepping outside of yourself has exponential gains both for you and the person and/or cause that you are serving.

From a professional point of view, volunteering is also a brilliant way to gain experience and participate in fields and skills that may interest you. For example, volunteering is a great way to stay sharp on your skills while you are between jobs, it is an excellent way to develop new expertise and refine current talents, and it is also an extraordinary way to demonstrate and hone your leadership skills. After all, if you can inspire and lead a group of people that are not paid to show up, then that is a true mark of leadership that employers can value! Refer to the Additional Resources section of the book for same great options of where to get started.

Chapter 17

The most incomprehensible thing about the world is that it is at all comprehensible.
— Albert Einstein

Sleeping, Breathing, and Pooping

It is often the simple things in life that we take for granted. Yet, these simple things are often among the most important. This chapter explores some of life's most basic bodily functions and the impact that neglect of attentiveness to these functions can have on our health and wellbeing.

Sleeping

We all know at least one overachiever; the type A personality that exists on adrenaline and caffeine. They claim they are too busy to sleep. Sleep gets in the way of their productivity and success. Even though I must admit that at times in my life I am guilty of succumbing to this irrational belief and behavior, the reality is, it is quite absurd. Whether professional success or optimal health is your primary ambition, the last thing you should be sacrificing is sleep.

As our head hits the pillow and our eyes begin to close, the forthcoming sleep promotes the release of anti-aging, human growth hormones. Sleep resets appetite controls, reboots our immune system, and allows for consolidation of learning. It prepares our system to take on a new day, to process information faster, and to be more alert and engaged upon waking. There is no amount of Red Bull® or Starbucks® coffee that can offer the same effects. Most Americans average only about six hours of sleep each night and men are frequently the worst offenders often sleeping less than six hours according to a survey conducted by the Centers for Disease Control and Prevention.[346] This is a cause for concern since a study presented at the SLEEP 2012 conference in Boston[347] found that middle age to older aged people who frequently get fewer than six hours of sleep have an increased stroke risk even if they are not overweight, even if they do not have a history of stroke, and even if they do not have an increased risk of obstructive sleep apnea or other sleep problems. Sleep-deprivation can also result in increases in systemic inflammation and in impairment of the immune system[348] leading to more frequent illness and less resilience in the face of disease.

Sleep can also be your friend or foe when it comes to achieving a healthy body composition. For years, scientists have understood that sleep deprivation increases levels of the hormone ghrelin which stimulates the appetite, and decreases levels of leptin, a hormone that sends a signal of satiety to the brain. When you do not get enough sleep, ghrelin levels rise making us want to eat more, and leptin levels drop, quieting our cue to stop eating.[349,350,351] These mixed messages can lead to overeating and fat gain.

A 2010 study elegantly illustrates how too little sleep can thwart our efforts when it comes to body fat loss.[352] Researchers monitored the body composition of participants on a calorie restricted dietary plan and found that compared to those that slept 8.5-hours, participants who slept only 5.5 hours a night decreased the proportion of weight they lost as fat by 55%, and increased their loss of fat-free body mass (including lean muscle mass) by 60%! This study therefore brings to light the concern that sleep deprivation can induce the loss of muscle mass and the retention of body fat. To add insult to injury, in addition to the metabolic alterations that lead to these detrimental changes in body composition, sure enough, (consistent with past studies of sleep and hunger) the researchers also found that those sleeping only 5.5

hours per night experienced increased hunger, which certainly does not help when one is trying to shed fat.

What if we have a genetic predisposition to weight/fat gain? A 2012 study from the University of Washington Medicine Sleep Center explored that very question examining the impact of sleep on our genes. By studying identical twins, the researchers found that adequate sleep can override the negative impact of genes that may contribute to weight/fat gain. The researchers were able to find differences in how much twins weighed based on their sleep duration. The more consistently the twin adhered to an optimal sleep schedule, the healthier their weight and body mass index (BMI).[353]

So how much sleep is enough? While there is no magic number, experts generally recommend that for most people, seven and a half to eight hours a night is the optimal time required for recuperative slumber. Although, if we cannot hit those numbers we may be able to make up the difference in our sleep debt in any given 24-hour period.[354] For example, some studies have suggested that napping for as little as six[355] to ten[356] minutes during the day may be sufficient to improve cognitive performance and minimize fatigue. Naps longer than thirty minutes may be helpful as well, but be prepared to deal with some grogginess upon waking.[357] If you have the time, a ninety minute nap may be your best bet as this allows the brain to go through a complete sleep cycle with minimal grogginess when you wake.[358] However, avoid naps that last longer than ninety minutes or naps past 4:00 pm, as these can begin to interfere with your nighttime sleepiness.

The best way to determine if you are reaching your optimal personal recovery needs when it comes to sleep is to listen to your body. Consider the following: Do you feel tired during the day? Do you sleep in on the weekends? Do you doze off when sitting down during the day to read or watch television? This is no joke. Researchers found that the risk of having a stroke went up two to fourfold in older adults who frequently fall asleep inadvertently during the day.[359] While the study did not consider individual psychological characteristics and stresses, it still reinforces the importance of adequate sleep.

The Bottom Line:
If you responded yes to any of the questions I just posed in the previous paragraph, then chances are you could use a good night's sleep.

I have listed below eight tips to improve your sleep hygiene to ensure rejuvenating slumber:

1. **Find a bedtime and stick with it.** Establish a routine; make sure you have a consistent time each day that you go to sleep and wake.

   TIP! If you tend to stay up late, commit to going to bed tonight even just 15 minute earlier.

2. **Avoid caffeine 4 to 6 hours prior to bedtime.** This may seem intuitive but for many of us, caffeine can be the culprit that keeps us awake at night. For me, if I have coffee after 3:00 pm I know I will be up and sleepless during the witching hours.

3. **Establish a pre-sleep ritual.** For me, this is a warm mug of ginger tea with a splash of almond milk. For you it might be a warm bath or shower or a few minutes of reading.

4. **Practice selective napping.** For some, a nap during the day for as little as 6 minutes can be rejuvenating. But if you have trouble sleeping at night avoid napping during the day. Even if you do not have disturbed sleep, limit daytime napping to no more than 90 minutes.

5. **If you cannot fall asleep after 20 minutes, leave the room.** Avoid tossing and turning all night. If after twenty minutes you still cannot fall asleep then get out of bed and leave the bedroom. Read a book, enjoy an herbal tea, or perform some quiet activity. Do not watch television or engage in intense work. In twenty minutes, you will be ready to hit the pillow in bed again.

6. **Avoid bringing worries to bed with you.** I find it helpful to have a journal or notepad by my bed to write down any ideas that come to mind so that they do not linger in my thoughts and distract me from sleep. Guided imagery or breathing techniques (try the activity described in the next section) can also be helpful to induce relaxation before slumber.

7. **Reserve the bedroom for sleep (and sex).** If you have a television in your bedroom, get rid of it. Associate the bed with sleeping.

8. **Avoid frequent all-nighters and shift work.** While this may be challenging for some, the benefit is worth it. New research is emerging that suggests the disruption to our circadian rhythm that occurs with shift work (working at night, sleeping during the day) may increase the risk of cancer and heart disease.[360]

Breathing

I once heard Dr. Andrew Weil say that the most important thing he can offer his patients is to teach them to breath. You might think how silly, if they could not breath they would not be in your office in the first place! Well, there is a difference between just breathing to survive, and deep breathing to thrive.

Deep breathing may help reduce blood pressure, relieve stress and anxiety, and even help induce sleep and manage pain by triggering the release of feel good endorphins. [361] It is as easy as 4-7-8 to learn.

Here is one common deep breathing technique taught by many healthcare practitioners, often referred to as the 4-7-8 breath.

4-7-8 Breath

1. Exhale completely through your mouth.
2. Close your mouth and inhale through your nose to a count of four allowing you belly to expand as it lets in the air.
3. Hold your breath for a count of seven.
4. Exhale completely through your mouth to a count of eight, allowing you belly to shrink in as the air is expelled.
5. This is one breath. Repeat the cycle three more times.

You will notice that this simple breathing technique will make you feel clearheaded and calm instantly. Try to practice it at least twice a day. If you feel a little lightheaded initially, do not worry, it will pass. As you practice this breath it will get easier. Practice this daily but also use it as first aid intervention when confronted by any of life's stressors; Employ this to relax before a presentation, an important meeting or conversation, or to calm down when feeling anger or anxiety. If you have trouble sleeping, use this simple breathing technique to help induce relaxation. You will be amazed at how affective this simple technique can be.

Pooping

A little maturity please! We all do it. Although, I think I have effectively convinced the men in my life that I do not poop and instead mine magically disintegrates. But my dysfunctional relationship quirks aside, pooping may still be a little taboo as far as polite dinner table banter goes, but it is a basic human function that can reveal a lot about your state of health and well-being. That bowel movement provides a wealth of information if you know what to look for.

This next recommendation is not pretty but it can save your life. Next time you have a bowel movement, take a look at the product of your efforts. What does it look like?

Here is a simple guide to help you interpret what your fecal matter is telling you.

Frequency:
➢ The average person has a bowel movement once or twice a day, but many people go more, and some go less frequently, as little as once or twice a week. In general, as long as it is normal for you, the frequency is not a cause for concern. Although, if you are going less than a few times a week or even less than once a day, it is likely an indication that you could benefit from increasing your dietary fiber intake by eating more foods such as vegetables, legumes, nuts, and/or whole grains. If you notice a dramatic change in the frequency or your normal bowel movements, visit your doctor to check it out.

Color:

- ➢ Normal poop has a light to dark brown color. This is mostly from the bile that has been produced in the liver and aids in the digestive process.

- ➢ The food we eat typically takes three days from the time we ingest it until it finishes its journey into the toilet. If it takes less time, it can appear a little green. This is generally not a cause for concern.

- ➢ If the poop does not contain bile it can look grayish. This may indicate a blockage at the bile duct or at the pancreas possibly by a tumor, so visit your doctor to check it out.

- ➢ If the stool is black, this can indicate bleeding in the upper intestines. Visit a doctor to check it out. A colonoscopy may be in order.

- ➢ Bleeding that occurs lower in the intestines, particularly in the colon will often impart a red or maroon color to the stool. This can be caused simply by a fissure (tear) and may not be a problem at all. It may also suggest hemorrhoids. If recurrent, visit a doctor to check it out.

- ➢ Temporary color changes can also be simply a product of what you eat: Medications like Pepto Bismol can turn the stool black. Beets and other red fruits and vegetables can turn stools a reddish color. Food dyes in processed foods, may also color the stool.

Shape:

- ➢ While a soft, S-shaped poop is considered the ideal, the size and shape of poop is rather irrelevant. Smaller, hard poops may reflect constipation while mushy poops or a complete lack of shape occurs with diarrhea.

Odor:

- ➢ Odor is not only normal, it is probably a good indicator that your gut is full of good for you bacteria that are keeping you healthy. An extra foul odor may occur in the presence of medical conditions such as Crohn's disease, malabsorption, or celiac disease.

Diarrhea:

➢ Diarrhea may just be from one bad meal or it may suggest the presence of a virus or bacteria. People with food allergies or food sensitivities may also develop diarrhea in response to exposure to that food item. Chronic diarrhea suggests malabsorption of nutrients which can lead to nutritional deficiencies. If diarrhea is recurrent, visit your doctor to check it out.

Constipation:

➢ Constipation can suggest that your fiber intake is too low, that you may not be drinking enough water, or both. Even medications or a drop in physical activity can cause it. It can also suggest a blockage in the intestinal tract. If this is an ongoing problem, visit your doctor to check it out.

Gotta Pee!

Ok, so one more taboo discussion here, because when you gotta go, you gotta go. Just like our bowel movements, our urine can also be a window into our health and physiologic function.

Urine gets its signature yellow color from a pigment call urochrome. This chemical is a normal end-product of hemoglobin breakdown from our blood and since the kidneys act as a filter for the blood, the urochrome colors our urine. The color of urine can vary from pale yellow to a deep amber hue, it simply depends on how concentrated the urine is. A darker hue is usually an indication that you are not consuming enough fluids. Conversely, if it is very pale you are either consuming an abundance of liquids or you may be on a diuretic.

Certain foods and drugs can impart a colorful hue upon our urine. Some medications can turn it blue or green, eating a lot of carrots may give it an orange tint, and water soluble vitamins such as vitamin B can make it appear bright yellow. If you see red, it could be from food or it could indicate blood. If there is blood in the urine and it is also cloudy, this could indicate an infection. When an infection is present you may also notice it is accompanied by a sense of urgency (having to rush to get to the bathroom) or pain. The pain can be with urination or you may feel it in your belly or even your lower back. The lower back pain can suggest a kidney infection so go see your doctor right away. Whether the urine is cloudy or not, in rare cases blood in the stream can also suggest bladder cancer. Either way, it warrants a visit to your doctor. If you have a hard time initiating a stream of urine or after you urinate you still do not feel as though you have completely voided, then this can suggest a blockage. In men this may indicate a benign enlargement of the prostate or it can also be a sign of prostate cancer. Either way, go see your doctor to check it out.

As a rule of thumb, if any unusual symptoms appear in or with your pee, and it lingers for multiple streams, go see your doctor to check it out.

Brushing your Teeth

What if I told you that proper oral hygiene can actually help prevent heart disease? You may think I am just marketing the latest dental gadget but this statement is absolutely true. Brushing teeth has always been treated as more of an aesthetic issue rather than a health promotion one, but our mouth is a critical portal to health and with neglect, it can become a portal to disease.

Poor oral hygiene has been associated with a higher risk of cardiovascular disease and low grade systemic inflammation.[362,363] In fact, it appears that systemic inflammation is the underlying mechanism that links oral health and cardiovascular disease. A study in Taiwan that tracked over 10,000 people for an average of 7 years found that those who had their teeth professionally cleaned at least once every two years were 24 percent less likely to have a heart attack and 13 percent less likely to have a stroke. The regular dental visits and oral hygiene reduced the growth of inflammation causing bacteria.[364]

The link between systemic inflammation and a variety of chronic diseases from Alzheimer's to certain types of cancer has recently been elucidated so it is plausible to extrapolate from these findings that proper oral health may be help prevent a variety of diseases that result from chronic, systemic inflammation.

Just as mom said, do not go to bed without brushing those teeth. When you wake, brush them again. Floss each day too. Bacteria in your mouth love sugar so keep cavities at bay by avoiding starchy foods and those with added sugars. And visit your dentist, at least once a year.

Sit Up Tall and Don't Slouch

Posture is another topic that has often been relegated to being more about etiquette and aesthetics than health and hygiene. However, sitting tall and not slouching can be a vital component of maintaining strength and mobility and preventing pain and degeneration as we age. Overtime, poor posture can lead to a cascade of problems including muscles imbalances, the early degeneration of joints, and general musculoskeletal pain and dysfunction. Poor posture can impact every joint in the body from the spine, hips, and knees to the shoulders, feet, and ankles. Poor posture may even be the reason you have headaches by days-end or the nagging pain in your neck, low back, or shoulders. The good news is that postural fixes are easy to make; they just require a little mindfulness.

Paying attention to your posture is worth the effort since good posture:

➢ Prevents our muscles from holding awkward positions that lead to fatigue, tension, and pain
➢ Maintains proper alignment of muscles and joints and prevent abnormal stresses or wear and tear of joints that can lead to degeneration or osteoarthritis
➢ Minimizes stress on the ligaments that keep our spinal bones in proper position
➢ Prevents muscle strain
➢ Prevents backaches
➢ Makes you look confident, and makes you look good. And when you look good, you *feel* good!

Here are some tips to help you maintain a healthy posture in all of life's static situations. Keep in mind that often when you first attempt to position yourself in a normal posture it may initially feel a little awkward. This is simply because your body is not used to it. The more you mindfully maintain these postures, the more your muscles, ligaments, and joints will adjust to the new position, and the more natural it will feel.

Correct posture while standing

Distribute body weight evenly to the front, back, and sides of the feet while standing. Place your feet slightly apart and have one foot positioned slightly in front of the other and knees bent just a little; not locked. Shoulders should be directly above the pelvis to help maintain the natural s-shape of the spine (verify you position by taking a look at yourself in a mirror from the side). Tuck in your belly (pull your belly button in towards your spine but keep breathing!) and tuck in your buttocks as well.

Troubleshooting: Avoid leaning to one side by putting all your weight to the left or right foot. Overtime this can contribute to muscle imbalances and pain affecting the hips, knees, lower back, and even the neck.

Also, avoid carrying a purse or bag on the same side every time. This habit may also contribute to muscle imbalances. Alternate carrying purses or bags from the left to the right side and avoid carrying anything that is too heavy. Do you really need all that stuff in your purse? Really?

Additionally, be careful with those high heel shoes. I must admit, wearing heels are my guilty pleasure so this is one instant in this book when I will tell you do as I say and not as I do! Heels above two inches can promote a sway back posture that puts a lot of stress on your lower back and can contribute to lower back pain and foot, ankle, and hip pain. Keep the heels under two inches or if you are a sucker for the four or five inch Christian Louboutins and Manolo Blahniks, bring a pair of flat heeled shoes to change into after you make your entrance!

Correct posture while seated at home or at work

Whenever you are seated, ears, shoulders, and hips should be aligned in one vertical line. Hips and knees should be comfortably positioned at angles of 90 degree. Shoulders should be relaxed, down and away from your ears and elbows should rest on an armrest and be positioned at an angle greater than 90 degrees.

If seated in front of a computer, position the monitor so that if you drew an imaginary line from your eyes to the monitor the line would just skim over the top of monitor. This will ensure you maintain your neck comfortably in a neutral position without the need to extend it upwards or flex it forward to see the monitor, which overtime can lead to neck strain and even headaches.

Wrist should be resting on the keyboard and on the mouse in a neutral position; not extended backwards or flexed forwards.

TIP! Ask your employer if they can provide you with an adjustable workstation (chair and desk). Foot rests and lumbar supports are inexpensive options to help maintain alignment if you do not have an adjustable workstation.

Troubleshooting: Avoid crossing your legs while seated or allowing your shoulders and head to lean, or protrude forward. Also, avoid lifting your shoulders up towards your ear. This is a common position one assumes when the arm rests of a chair are set too high, or when a key board is too high on your desk. Overtime, this can lead to fatigue, tension, and pain in those muscles.

Correct posture while driving
Good posture while driving not only helps prevent aches and pains but it also can minimize the risk of, and the extent of injuries should you experience a collision while driving.

Sit straight and place your buttocks and back directly against the seat, with your knees level with your hips. Take advantage of the car's lumbar support and sit directly against it to support your spine. If your car does not have an adjustable lumbar support, invest in a portable one, particularly for long distance driving.

Sit at a comfortable distance from the steering wheel. Sitting too far can cause you to lean forward and this type of reaching can increase pain in the low back and increase stress on other joints. Sitting too close can increase your risk of injury from airbags in the event of an accident. Consider placing at least 10 inches between the center of the air bag cover and your breastbone. Compromise this position with placing the seat at a distance from the gas pedal that allows you to compress the pedal while still maintaining a slight bend in your knee. Knee should be at roughly 120 degrees. Thighs should be as far apart as is comfortable and the left foot should be resting flat on the floor. This helps increases support to the pelvis.

Troubleshooting: Ensure you are not sitting on anything that can throw your spine out of alignment. Wallets are common culprits for this as are chunky coats for those of you residing in cooler climates.

And do not forget; always wear your seat belt!

Correct posture while lifting
Always keep the object you are lifting as close to your body as possible. Squat down by bending at your knees not at your waist. Rise up with the object by engaging the muscles in your legs to push yourself up as your knees and hips straighten. Your back should be upright and in a neutral position the entire time. The goal is to pick-up the object while maintaining the S-shape to your spine (see standing posture above). Tighten your stomach (pull your belly button in towards your spine) but keep breathing. This will help support your lower back as you lift.

Troubleshooting: Twisting one's back while lifting is a sure-fire way to injure a vulnerable back. If you need to turn, turn by moving the position of your feet, not by twisting your back.

Correct posture while sleeping
Most of us sustain our posture at rest for at least six hours a night so proper sleep posture is essential for helping prevent neck and back pain. The optimal sleep position is lying on your back. This position helps you maintain a neutral position to the spine and offers an extra bonus of helping to prevent facial wrinkles caused by faces mashed against pillows! Use a small pillow that can support the natural curve of your neck without causing your chin to jut forward. If you have back pain, place a pillow beneath your knees to help further reduce the stress on your lower back.

Troubleshooting: If you snore, sleeping on your back can sometimes make the problem worse. Lying on your side will be a preferred position to keep your airway open. If you have acid reflex then place a large wedge pillow to lift up your torso (not just your neck) to minimize night time reflux. Better yet, if you snore or if you suffer from acid reflex, see your doctor to learn about what you can do to treat these conditions and to ensure they are not signs of more serious underlying health problems. Snoring may indicate the presence of sleep apnea, a breathing disorder that can contribute to daytime fatigue, high blood pressure, obesity, and even stroke and heart failure. Barrett's esophagus is caused by ongoing acid reflux and its presence can increase the risk of developing esophageal cancer.

Sleeping on your side is the next best thing to sleeping on your back. Place a small pillow between your knees to keep your hips in a relaxed and neutral position. Use a pillow that is the width of the distance from the tip of your shoulder to the base of your neck. This will ensure your head and neck remain in a relaxed and neutral position all night.

Troubleshooting: Unless you are in utero, avoid tucking yourself into a tightly curled side-lying fetal position. This can place undue strain on your muscles and joints as you sleep. If you have spinal arthritis or back pain, this can contribute to pain in the morning upon waking.

Special consideration: If you are pregnant, sleep on your left side; this is optimal for blood flow. A body pillow can also be helpful to support hips, low back, and arms.

If you are accustomed to sleeping face down on your belly, it is time to break the habit. The face down sleep posture puts excessive strain on your neck and back and contributes to facial wrinkling. Especially if you are also using a pillow, the latter is simply adding flames to the fire by placing additional strain on your neck. To break the habit, try this silly but effective trick. Lay down to sleep on your back or side and place two tennis balls in the pockets of your pajama pants. If you instinctively roll onto your belly at night, the tennis balls will stop you! After a few nights, your body will slowly accommodate to your new sleeping posture.

Prevention and maintenance

Visit a doctor of chiropractic to assess your posture. A chiropractor can identify muscle imbalances and provide you with activities that will help correct them. Chiropractors can also help restore motion to any joints that are causing pain and/or limiting mobility in your spine or elsewhere in the body. You will be amazed at how good it can make you feel! To find a licensed chiropractor in your area contact your local association. I have listed select national and international chiropractic associations in the resource section at the back of this book.

A final word about posture: No matter how great your posture or alignment is, avoid remaining in one static position for too long. Plan to change positions frequently throughout the day to avoid muscle fatigue, spasm, and pain. If driving, take a break every hour to step out of your car and stretch. If you are at work, set a reminder for yourself to stand up and stretch every 30 minutes. A good trick is to establish a rule that each time the phone rings, you can stand up to take the call. Not only will standing help you sound more confident on the phone, it will help prevent undue physical strain that comes on from prolonged seated postures.

Chapter 18

You have your way. I have my way. As for the right way, the correct way, and the only way, it does not exist.
— Friedrich Nietzsche

Accommodating Food Sensitivities

One of the beauties and complexities of humanity is that we are all different. We each have our unique quirks and peccadilloes that are charming to some, annoying to others. Our health is no exception. The one-size-fits-all approach to health care is rapidly fading. Instead, a more personalized approach to health and wellness is emerging; an approach that celebrates and caters to these differences among individuals and tailors treatment and care to meeting the unique needs of each person.

In the context of food, sensitivity to certain dietary components is being recognized as a common trigger for everything from headaches to muscle pain, behavioral problems, and digestive difficulties. Frequent exposure to such food in susceptible individuals may also contribute to low grade systemic inflammation. These days much attention has been directed towards the issue of gluten sensitivities. Many people have reported sensitivities to gluten and are opting to avoid consuming it all together. Since this has become such a prevalent concern, I will discuss gluten sensitivities in greater depth later on in this chapter. In the meantime, gluten is not the only food component that has the potential to cause undesirable reactions in certain individuals. Foods and food components including dairy, soy, sulfites (and other food additives), and refined sugars also have been implicated as potential triggers. So how do you know if you are one of the people whose aches and pains are in response to a food sensitivity and therefore, that require a modification to your manner of eating?

Researchers are still gathering convincing evidence to establish standardized approaches for food sensitivity testing, in the meantime, one of the best and most simple ways to see if you have sensitivity to a food or food component is by an "elimination diet". I know, I know! I used the four letter word, "diet"! However, the elimination diet is different, so I will momentarily break my own rule to help you understand how to implement this helpful technique for identifying hypersensitivities to select foods.

The Elimination Diet

First of all, the Elimination Diet is not a dietary strategy that is intended for everyone. It is however, beneficial if you have generalized aches, pains, digestive distress, rashes, fatigue, headaches, or other symptoms that have not responded to conventional medical interventions. This is for someone that has had their symptoms evaluated previously by a doctor, red flags (including cancer, infection, fracture, or dislocation) have been ruled out, yet an effective management approach to reducing their symptoms has not yet been found.

> **Important:** While the elimination diet can be implemented alone, I strongly encourage you to embark upon this dietary intervention with the support of an experienced health care practitioner who can help monitor your response and progress.

In people with food sensitivities, consuming certain foods can trigger potentially adverse effects. As discussed in chapter 3, these sensitivities are different from a food allergy. An allergy to a food item typically provokes symptoms within minutes to hours and the symptoms can manifest in mild symptoms such as a rash or diarrhea or as anaphylaxis, a life-threatening type of allergic reaction. Food allergies are identified through lab testing. People with food allergies must eliminate the provocative food or food component completely.

With food sensitivities, symptoms can take hours to days to show up and may manifest as a variety of vague disorders or symptoms including: dermatitis, sinus congestion, fatigue, abdominal pain or discomfort, joint inflammation, skin rash, mood swings, indigestion, or headaches. The foods and food components most often implicated include dairy products, eggs, soy products, peanuts, shellfish, refined sugars, and gluten.[365] Lab testing may one day be useful for identifying food sensitivities but these innovative approaches still need to be validated in clinical trials before they can be deemed sufficiently reliable and recommended for widespread use by healthcare practitioners. In the meantime, the elimination diet and subsequent challenge phase, is commonly used for identifying food sensitivities.

It is worth noting that a variety of health conditions are currently being investigated to determine whether food sensitivities play a role in provoking symptoms of the disease. Many, but not all patients with conditions including migraine headaches,[366] ADHD,[367] and rheumatoid arthritis[368] have been reported to benefit from an elimination diet. While this still remain a relatively new area of research, a growing body of evidence shows that food sensitivities may contribute to a wide range of symptoms and diseases. Since this is a safe intervention with a potential for a significant benefit, many integrative healthcare practitioners recommend at least trying an elimination diet when your condition does not respond adequately to conventional methods of care.

So what is the elimination diet? Here it is in three easy steps:

Step 1
Planning: The first step is to determine which foods to eliminate. If you suspect one particular food, then only that single food will be eliminated. If there is a food you tend to eat all the time such as for example tomatoes, try eliminating that food to see if it is the culprit. If you suspect a specific food component such as gluten, then all foods

that contain that food component will need to be excluded. If you are uncertain which food to eliminate, the most common dietary triggers include: gluten (a protein found in wheat and other grains), dairy products, eggs, soy products, peanuts, shellfish, caffeine (coffee, tea and soda), alcohol, nightshade vegetables (tomatoes, eggplant, potatoes, sweet and hot peppers), food dyes and additives (in processed foods), and refined sugars. Additionally, in some cases beef, chicken, pork, beans (including peas and lentils), citrus fruits, seeds and nuts can be eliminated as well.

Plan to eliminate these foods for a minimum of 14 days but ideally, for 4 weeks. Even if you choose to go all out and eliminate all the potential triggers I have listed above, it is not as bad as you might think. It still leaves on your menu various animal proteins such as fish, lamb, turkey and wild game, rice and buckwheat are permitted, as are most types of fruits and vegetables, almond and coconut milk, and herbal teas.

Special consideration: For some diseases and health conditions, there are specific foods that have been identified as common triggers. For example, many people that suffer from migraine headaches notice that foods such as aged cheeses or sauerkraut can provoke their symptoms. These types of foods contain histamines which have been implicated as common triggers of migraine headaches in susceptible individuals when consumed in large quantities.

Another common example is with Irritable Bowel Syndrome (IBS). Many individuals with this condition find that their symptoms are provoked when they consume specific types of carbohydrates. These types of carbohydrates are referred to by the acronym **FODMAP** (Fermentable Oligo-Di-Monosaccharides and Polyols). FODMAPs are select carbohydrates that are not always digested or absorbed well and when consumed by people with IBS can lead to gas, bloating, cramping, and/or diarrhea. These FODMAP foods include: fructose, lactose, fructans (including wheat, onions and garlic), galactans (beans, lentils, and legumes such as soy) and polyols (can be found in sweeteners containing sorbitol, mannitol, xylitol, maltitol, and in stone fruits such as avocado, apricots, cherries, nectarines, peaches, and plums).[369] While many of these foods are healthy for the rest of us, in those suffering with IBS they are often triggers that may need to be eliminated from their food plan, even if just temporarily to allow the body to heal. These types of disease or condition specific elimination diet plans are rather complex and beyond the scope of this book. Speak with an experienced healthcare provider to learn more about common dietary triggers for select medical conditions.

Step 2
Elimination and monitoring: This is the *avoidance phase* when the elimination of suspect foods begins. For the greatest success, keep a symptom log or journal throughout the elimination diet. Record how you are feeling each day and the symptoms you are experiencing, if any. If symptoms decrease during this avoidance phase it is possible that the food(s) that were eliminated were contributing to the symptoms. Remember: eliminate the potential food triggers for a minimum of 14 days but, ideally for 4 weeks.

Step 3
The challenge phase (reintroducing foods): This is the most important phase of the elimination diet. Symptoms of many chronic diseases relapse and remit spontaneously, so this final step of reintroducing the eliminated food(s) helps us learn whether that food was truly the culprit. In other words, this step helps us determine whether the symptoms just went away coincidently during the avoidance phase – it was simple a good few weeks as is common with certain health conditions – or, was it really the food. If the symptom(s) resolved during the avoidance phase but they return now when you reintroduce one of the suspect foods, then we have reasonably good evidence that food item is likely the culprit.

The challenge phase should be approached as follows: reintroduce one eliminated food at a time. On day one, only consume a small quantity of the eliminated foods at first (perhaps at breakfast) and then, consume a relatively larger serving at a subsequent meal on the same day. Monitor how you feel that day and log your response in your journal. Pay attention for any symptoms to reoccur. Symptoms of food sensitivities may take a few days to reappear so if you eliminated more than one food or food component, wait at least 3 to 4 days before reintroducing the next eliminated food. Continue this pattern until each eliminated food has been subject to this challenge.

If the symptoms reoccur from one or more food items, continue to eliminate that food for at least 3 to 6 months. Then, attempt to reintroduce the food again. Some evidence exists that after the food is avoided for an extended period of time, the intolerance may no longer be found. If on the other hand, even after 3 to 6 months of avoidance the symptom returns with exposure to that food, then it is reasonable to avoid that food altogether.

> **Precaution:** A food leading to an anaphylactic reaction (severe allergy) should <u>never</u> be reintroduced. Furthermore, the elimination diet is not recommended if you have ever had an eating disorder such as anorexia or bulimia. If you have *ever* suffered from one of these disorders, then speak with your doctor before attempting an elimination diet.

Understanding Gluten Sensitivity

These days it seems as though almost everyone is claiming an allergy or sensitivity to gluten. The reality is that very few people have a *true* allergy to this protein that is found in grains such as wheat, barley, rye, and spelt. Celiac disease is also relatively rare affecting only about 1% of the general population.[370] Celiac disease is not an allergy per se but rather an autoimmune disorder in which the consumption of gluten leads to damage of the lining of the small intestines, severe gastrointestinal distress (pain, nausea, vomiting, diarrhea and/or constipation), improper absorption of nutrients and consequently, malnutrition in those afflicted, coupled with potentially life threatening complications. In patients with celiac disease, gluten consumption must be avoided completely.

Gluten sensitivity is different. As described earlier in this chapter, those with a hypersensitivity to a food or food component (such as gluten) can consume it in small amounts but it can lead to vague and bothersome symptoms from headaches, diarrhea, and anemia, to depression, rash, fatigue, and joint pain.[371] It is neither an actual allergy nor an autoimmune disease however in some cases the symptoms that result can still be extremely troublesome.[372,373] In fact, excessive consumption of gluten in those who are sensitive to it has even been suggested to have a link to weight gain, obesity, and systemic inflammation.[374,375,376,377] As there is no specific blood test at this time that can definitively detect a sensitivity to gluten, gluten sensitivity is generally identified through what is considered a diagnosis of exclusion, (rule out all the other worst possible causes of each symptom and this is the diagnosis that remains) and by using an elimination diet and challenge as described earlier in this chapter.[378]

People with gluten sensitivity experience an improvement in their symptoms when they adhere to a manner of eating that excludes gluten. Some critics argue that in certain cases, the reported benefit may simply be a product of the placebo effect. In response to that criticism I say, *so what?!* In this case, placebo is the safest, cheapest, and best type of medicine, so bring it on! In reality, in many cases the placebo effect can be avoided by implementing the elimination diet and challenge in a blinded manner. This can be accomplished by a controlled exposure to gluten after a period of elimination when the patient does not know that the food they are consuming is a source of gluten. This type of blinded challenge needs to be accomplished with the guidance of an experienced health care provider.

So, why the recent increase in cases of gluten sensitivity? The truth is, while many theories abound, the reason why so many of us seem to have a hard time tolerating this protein remains unclear. Several experts have suggested that the reason for the prevalence of gluten sensitivities these days is that the wheat of today is not the same wheat of yesteryear. Most commercially available sources of wheat sold these days are the product of a process called *hybridization*. Since the fifties, scientists have been cross-breeding wheat to improve its strength and resilience. While technically considered a natural process, hybridization of wheat leads to genetic changes in the grain and introduces proteins into the wheat that were not found in the parent plant. These proteins may help the grain become hardier during growth but there is concern that they are difficult for humans to digest. Additionally, these grains also contain significantly more gluten then the same wheat product did a generation ago.[379,380,381,382] Some experts suggest that the process of hybridization has created in effect a 'super gluten' that is more amenable to disrupting intestinal permeability and provoking an inflammatory response in susceptible individuals.[383]

An alternate school of thought suggests that the increase in cases of gluten sensitivity may simply be another byproduct of the typical excess in our modern food plans. Many processed and fast foods from cereals and sausages to soups and ice cream can contain gluten as it is often used as a protein filler even in processed foods that do not contain wheat. Studies looking at populations in Europe, found that the mean consumption of gluten generally falls within 10 to 20 grams a day, but many individuals consume in excess of 50 grams a day of gluten![384,385] Many of us may simply have not adapted to tolerating this excessive quantity of gluten in our food supply.

Similarly, the prevalence of gluten in our food supply has led to young children being exposed to gluten-containing foods very early in development. This also may lead to intolerance. A study published in the Journal of the American Medical Association found that infants exposed to gluten in the first three months of life had a fivefold increased risk of developing celiac disease, compared with children exposed at 4 to 6 months.[386]

Finally, could it be that gluten is the trigger, but not the cause? Many experts express concern that perhaps gluten alone is not the problem but rather the plethora of other contaminants and additives in processed foods that are damaging our intestinal lining and making us more vulnerable to the effect of gluten and other food components. There is also concern that perhaps the overuse of antibiotics is disrupting our gut flora and making us more susceptible to the effect of gluten[387] or that excessive exposure to gluten may itself disrupt the balance of healthy bacteria in our gut and this in turn, may render us vulnerable to symptoms and disease.[388]

At this time, it seems there are more questions and theories than answers when it comes to understanding the prevalence gluten sensitivity. While the reason may remain unclear, the improvement reported by many people when they remove sources of gluten from their intake is real. Furthermore, it is now being taken seriously by the medical community. In fact, a new term has recently been coined to describe this sensitivity: *Non-Celiac Gluten Sensitivity* (NCGS).

The Bottom Line:

If you think you are sensitive to gluten, then follow the steps outlined in this chapter to complete an elimination diet followed by a gluten challenge. If you see an improvement in your symptoms (and a provocation of symptoms during the challenge phase) then a gluten free manner of eating may be just what the doctor ordered.

If you are sensitive or allergic to gluten, the following is a list of some common food sources of gluten to <u>avoid</u>:

- Wheat
- Barley
- Rye
- Spelt
- Bulgur
- Durum flour
- Farina
- Graham flour
- Kamut
- Semolina
- Spelt
- Triticale (a cross between wheat and rye)
- Malt, malt flavoring and malt vinegar are usually made from barley and should also be avoided
- Oats (While pure oatmeal does not contain gluten, many oats on the market have been cross-contaminated with wheat, barley, and/or rye. Therefore, unless an oat product explicitly indicates that it is *gluten free*, it is generally advisable for those sensitive to gluten to avoid oats.)

Unless labeled as "gluten-free", <u>avoid</u> the following as well:

- Beer
- Pastas, cereals, breads, matzos, and croutons
- Cakes, pies, cookies, candies, and crackers
- French fries
- Salad dressings, gravies, and sauces, including soy sauce
- Imitation meat or seafood
- Processed luncheon meats
- Seasoned rice mixes, soups, and soup bases
- Seasoned snack foods, such as potato and tortilla chips

Some great <u>gluten-free</u> options include:

- ✓ Quinoa
- ✓ Amaranth
- ✓ Arrowroot
- ✓ Buckwheat
- ✓ Flax
- ✓ Millet
- ✓ Rice (including: basmati, brown rice, and wild rice)
- ✓ Sorghum
- ✓ Soy
- ✓ Tapioca
- ✓ Teff

By the way, I am sure you know this by now but keep in mind that just because a food product is labeled as gluten-free, *does not mean that it is healthy*. Read the rest of the label first and *then* decide if it deserves real estate in your pantry and in your belly.

Chapter 19

Turn your wounds into wisdom.
— Oprah Winfrey

Preventing Pain from Getting in the Way

As a chiropractor, I understand the debilitating hurt and frustration that pain can bring. There is nothing worse than seeing a patient who is actively taking steps towards living a healthier life suddenly be stopped in their tracks by joint pain, headaches, or muscle pain. The question is what is the quickest, safest, and easiest way to get back in the game after being sidelined by pain?

A major challenge is the fact that there is no simple, one size-fits-all solution for treating pain. Pain is complex; often the underlying cause is multifactorial and consequently, so is its management. Therefore, the first thing you need to do when experiencing any new or ongoing pain is to see a doctor to get the condition evaluated. In general, if a pain persists beyond one day, a visit to your doctor is appropriate. Do not wait and hope it will get better on its own or just attempt to sleep it off for a few days. This can make it worse. Most importantly, do not borrow your friend's pain medication.

In the best case pain is a nuisance; in the worst case it is debilitating, but it can also be protective. It alerts us to stop activities that may be harmful to us and protects us from causing further trauma or injury to a vulnerable part of our body. Pain and its frequent companion, acute inflammation, are therefore not always bad. In fact, acute inflammation (refer to chapter 5 for a reminder of the difference between acute versus chronic inflammation) is the body's means of self-protection and healing. The cardinal signs of inflammation: *rubor,* redness; *calor,* heat or warmth; *tumor,* swelling; and *dolor,* pain; are all a part of the body's innate response that set the stage for the healing process to begin, allowing us to recover from injury.

While your body does a remarkable job healing itself, as I mentioned before, any pain that is new and/or persistent, is worth paying a visit to your doctor. Your doctor's most important task will be to rule out any serious "red flags". The term *red flag* is common medical jargon referring to any sign or symptom that may suggest the presence of a very serious health condition that may pose a threat to life or that may result in irreversible disability or damage. Most often, these red flags can signal the presence of conditions such as cancer, infection, fracture, joint dislocation, aneurysm, or stroke. Once these red flags are ruled out, meaning there is insufficient clinical evidence to support the presence of one of the serious conditions described above, that is we gain a critical tool in the healing process: *peace of mind.*

For many people, muscle or joint pain immobilizes us because we are afraid that with one wrong move we may cause ourselves additional harm. Ironically, the problem with being immobilized by this fear is that for many musculoskeletal conditions, the lack of movement may actually do more harm than good. For example, for many years doctors believed that bed rest was good for back pain; however, we now know that this is not the case.[389] For certain conditions, prolonged bed rest and immobilization can actually inhibit healing.[390,391] For most muscle and joint pain, even arthritic pain, controlled movement is not only safe, it is actually *therapeutic.*[392,393,394]

ACTION STEP: If you are sidelined from any activity, dealing with chronic pain or recovering from an injury, in addition to performing your prescribed rehabilitation under the supervision of a licensed healthcare practitioner, talk to your doctor about participating in an activity that uses *other* areas of your body as well. Have you suffered a shoulder or wrist injury? Go for daily walks. Is it your knee that is bothering you? Try a seated upper body weight training class. It is your ankle? Go swimming. You will be surprised how good the movement makes you feel and how well remaining active in whatever manner you can, will help you recover.

Avoid Being Defined by a Diagnosis

The most common types of musculoskeletal conditions that inhibit activity are injuries and disorders affecting the neck, back, knee, ankle, and other joints. When it comes to diagnosing the cause of these conditions, it is common for doctors to arrive at a diagnosis without fully explaining it to their patient. The patient is then labeled with a condition, but the doctor may not always provide an explanation as to what that diagnostic "label" really means in terms of its impact on the individual's function and ability. This is most often an unintentional oversight; time-pressured practitioners often provide only brief explanations if not questioned further by their patients. This can leave some patients with a very limited understanding of their condition and with little knowledge about how best to manage it at home.[395] One study conducted at Northwestern University found that 80% of patients discharged from emergency room care did not know what to do to manage their symptoms at home and 14% could not accurately describe their diagnosis.[396]

Part of the problem may be that some healthcare providers become desensitized to these diagnostic labels and other medical jargon so they may occasionally lose sight of the profound impact these words can have on their patients. Remember that for doctors, identifying the diagnosis is paramount, as it is a means of understanding and characterizing a state of disease and determining an appropriate course of treatment. However, when communicating diagnoses to patients, the complete psychological impact is not always adequately considered.

Some doctors are guilty of throwing medical terms around too freely without adequate explanation, seeming to forget that there is a human being attached to that diagnosis that does not share the same degree of understanding of that condition. As patients, we can be greatly affected when we are labeled with a diagnosis. We may associate that diagnosis with a condition that caused a friend or loved one to suffer or perhaps we associate it with something upsetting we saw on a television show or in a film. Thus, simply stating the diagnosis without adequately communicating what that condition *really* means for that person, often spurs unnecessary fear in those bearing the label. In turn, the diagnosis can become somewhat of a self-fulfilling prophecy. There is a powerful psychological response to being told you have a disease or a condition and this response can at times, feed the disability. A person can become defined by their diagnosis and immobilized by fear which can make the situation worse. Interestingly, even though I am a doctor who knows exactly what all of these diagnostic labels and medical jargon mean, all bets are off when I am the one in the patient role! In those moments I seek the same explanation and reassurance that any patient needs. The comforting reality is that the diagnosis merely characterizes a condition, it does not define the individual.

Studies on lower back pain (LBP) offers us a good illustration of why we need to avoid putting too much weight into a diagnostic label and instead, focus on what we can do to assume control over the condition. The fact is that when it comes to LBP, it is actually very challenging to arrive at a true diagnosis. Even though LBP is one the most common causes of disability in Americans under 45 years of age and one of the most common reasons people go to the doctor,[397] studies exploring the cause of LBP still have not found a clear link between risk factors, the anatomical structure that is injured, and the symptoms a person experiences.[398] This speaks to the complexity of these conditions and leads to a challenge establishing a proper diagnosis. In fact, often times once red flags are ruled out, many practitioners simply describe LBP as *non-specific,* meaning that no specific cause of the LBP has been identified.

The reality is that only 1% of LBP is ever caused by serious pathology requiring surgery, only 1% is ever caused by specific spinal disease requiring medical intervention, and only between 5% and 10% of the cases of LBP involves serious irritation of the spinal nerves.[399] This means that for almost 90% of LBP we do not have a clear diagnosis with predictable signs and symptoms. Yet, often doctors will fail to explain this to patients and furthermore, will still provide patients a specific diagnosis without offering adequate clarification of what it really means. Many spinal diagnoses can be frightening to hear, particularly when not put into an appropriate context. Regrettably, too often doctors neglect to mention that regardless of what "label" is given to their low back pain condition, as long as the red flags have been ruled out, safe, controlled movements are good and palliative! Without this reassurance, many patients may be immobilized by the fear of doing more harm and subconsciously use that as justification *not* to participate in activity, thereby making things worse.

Degenerative disc disease and osteoarthritis of the spine (known as spondylitis) are two examples of very common diagnoses of spinal conditions. By name they both sound terrible and frightening, but in reality, their presence may or may not result in any noticeable signs, pain, or dysfunction. So, in and of themselves their presence is not a cause for concern or a reason to limit one's participation in an active life. Quite the opposite in fact: remember movement is therapeutic! Often not explained to individuals diagnosed with these conditions is that in most cases there is a minimal to a nonexistent correlation between their symptoms and their findings on imaging studies like CT scans or MRIs.[400,401,402] MRI studies frequently find signs of both these diseases *incidentally* in patients that are being evaluated for something completely different.

These diagnoses are therefore not a cause for fear or a fool proof prediction of pain or disability to come. Like most musculoskeletal diagnoses, they are labels to help us characterize a state of being of the body and in some cases to help inform steps we can take to prevent them from progressing or manifesting in pain. I have seen labs, x-rays, and MRIs of patients that would suggest that they are bedridden, but they are pain free and running marathons! Conversely, I have also seen labs, x-rays, and MRIs of patients that look like the perfect textbook model of health, and yet that person can barely get up in the morning due to musculoskeletal pain. Clearly, the diagnosis alone does not define the state of one's health.

The Bottom Line:
Musculoskeletal pain and disease is complex and multifactorial so a diagnosis alone does not define ones state of health. Therefore, *do not allow the diagnosis to define you.* Instead, use the diagnosis as a *reason* to

participate in therapeutic activity to support healing and recovery and not as the excuse to avoid it.

ACTION STEP: If you have been diagnosed with any musculoskeletal condition and you feel that your doctor has not offered you sufficient information about the diagnosis and how you should manage it, it is time for you to take the initiative and *ask*. Ask questions such as: *which activities will be the best to support my recovery and/or prevent the progression of the condition? Which movements are most palliative? Which movements should I avoid?* Together, work with your doctor to establish an activity plan that will support your recovery.

NOTE: If your doctor does not have *specific* answers to these questions, then ask him or her for a referral to a practitioner that does.

If You Ever Take Pain Pills, Read This.

The most common reaction for most us at the first sign of pain is to reach for an over the counter pain reliever. If you use or have used this class of drugs then you are not alone; non-steroidal anti-inflammatory drugs (NSAIDs) are one of the most commonly prescribed drugs in the United States.[403] For many, NSAIDs are a common first line of defense following the onset of injury and pain. It is important to understand that even though these drugs are available over the counter and without a prescription that does not mean they are always safe.

All drugs have side effects, even over the counter ones. Therefore, when we make a decision to take a medication we need to be certain that the benefits outweigh any potential risk. When it comes to pain medications, the benefit is naturally a reduction in pain but the side-effects can be severe and often are not sufficiently considered. All NSAIDs including low-dose aspirin, common over the counter drugs such as ibuprofen (Advil®), naproxen (Aleve®), and aspirin (Bayer®) as well as prescription medications like rofecoxib (Vioxx®), celecoxib (Celebrex®) and etodolac (Lodine®), have the potential to damage tissues of the gastrointestinal tract anywhere from the mouth to the anus. Damage can range from an obvious ulceration to microscopic blood loss that leads to anemia over time. Pardon me for being so graphic, but the worst case scenario from taking NSAIDs is gastrointestinal bleeding leading to death, so it is important to be aware of this risk. Before you dismiss this as a rare impossibility, consider that according to available reports, deaths attributable to NSAIDs have varied from 3,200 to higher than 16,500 deaths per year in the United States.[404,405]

NSAIDs have also been linked to increased cardiovascular disease risk[406] which is ironic since they have often been advocated as an ally against cardiovascular disease due to their anti-inflammatory effects. However, a recent study has suggested that taking NSAIDs for prolonged periods might gradually increase a person's risk of heart attack and stroke by causing a progressive hardening of the arteries.[407] Other trials have shown that some NSAIDs may be safer than others when it comes to cardiovascular disease risk. For example, a Canadian study reported that of the medications they studied, ibuprofen and naproxen were the least likely to increase the risk of heart attacks and coronary heart disease death.[408]

Another startling side effect of NSAIDs is that while they are effective at reducing pain, they do so at a great cost to the healing process. NSAID use has been shown to delay and inhibit the healing of muscles, ligaments, tendons, and cartilage. This can contribute to incomplete healing and decrease in the resilience and recovery of these tissues.[409,410] This informs us that there is a major difference between pain relief and healing and thus, begs the question: *is there a better way?*

In fact, several natural follow-up questions emerge as we learn more about this class of drugs. The major questions are: *should people continue to take NSAIDs? If so, what are the precautions? Which NSAIDs are safest for people with high cardiovascular risk?*

ACTION STEP: Speak with your doctor to find out the correct answers for *you*. Find out if you are at risk for any of the common side effects of NSAIDs. If, with your doctor's guidance, you choose to take NSAIDs, *always* take them with food to minimize the gastrointestinal complications. If you are taking NSAIDs for a mild injury, see if you can delay taking it for at least the first 24 to 48 hours so as not to inhibit the healing process.

The Bottom Line:
NSAIDs have their place. They are effective at managing pain, when necessary. With regard to risk of gastrointestinal bleeding or cardiovascular disease, they appear to be safe when taken *short term* and ibuprofen and naproxen appear to be the safest choices for those at high risk of cardiovascular disease. Clearly, more research is needed to help doctors make the best choices about how to use these drugs safely. In the meantime, consider talking to your doctor about some potential alternatives for pain relief that may benefit you since many options are available these days.

Noninvasive Approaches to Pain Management

When it comes to musculoskeletal pain, when we look to the scientific evidence, conventional treatments such as anti-inflammatory medications have actually been shown to have *limited* benefit in improving outcomes.[411] Physical activity programs have been shown to prevent recurrences of back pain, but there is conflicting evidence as to whether or not activity should be prescribed as *a standalone* treatment.[412] A review published by the Agency for Healthcare Research and Quality, found that complementary and alternative therapies (CAM) for back pain (such as acupuncture, massage, and chiropractic manipulation) provide a greater, albeit modest, benefit by reducing pain and/or disability as compared to usual medical care (such as anti-inflammatory medications and exercise), physical therapy, or no treatment.[413]

CAM therapies, such as chiropractic care, are also a wonderful adjunct to conventional medical care as illustrated in a 2013 study published in the respected journal, Spine. The randomized controlled trial demonstrated that active duty military personnel receiving chiropractic manipulative therapy combined with standard medical care experienced significantly greater reductions in their back pain and improved physical functioning when compared to those receiving standard medical care alone.[414] In a 2014 systematic review of the literature that I completed with some of my colleagues, we found a similar benefit to integrative care. Based on our review of the clinical trials completed to date, integrated therapy which includes spinal manipulative therapy combined with exercise therapy and acupuncture combined with conventional medical care or with exercise therapy, appear to be more effective than select single therapies alone for treating LBP.[415] Furthermore, it is important to note that CAM therapies have been shown to be remarkably safe[416] and cost effective[417] and there is great patient satisfaction associated with their use.[418,419]

In recent years, more and more evidence is emerging to support the benefits of CAM therapies for musculoskeletal pain relief. For example, a 2012 study funded by the National Institutes of Health tested the effectiveness of different approaches for treating mechanical neck pain. Participants received either spinal manipulative therapy from a doctor of chiropractic, pain medication (over-the-counter pain relievers, narcotics, and muscle relaxants), or physical activity recommendations. After 12 weeks, about 57 percent of those who met with the chiropractors and 48 percent who engaged in physical activity reported at least a 75 percent reduction in pain, whereas only 33 percent of the people in the medication group reported pain reduction. After one year, approximately 53 percent of the chiropractic care and physical activity group participants continued to report at least a 75 percent reduction in pain; compared to just 38 percent pain reduction among those who took medication.[420]

While CAM therapies can help with managing pain, they also can support restorative healing of damaged tissues and promote overall health. For example, a 2010 study found that patients seeking CAM care for back pain also derived additional benefits that included "increased hope, increased ability to relax, positive changes in emotional states, increased body awareness, changes in thinking that increased the ability to cope with back pain, increased sense of well-being, improvement in physical conditions unrelated to back pain, increased energy, increased patient activation, and dramatic improvements in health or well-being".[421]

There is no longer a question as to whether chiropractic, acupuncture and oriental medicine, massage therapy, and nutrient and herbal therapies are viable treatment options for musculoskeletal pain and overall health management. In many cases, there is evidence of their efficacy as standalone therapies or in combination with conventional medical care. In the Additional Resources section of this book I have included a list of professional associations to help you find a licensed

CAM practitioner in your area. Visit one directly or talk to your other healthcare providers to see which one(s) may be right for you.

The Bottom Line:
Whenever musculoskeletal pain is limiting activity and red flags have been ruled out, it is time to work with a CAM healthcare provider such as a chiropractor and/or acupuncturist to help you get the pain under control, address the underlying cause of the condition, and help restore your quality of life. Pain medications should be taken with caution, on the advice of your medical doctor, only temporarily while symptoms are severe.

NOTE: While your goal may be to prevent dependence on medications, never stop taking a prescribed medication without speaking with your medical doctor first.

A Primer for Self-Care

I have included below a "first aid" guide to help get you through the first few days of an acute musculoskeletal injury or flare-up safely. I have also included strategies for self-care of chronic pain including descriptions of safe and therapeutic movements that can facilitate your healing and recovery.

> **Important:** If you experience any of the following, be sure to see your doctor as soon as possible before resorting to managing the pain on your own.
>
> - ➤ Your pain is severe;
> - ➤ Your pain is from a fall or an injury;
> - ➤ Your pain is getting worse or not getting better over time;
> - ➤ You have had cancer;
> - ➤ You have any of the following along with back pain: trouble urinating; weakness, pain, numbness, or tingling in your legs, fever, or unplanned weight loss.

First 24-48 Hours Following Injury:

Ice is a great first line of defense for reducing pain. Its greatest benefit comes from the fact that it is a natural analgesic. Ice helps minimize the perception of pain and may also reduce inflammation.

NOTE: Some experts these days are suggesting that the application of moist heat may actually be a better first line of defense than ice to expedite the healing process for musculoskeletal injuries. The rationale is that ice limits blood flow to the area and this in turn may delay recovery.[422] Heat on the other hand, will increase blood flow to the affected area which may promote quicker healing. With this in mind, some experts now suggest using METH with acute injuries. No, not that kind of meth! METH: Movement, Elevation, Traction, and Heat. This is in contrast to other experts who suggest the use of MICE to promote healing: Movement, Ice, Compression, and Elevation. In my clinical experience using ice as an analgesic can prevent or minimize the use of pain medications so I still recommend it as a means of managing acute pain. If the pain is tolerable, then you can opt to forgo the ice and use a moist heat pack instead. But if the pain is bothersome, use the ice before popping a pain pill. A combination of ice and heat is also a good strategy. For example alternate using the ice for managing the pain and using the moist heat if the area feels tight or stiff.

If using ice, apply it to the affected area for 10 to 15 minutes at a time, until you feel each stage of "CBAN":

> C-cold
> B-burn
> A-ache
> N-numb

Once you reach the point of numbness, remove the ice. Allow the body to restore normal temperature then reapply the ice to manage pain as needed.

For Chronic Pain:

Moist heat is helpful for managing long standing pain and stiffness but you can also try a topical application of capsaicin. Capsaicin is the component of hot peppers that make the peppers taste spicy hot. When we apply capsaicin to our skin, it produces that same warm feeling. These days you can find capsaicin within easy to apply patches at any drug store. The patch is placed over the affected area and the capsaicin within the patch creates a warming sensation as it is applied to the skin that can offer hours of calming pain relief. This is a great option for people dealing with chronic pain caused by osteoarthritis or muscle pain.[423] The only consideration is that if you have an allergy to capsaicin the patch could be irritating. So, if you have a known allergy then these patches should be avoided, or if an irritation occurs, discontinue use.

Healing Through Movement
Whether you are a fan of MICE or METH, all experts agree that safe, controlled movement is an important part of the healing process. For back or neck pain two great first aid movements are head retraction and the pelvic tilt.

For Neck Pain: Head Retraction
In a seated posture with your head in a neutral position, put your finger on your chin. Push your head back (retract it) without tilting your head up or down. Then, allow it to come back to its neutral position. Repeat this 10 to 15 times, three times each day within a pain-free range of motion. When this movement is completely pain-free, progress to adding controlled neck rotation.

To add rotation, when your head is retracted, turn your head slowly to look to the left. Come back to the neutral position, and then do the same thing toward the right. Then come back to the neutral position. Repeat this to each side 10 to 15 times, three times each day.

NOTE: If there is pain in any position do not stop the activity, simply pull back to the point before the pain began and only work within that pain-free range of motion.

For Low Back Pain: Pelvic Neutral
To find your neutral pelvic position, begin by lying on your back with your knees bent to 45 degrees so your feet are resting flat on the bed or floor. Put your hand beneath your low back. Flatten your low back by bringing your lower back towards the floor or your hand that is resting beneath it (imagine pulling your belly button in towards your spine). Then, arch your back as much as you can. Now picture the midpoint

300

of these two extremes and assume that position. The midpoint is your *neutral pelvic position*.

NOTE: if there is pain at this midpoint position, tilt your pelvis forwards or backwards slightly (5 to 10 degrees) to find a neutral position in which there is no pain or the least amount of pain. This neutral pelvic position is a *safe* position for your back when in pain. Assume this neutral pelvic position pulling your belly button in towards your spine, to protect your back whenever changing posture, moving, lifting, sitting, or standing.

For Low Back Pain: Pelvic Tilt
Tilt your pelvis forward as far as you can (arching your back) and then slowly tilt it backwards as far as you can (flatten your low back). Use a slow controlled movement beginning with just 5 to 10 degrees of motion and progressing as much as you can within a pain-free range of motion. This will help gradually increase movement in your lower back and help with recovery. Repeat this 10 to 15 times, three times each day. The pelvic tilt can be performed seated or when lying on your back.

NOTE: Let pain be your guide. If you can only rock the pelvis forward or back 5 degrees without pain then limit your movement to within that range. If you can rock it 20 degrees forward and 10 degrees backwards then that will be your therapeutic range of motion.

Always remain within a pain-free range of motion. As your condition improves, this range will progressively increase.

Changing Positions While Experiencing Lower Back Pain:

Moving from a seated to standing position
Place your feet flat on the floor, about shoulder width apart. Bend at your hips, not at your back by hinging forward at your hips, chest out, and nose over toes. Push yourself up using your legs with your weight in your heels and using a hand support to assist you. Do not bend your back; maintain a neutral position the entire time with your bellybutton pulled in towards your spine.

Moving from a standing to seated position
This is essentially the opposite of the above. Stand in front of the seat, feet about shoulder width apart. Then bend at your hips, being sure not to flex your back, and bend your knees to lower yourself down towards the chair remembering to keep your bellybutton pulled in towards your spine to help support your lower back.

Moving from a lying to standing position
The key here is not to bend or twist your spine. First, pull your bellybutton in towards your spine. This helps stabilize your back. Shift your hips so you are lying on your side and then shift your shoulders to follow. Use your arms to push from the bed and allow your legs to act as a pendulum to swing you into a seated position.

Foods that Support the Initial Stage of Healing

Hippocrates, the father of medicine, said it best when he famously proclaimed: "Let food be thy medicine and medicine be thy food." Select foods can be excellent allies to support healing. As discussed earlier in this book, certain foods have known anti-inflammatory properties meaning the can help modulate the inflammatory responses within our body establishing an environment that is most conducive to healing.[424] Conversely, other foods have pro-inflammatory properties that may delay healing. In general, eating foods high in trans-fats, saturated fats, and omega-6 fatty acid rich vegetable oils will result in a *pro*-inflammatory state, while eating monounsaturated fats and omega-3 fatty acids will be *anti*-inflammatory.[425] Choosing to emphasize consumption of foods with known anti-inflammatory properties while reducing intake (or avoiding) foods with pro-inflammatory effects may support the healing of acute injures and may also help reduce symptoms of chronic conditions like osteoarthritis.[426,427]

The chart that follows identifies select anti-inflammatory foods, herbs, and spices that support healing and that should be consumed while recovering from injury. The column on the right lists common foods with pro-inflammatory properties. While you are likely minimizing or avoiding intake of some of these foods anyways as part of your new manner of eating, other pro-inflammatory foods listed are generally considered very healthy (such as the nightshade vegetables), so intake of these foods should only be minimized while recovering from injury or if trying to reduce hs-CRP levels. As long as hs-CRP levels are within normal limits (refer back to chapter 5 if you need a refresher on hs-CRP), and as long as you do not have a hypersensitivity to any of these foods, which can be determined by an elimination diet (refer to chapter 18), then you can resume inclusion of those foods into your manner of eating after you recover from your injury.

NOTE: If you have a food allergy or sensitivity to one of the foods listed in the anti-inflammatory column, then that food should be avoided since food sensitivities often trigger inflammation.

Select foods, herbs, and spices with anti-inflammatory properties *(increase intake)*	Select foods with pro-inflammatory properties *(limit intake)*
Onions	Sugar
Garlic	Grain-fed, non-organic meats
Cruciferous Vegetables including Broccoli, Brussels sprouts, kale, and cauliflower	Common Cooking Oils: Safflower, soy, sunflower, corn, and cottonseed oil
Ginger	Trans fats
Rosemary	Red (especially grain-fed) and processed meats
Turmeric	High fat dairy (feta and grating cheeses, such as Romano and Parmesan are ok)
Cinnamon	Refined grains including white rice, white flour, white bread, pasta, and pastries
Oolong, white, and green tea	Alcohol
Nuts including walnuts, almonds, and hazelnuts (not peanuts)	Artificial food additives including aspartame, MSG
Sardines	Processed foods
Wild Alaskan salmon	Candies and cookies
Black cod	Boxed cereals (except oatmeal)
Avocado	Fried foods including French fries, egg rolls, etc.
Extra virgin olive oil	Tortillas, popcorn, and chips
Whole grains such as brown rice, quinoa, and bulgur wheat	Jams and fruit juices (choose the whole fruit instead)

Berries	Caffeine
Kelp	Nightshade vegetables:
Tofu and tempeh	Substances in these foods called
Legumes including lentils, garbanzo beans, and peas	alkaloids, can be pro-inflammatory in *susceptible individuals* only. These foods include: potatoes (not sweet potatoes), tomatoes, eggplant, sweet and hot peppers, tomatillos, pepinos, pimentos, paprika, and cayenne peppers.

Mind-Body Healing

Another wonderful ally to support healing is your mind. Remember, what we discussed in chapter 15? Practice the deep breathing techniques (4-7-8 breath) you learned in that chapter to help assume power over the pain. Also, invest in a great guided imagery recording that is designed to help with managing pain and supporting healing. I encourage you to explore the final section of the book where I include some great resources. Guided imagery and other forms of meditation and mind-body healing are a fantastic tool to distract your attention away from the pain and to harness the power of thought to stimulate healing.

Assembling Your Team

It is now well established that the complex healthcare needs of individuals exceed the capability of any one individual healthcare discipline.[428,429,430,431,432] If you are dealing with either acute or chronic pain, surround yourself with a capable team of healthcare professionals that will be your partners on your healing journey.

At the very least, your healthcare dream team should include a medical or osteopathic doctor (M.D. or D.O.) and a doctor of chiropractic (D.C.). Find a medical or osteopathic doctor who is a proponent of integrative medicine and find a chiropractor that can help you recover by addressing not only your symptoms, but also the underlying cause of your pain. This may include structural or muscular imbalances, poor ergonomics, and/or poor form or improper technique during sport.

Chiropractors are also trained in a variety of treatment options to help you recover including manipulation, mobilization, physical therapy and rehabilitation, and nutritional counseling.

Additionally, align yourself with a qualified nutritionist - a certified nutrition specialist (C.N.S.) or a registered dietician (R.D.) - to offer personalized nutritional support, and an acupuncturist/oriental medicine practitioner (LAc., M.A.O.M., or D.A.O.M.) and massage therapist (L.M.T.) to help restore balance to your body and help manage pain.

Consider also visiting a naturopathic doctor (N.D.) who are trained in many facets of natural medicine, and a certified Ayurvedic practitioner to gain a novel perspective on your overall health. If you are unfamiliar with Ayurveda, consider this: some of the top medical centers in the U.S. such as Scripps Center for Integrative Medicine and University of Maryland Center for Integrative Medicine are now offering training in Ayurveda for medical doctors to aid in their prevention, diagnosis, and treatment of disease.

Refer to the Additional Resources section of the book to find links to associations that can help you locate practitioners in your area who possess the appropriate certifications, licensing, and credentials for their discipline.

Chapter 20

Just because you're not sick doesn't mean you're healthy.
— Author Unknown

Know your Numbers

There is no doubt that prevention is the best medicine, and adhering to the *manner of living* outlined in this book is a powerful and evidence-based means of preventing disease. However, there are times that despite our best efforts, we may still be vulnerable to the onset of disease. Fortunately, contemporary medical science is bursting at the seams with innovative ways to help us understand our current state of health and identify silent risk factors for disease. Amazing screening tools now exist that allow us to look into a veritable crystal ball and identify conditions and diseases that we may be at risk for well before these conditions rear their ugly face with overt sign and symptoms. This knowledge is powerful as it arms us with the ability to intervene early to help delay and ideally, to prevent or even reverse the progression of disease.

Monitoring our blood pressure measurements and cholesterol levels are examples of some common screening tests that we are all familiar with. Early in this book we explored the importance of measuring our waist circumference, body fat, and hs-CRP as additional markers of our health and risk for disease. While each of these tests are incredibly important and an essential part of monitoring your health, these days there are even more tests at our disposal that you may not be as familiar with, but that can help predict our health risks for many diseases earlier and more effectively than ever before. Since some of these are new and not yet a part of standard health screening procedures, you may need to ask your doctor for these tests by name and ask them if the test would be right for you.

Recommended Preventive Screenings Tests

Look at your annual check-up at your doctor's office not as a dreaded occasion for someone to poke and prod you, but rather as a visit to an evidence-based fortune teller that can help you gain a glimpse into your future state of health! No matter what our age or current state of health, modern science has provided us with a gift of a veritable crystal ball of screening tools that can offer us important information that may help predict our future health. Armed with this knowledge, we can choose to act; to incorporate more healthy behaviors into our daily routine, and/or change destructive behaviors before they become a significant problem.

Not convinced you want to see your health future? Believe that ignorance is bliss? Then consider this: If screenings reveal a problem, a risk factor for disease, then with few exceptions it is always easier to prevent and/or manage a condition when it is detected early then once it has progressed. Other than with musculoskeletal injuries, pain and other overt symptoms are often the last things to manifest when something is going wrong. Therefore, if we wait until our body flashes overt red flags and warning signs, it is sometimes too late or at best, much more difficult to effectively manage or reverse a disease process.

In the pages that follow, I have assembled a to-do list of select important screening tests for all ages and stages of adult life. Please keep in mind that this list is not comprehensive nor is it intended to replace the advice of your doctor. Speak with your doctor to establish an appropriate screening plan and schedule that is right for *you*. However, if he or she does not recommend one of the tests listed, ask *why not?* A discussion on the pros and cons of select screening tests is

308

appropriate to determine what is best for meeting your personal healthcare needs. If he or she is not familiar with one of the screening tests described below or simply does not offer them, feel free to ask for a referral to another practitioner or contact another healthcare provider yourself.

Remember: *you are in charge of your own health.*

NOTE: Before we proceed to listing all the screening tests, it is important to put screening tests and disease risk into perspective. When a screening test identifies a risk factor for disease, it means either:

a) the chance of developing a particular disease within the next few years or within one's lifetime is higher than for others who do not possess that same risk factor, or

b) a person may *already have* a disease and does not know about it yet; they are not yet showing obvious symptoms.

Screening tests help us to identify these early indicators (risk factors) of disease and empower us with the ability to take action to mitigate the risk. But it is important to keep in mind that not all risk factors are a guarantee that you will develop that disease or that the disease will impact your quality of life or lifespan. So before you take action in response to the findings of a screening test, it is imperative that you first explore all the pros and cons of intervening.

For example, if the risk factor you identify is an increased waist circumference, elevated blood pressure, or an elevated hs-CRP and the intervention proposed is to improve your *manner of living* then go for it! The benefits of that intervention far outweigh any risks! But, if the proposed intervention is an invasive therapy such as for example, surgery to remove a mass found on the prostate during a prostate cancer screening test, then potential risks versus benefits of that intervention and all other management options should be carefully considered and discussed with a team of healthcare providers before any action is taken. As remarkable as modern medicine is, it is still not a perfect science or infallible and in some cases and for some individuals, the interventions can be worse than the disease itself, especially when considered from a quality of life perspective. In the example noted, surgery to remove the prostate carries a high risk of permanent erectile dysfunction and incontinence and is not even a guarantee that it will prolong a man's life. In fact, a study published in the New England Journal of Medicine found that prostate cancer surgery did not prolong survival any better than mere observation.[433] Prostate cancer is often a slow growing cancer so it may never spread during a man's lifetime and in fact, in many cases a man eventually dies of other conditions completed unrelated to the prostate cancer. Thus, particularly in older men and in those without any other obvious symptoms, sometimes the best decision is simply to monitor the condition and avoid surgery.

The Bottom Line:
Overall, a good strategy to employ when a screening test reveals a risk for disease is: 1) discuss with you doctor the significance of that risk and determine how strongly is it associated with the disease in question, 2) determine what are the risks and benefits of action versus inaction in response to that risk factor, and 3) if treatment is required, exhaust all viable, evidenced-based, noninvasive management options first before resorting to any invasive interventions.

Men and women under the age of 40

SELECT SCREENING TESTS
Blood pressure (regular monitoring)
Complete blood test for liver, kidney, and thyroid function
Cholesterol and Lipid Screening stating at age 20. Ask for your doctor to include a cholesterol particle size test known as the NMR lipid profile. This test not only identifies the number of LDL, HDL and triglycerides it also determines the size of select particles. Small, dense LDL particles are considered more dangerous and increase associated health risks.
Liver Function Tests (LFT): This can be a marker for excessive junk food consumption as levels have been shown to increase in as little as four weeks in those who consume high amounts of fast food.[434] Overtime, elevated LFTs can indicate liver disease and risk of cardiovascular disease.[435]

Complete nutritional analysis
Skin cancer self-test: once a month, look over your skin for any changes. See your doctor once a year for a more thorough test.
Fasting glucose test if you have risk factors for diabetes
Hemoglobin A1C (measures your average blood sugar over 2 to 3 months; more accurate than the standard fasting glucose test). Test if you are overweight and have risk factors for diabetes or heart disease.
Fasting insulin test: Level of insulin will often increase even before glucose and Hemoglobin A1C, so this can be an early marker for diabetes.
Lipoprotein(A) this is a test for a protein that attaches to LDL cholesterol and encourages it to infiltrate the walls of our coronary arteries. It is inherited and is a powerful predictor of heart disease, particularly in younger people. Test if you have risk factors for heart disease, even if your cholesterol is normal.
Spinal and postural assessment (including identifying muscle imbalances) by a Chiropractor. Postural and joint alignment assessment can be an effective crystal ball to predict risk of musculoskeletal injury. If imbalances are found, your chiropractor can design treatments and/or workouts to help restore proper balance to muscles and joints to minimize future risk of injury.
Dental screening by a dentist
Waist circumference measurement
Body fat percentage measurement
C-reactive protein test: ask your doctor to add it to your annual blood work
Vitamin D: ask your doctor to add testing of 25-hydroxyvitamin D to your annual blood work
Apolipoprotien E (ApoE): Genetic marker (only need to check this once) that reflects an increased risk of heart disease[436] and Alzheimer's disease.[437] Its presence indicates a need for more aggressive lifestyle change interventions to reduce risk.

Women under the age of 40 add:

SELECT SCREENING TESTS
Breast self-exam once a month
Clinical breast exam by a physician, annually
Cervical cancer screening: (Pap test or Pap smear) begin as soon as you become sexually active.

Men under the age of 40 add:

SELECT SCREENING TEST
Testicular self-exam once a month

Men and women over the age of 40

SELECT SCREENING TESTS
Continue self-tests and screenings recommended for those under 40
Colorectal cancer screening using a digital rectal exam with a fecal occult blood test, sigmoidoscopy, or colonoscopy
Cholesterol and Lipid Screening: Ask for your doctor to include a cholesterol particle size test known as the NMR lipid profile. This test not only identifies the number of LDL, HDL and triglycerides it also determines the size of select particles. Small, dense LDL particles are considered more dangerous and increase associated health risks.
Complete nutritional analysis
Carotid Ultrasound for assessing stroke risk
Echocardiogram for heart murmurs
Initial electrocardiogram (EKG) to detect early changes and for future reference
Urine cytology for bladder cancer
Hemoglobin A1C (measures your average blood sugar over 2 to 3 months; more accurate than the standard fasting glucose test)
Lipoprotein(A)
Endothelial Function Test (EndoPAT) analyzes the inner lining of blood vessels (endothelium) and the ability of these vessels to dilate. Endothelial dysfunction can be the *first sign* of vascular disease. Good news is that it is receptive to improvements in your manner of eating and living.

Spinal and postural assessment (including identifying muscle imbalances) by a Chiropractor. Postural assessment can be an effective crystal ball to predict risk of musculoskeletal injury. If imbalances are found, your chiropractor can design workouts to help restore proper balance to muscles and joints to minimize future risk of injury.
Dental screening: This is not just about appearances; gum disease can increase systemic inflammation and risk of heart disease.
Waist circumference measurement
Body fat percentage measurement
C-reactive protein test: ask your doctor to add it to your annual blood work
Vitamin D: ask your doctor to add testing of 25-hydroxyvitamin D to your annual blood work

Women over the age of 40 add:

SELECT SCREENING TESTS
Cervical Cancer screening (Pap test or Pap smear)
Bone mineral density scan. Over age 65 or younger if you have risk factors for osteoporosis.
Breast cancer screening. Includes regular breast self-exam, clinical breast exam by your doctor, and mammography for women 40 years of age and older or younger if you have a family history. NOTE: Mammograms have lately become the subject of significant controversy. A 2014 study suggests that they may not be more reliable than a clinical breast examination in decreasing breast cancer mortality.[438] But, careful not to throw the baby out with the bath water. While mammograms may not have the impact that we hoped, it is important to talk to your doctor to decide whether this screening test is right for *you.*

Men over the age of 40 add:

SCREENING TESTS
Prostate cancer screening. Annual digital rectal exam (DRE) and prostate-specific antigen (PSA) blood test for men 50 and older or younger if you have a family history. NOTE: Similar to mammograms, PSA blood tests are also the subject of significant controversy. Several studies question the reliability and usefulness of this test citing frequent false-positive results that may lead to negative psychological effects, over-diagnosis, and unnecessary interventions and treatment.[439] That said, the PSA test may still be of value in certain cases and for tracking trends in your PSA levels over time so men, talk to your doctor to decide whether this screening test is right for *you*.

Chapter 21

Watch your thoughts for they become words.
Watch your words for they become actions.
Watch your actions for they become habits.
Watch your habits for they become your character.
And watch your character for it becomes your destiny.
What we think, we become.
— Margaret Thatcher

Like Brushing your Teeth

The challenge with adopting a new habit or refining an old one is making the new habit stick. Remember, your new *manner of living* is for life. Gone is the temporary, transient mindset that permits us to revert back to hurtful habits after reaching some arbitrary goal. The goal of adopting a new *manner of living* is not one stop on your life's journey; *it is the journey.*

This chapter shares with you some important thoughts on how to make maintaining your new *manner of living* even more realistic and sustainable through the decades to come.

Realistic Expectations

Whenever you try to make a change in your life it helps to understand how human beings in general, adapt to change. This understanding helps prevent you from setting unrealistic expectations and setting yourself up for failure. We tend to be a society that seeks instant and immediate gratification. And for the most part, we have engineered a modern existence that caters to this whim. We do not need to hike miles to get to the market or to a friend's home, we do not need to sow and toil the land for our food, gone are the days of walking miles in the snow to school, and we have almost all but forgotten the time when one had to stand up from the couch and actually walk to the television to change the channel. No doubt, instant gratification can set the stage for an easy and satisfying existence. However, when it comes to behavior change, this type of immediate expectation is unrealistic and can be destructive.

The Process of Behavior Change

During the late seventies and early eighties two behavioral science researchers Drs. Prochaska and DiClemente, published extraordinary research exploring the process of human behavior change.[440] They determined that when we adopt a new behavior we generally move through five steps in the process of adopting that new habit. The model they developed is referred to as the Transtheoretical Model of Behavior Change. You might have heard of it before as the "stages of change" model.

The five stages of change are as follows:

1. Precontemplation
2. Contemplation
3. Preparation
4. Action
5. Maintenance

Let's explore each stage further.

Understanding the Five Stages of Change

Precontemplation: Just as it sounds, precontemplation is when one is not yet even considering change. In this stage, you may be unaware of a need for change or in denial of the need. When someone is in this stage, it is hard to convince them of a need to change. If you know someone that is stuck in this stage, the best strategy is not to point out the harm; but rather to help them identify the benefits of change. Someone in this stage needs to see for themselves that there may be an advantage to making different choices.

Contemplation: This is the stage when one recognizes a need to change. If you are in a contemplative stage, you are thinking about making a change in your life but have not yet taken action. This stage is characterized by ambivalence. One may see a need to change but does not yet acknowledge that the benefit of change outweighs the comfort of staying the same or that the benefit justifies the perceived amount of effort and sacrifice required to make that change. The goal in this stage is to find a compelling reason and a motivation to change.

ACTION STEP: If you feel stuck in the contemplation stage for one or more behaviors, then take a few minutes to do the following: Identify the behavior you want to change (for example: overeating, binge eating, smoking, checking emails constantly, biting nails, etc.). Now, write down that behavior. Next, list out ALL the negative things associated with that behavior from the most trivial (for example: my dog leaves the room when I smoke) to the most profound (for example: I am scared I will not be able to dance at my daughter or granddaughters wedding if I keep smoking). Be specific and personal with each item, and identify at least ten items for this list. Next, create another list of ALL the positive aspects of changing this behavior, once again from the seemingly trivial benefits (for example: I will have more money if I stop buying cigarettes) to the most profound and meaningful (for example: I will add years to my life, I will have more energy to do the things I enjoy with my partner). Once again, you should identify *at least* ten items for the list and be specific with each item. Now, each time you feel an urge to engage in that behavior, pause for just one minute. Delay that "gratification" and direct your attention away from the temptation - just for one minute - by simply contemplating the items on your lists. To make this practical, keep the list somewhere so you can see it daily as a frequent reminder of your motivation to change. Share it with a supportive friend that you can reach out to and call, or write down some of the items that are your key motivators and post them on you fridge door, or tape them to your cigarette case (if you smoke), your computer monitor, or mirror.

Preparation: By reading this book, you are at least in the stage of preparation when it comes to improving your overall *manner of living*. This is the stage when we not only recognize a need to change and have a willingness to change, but we also begin to gather information to help support making that change. The move from the preparation stage to the action stage that follows happens simply by taking that first step forward towards your goal. That first step marks the transition point between thinking and talking about change to actually *doing* something to make it happen.

Action: The action stage refers to the point when we are implementing the change. If you have implemented any of the information, tips, recommendations or action steps in this book, then congratulations! You are in the stage of action. If you are still in the preparation stage, then commit to taking *just one* step forward today. Try a new food from the list in chapter 5, incorporate a little more movement into your day as suggested in chapter 14, breathe deeply as you learned in chapter 15, or see your doctor to get any pain checked out as discussed in chapter 19. Just one step forward and you are in action! Each day, plan and choose to incorporate at least one more step forward.

Maintenance: This final stage of maintenance refers to when we have incorporated the desired change into our daily routine. That desired change has now became our new normal. When we are in the maintenance phase we have adopted a new *manner of living*.

While the above five stages appear to follow a natural progression, there is one critical fact that you must realize and accept as you read on. As Drs. Prochaska and DiClemente found, rarely do humans progress through these five stages in a linear, sequential manner. In fact, most commonly it is quite the contrary. Typically, as we progress from one stage to the next it is expected that there may be times in life when we move from action back to contemplation or even from maintenance back to precontemplation. The important thing to recognize is that not only is this ok, it is actually *normal*.

We all have times in our life where we may veer off course slightly. When unexpected life events may take precedence. Again, this is normal. Never let it dampen your spirits. The goal is to simply resume the action and maintenance phase as soon as you can; the next hour, the next meal, the next day, or even the next month. In fact, be prepared to veer off course once in a while but rest assured that this is normal so it should not discourage you. Resume your new behaviors, your *manner of living*, as soon as you can; no guilt, no regrets.

318

Remember when as a child your mother made you brush your teeth? You hated it, dreaded it, you may have even lied about doing it. It is funny though, overtime few adults can imagine waking up and forgoing the act of brushing their teeth. It becomes habitual, necessary, and almost as natural as breathing. As you grow up, it is hard to imagine not doing it. That said, I suspect most of us have had at least one morning where we did not brush our teeth right away. How did you feel that morning? You may have felt an icky and unclean taste in your mouth; a hesitance to be sociable and engaging since you feared your breath could destroy a small plant. You hurry to the nearest toothbrush to restore the fresh mouth feel that you have grown accustomed to since that moment as a child when mom told you to brush your teeth.

Brushing your teeth is the perfect illustration of how adopting a new behavior works and embracing your new *manner of living* is very similar. The first few days or weeks may feel forced; more of a conscious effort and at times, perhaps even somewhat of a struggle. But as you progress and as days pass, it will become more and more second nature. Your activities and the choices you make with regard to the food you eat will become less forced and more natural. Eventually it *will* become your new normal. Sure there will be days that you do not have your toothbrush at hand; there may be days when you may make lousy food choices, you may even revert back to some old habits, but just like brushing your teeth, this will feel off; a feeling that will encourage you to resume your new *manner of living* as soon as you can.

It is now time for the 80-20 rule.

The 80-20 Rule

The 80-20 rule is a rule that I rarely divulge to patients until I feel they are secure enough in their new habits to hear it. It is like the Jewish mysticism of Kabbalah, or "the force" for you Star Wars junkies; you can only learn it when you are ready. After reading this book dear reader, I feel as though I can let you in on this secret - the secret to sustaining your new *manner of living* for life.

Ready?

Here goes.

The secret for sustaining your new *manner of living* for life is to live literally by the book 80% of the time, but 20% of the time permit real life to happen. Allow me to explain. Most traditional approaches to losing fat or even lifestyle change in general fail because they are approached as an all or nothing proposition. On the flip side, the mantra *everything in moderation* is flawed as well, since it permits us to justify any behaviors without consequence, as long as it is in moderation. What the 80-20 rule dictates is that 80% of the time you should be purposeful and consistent with adhering to the new *manner of living* you have adopted. But allow yourself the freedom and flexibility so that 20% of the time, you can and should permit real life to happen (remember dessert for dinner?) and accept that it is perfectly fine.

Accept and expect that 20% of the time we can choose to deviate from our course intentionally (think vacation or birthday celebration), sometimes we are forced to temporarily veer off course due to stressors in life that are out of our control (such as illness or the loss of a loved one), or quite simply there may be times that we do not have access to healthy food options. This is not a cause for stress, guilt, or regret. Quite the contrary! This is a part of your *manner of living* that helps make it realistic, sustainable, *and* effective. As mentioned before, our body is very forgiving and resilient. Our body can accommodate such deviations from time to time without any harm. By accepting that the goal is not perfection but rather resilience, we permit these exceptions to take place without allowing them to derail us. In fact, they help strengthen us.

Reinforcing Resilience

At the end of the day, adhering to your new *manner of living* is really about finding resilience. Being able to respond to tough days, good news, and all the extreme emotional and physical challenges and gifts that life presents to you without allow them to overwhelm and unravel you.

320

Control of Your Destiny: The Life Checkbook

Your *manner of living* is about being informed, self-aware, and empowered in all that you do. You are no longer a passive participant in your own life; *you* define your needs and your next steps. In the pages of this book I hope I have offered a road map to help guide your decisions when it comes to food, movement, stress, and health. But ultimately, the choice is yours. You are in control. To support this notion, I leave you in this chapter with one final thought.

Imagine a giant checkbook; *your life's checkbook*. Imagine it is tied to an account that is your life. It is finite, and how you spend the investment is up to you. Sure there are some forces outside of your control that impact your investment, but these only exert a minimal influence. Some of the choices we make like smoking, being sedentary, or frequently overeating may require a significant withdrawal of time from our life's account. Other choices such as eating real food, laughing, and participating in enjoyable physical activities can actually increase our savings!

Each day you cash out the checks with the choices you make. The question is: will you spend the investment mindlessly or will you choose to grow you savings?

That choice is up to *you*.

Chapter 22

You cannot plough a field by turning it over in your mind.
— Author Unknown

Bringing it all Together: the Action Plan

Within this final chapter of this book, <u>you become the author</u>. To put your new *manner of living* into practice you must first personalize it and to do so you need to start by defining two things:

1) Your personal goal(s) and
2) Your action plan

These are two specific things that I cannot tell you. Even if you visited me as a patient in my practice, one-on-one, I could advise and support you, but I could not do this work for you. This part is entirely up to *you*. Ask yourself, what do you prioritize? What do you value? What motivates you? What are your *perceived* obstacles and barriers to change? What needs to happen, what steps do you need to take to overcome these obstacles or barriers? The answers to these questions are personal and are entirely up to *you*.

These next few pages are designed to help you script your goals and your action plan. This process will allow you to identify the steps you need to take to put your new *manner of living* into practice. I will guide you through this process. This is also a time for you to reflect on and draw from all the information I have outlined for you in this book. As I once heard the brilliant researcher and physician, Wayne Jonas, MD remark: "You can't predict the future, but you can create it". It is now the time to create *your* future. It is time to establish a plan for how you choose to allocate the checks connected to your life.

ACTION STEP#1: Set aside a moment to contemplate in silence and ask yourself, *what are the top three goals that I desire to achieve in order to enhance my manner of living?* <u>Do not skimp on this step</u>. The process of explicitly and specifically defining and writing out your goals is critical as it establishes some of your key destinations on this journey. Think grand here; long term, lofty goals! This is the time to think big picture but also ensure your goals are tangible and measurable, ambitious yet attainable. Additionally, include a timeline to define *when* you expect to achieve each goal.

Now, put everything aside, and take some time to think about your goals. As you reflect on this, refer back to chapter 2 where you wrote down your body fat percentage, waist circumference, and waist to height ratio. If those measurements place you at increased risk for disease, you may choose to include improving those measures as one or more of your goals. You may also wish to adopt or adapt one or more of the goals that I outlined throughout the book.

As soon as you arrive at a clear decision, write down three goals that are important to you.

Next, consider each of the three goals and make a decision which one is your *top* priority. To help you decide which one to prioritize, consider not only the benefits of achieving that goal but also the consequence of *inaction*. Take a moment and reflect on what would happen if you did *not* achieve that goal. If you continue on the current path, where will the road take you?

Once you have selected the goal that is the most important to you at this point in your life, then that is the goal you will begin working towards, beginning today.

The next step is to take that big picture goal and ensure that it is specific enough so that you can clearly determine when you have achieved it. A goal such as "I want to lose body fat" is far too vague. A better way to describe that goal would be as follows: instead of writing that your goal is to "lose body fat", you can write that your goal is "to achieve and maintain a waist circumference of 35 inches and decrease my body fat percentage by 10% by my 56th birthday on August 8th of this year by increasing my daily physical activity, by improving my lifestyle habits, and by improving the quality of food I consume." Remember, the goal needs to be specific, realistic, and measurable and include a timeline for achievement.

ACTION STEP#2: Beneath the clearly defined goal, explicitly describe what achieving that goal will mean to you. Consider, why is this goal important to you? How will you feel once you have achieved that goal? What is the benefit of achieving it? How will it change your life for the better? Write down everything that comes to mind. There is no right or wrong response; this is all about you and your motivation for change. This is the most personal part of this process and it is also the most meaningful. This step is about understanding and acknowledging your reason for making positive changes in your life. The process of change is not always easy, at times it may feel uncomfortable, but these reasons that you will define right now are what makes the journey worthwhile. Additionally, as you progress in your new *manner of living*, if you ever feel discouraged, turn back to this list to remind yourself why this is a worthwhile pursuit.

Example:

My goal: *To achieve and maintain a waist circumference of 35 inches and decrease my body fat percentage by 10% by the August 8th of this year by increasing my daily physical activity, by improving my lifestyle habits, and by improving the quality of food I consume.*

What achieving my goal will mean to me: *I will have more confidence, more energy, I won't get tired so easily, it will help my arthritis and knee pain so I can*

325

walk and play with my grandchildren without getting exhausted or without as much pain, and I will be healthy enough to dance at their wedding. I will reduce my chance of having a heart attack at the age of fifty like my father had. It will reduce the fear I associate with my current state of health. I want to be a role model for my children. I don't want to become dependent on medications as I age. I want to travel during retirement; I want to see the world, not the inside of a hospital.

ACTION STEP #3: Did you know that by the time most athletes win the Stanley Cup or the Super Bowl they have likely visualized that win in their mind's eye hundreds of times? Visualization is a powerful tool to help make our goals or dreams become a reality. This next action step is simply to take a moment to close your eyes and create a vivid picture in your mind of what achieving your goal will look like. Do not stop there. Also consider what it will feel like to have achieved the change you desire; embody the emotions and meaning that you described in Action Step #2. Once the image becomes clear and the emotion it evokes is genuine, then take a snap shot in your mind of that picture, while also capturing the feelings associated with it. Bring this image back into your mind's eye at least once a day to remind yourself of what you are working towards and how good it feels.

TIP! Identify a symbol to represent the image of your success. It can be a picture, an inspirational song, a mantra, or a poem. Identify some symbolic representation of your image of successful attainment of your goal that you can use to evoke the feelings and the picture you just described. Place the poem or picture somewhere you can see it often to draw inspiration from it. Perhaps select an inspiring song that you can make into your phone's ring tone so it plays when you least expect it as a reminder of your goal and to evoke that great feeling and inspiration toward attainment of your goal.

Now that you have clearly identified your upcoming destination – your goal – along with your reasons for embarking upon this journey, the next phase is to create your road map, the action steps you will need to get you to your destination. Remember, it is direction and action that will get you to your destination; not merely intention. In this book I have offered a wealth of resources to support your journey, but this is the time for you to personalize it so you can implement it. Consider, what are some of the perceived obstacles that are preventing you from reaching your goal? Now, *transform each obstacle into an action.*

ACTION STEP#4: Beneath your goal, list at least ten specific action steps you need to take to reach your goal. Make each action as *specific* and *measurable* as possible and again, include a *timeline* to commit yourself to achieving that action by a specific date. Keep in mind, the timeline is not the end point; that behavior should continue indefinitely as part of your new *manner of living*. The timeline merely ensures you remain on track; otherwise it is easy to become derailed by life's competing priorities. Refer to the tips and information that you have learned in this book to inform each of your action steps. To assist you further, refer to the example that follows.

Example:

My Goal:
I will achieve and maintain a waist circumference of 35 inches and decrease my body fat percentage by 10% by the end of this year by increasing my daily physical activity, improving my lifestyle habits, and by improving the quality of food I consume.

What achieving my goal will mean to me:
I will have more confidence, more energy, I won't get tired so easily, it will help my arthritis and knee pain so I can walk and play with my grandchildren without getting exhausted or without as much pain, and I will be healthy enough to dance at their wedding. I will reduce my chance of having a heart attack at the age of fifty like my father had. It will reduce the fear I associate with my current state of health. I want to be a role model for my children. I don't want to become dependent on medications as I age. I want to travel during retirement; I want to see the world, not the inside of a hospital.

The symbol of attainment of my goal:
The theme song from the film Rocky!

My Action Plan: *The action steps that will lead me to my goal*
Sample action steps related to dietary pattern
I will only eat at the dining room table this week
I will not watch TV while eating dinner this week

I will try Brussels sprouts this week
I will cook dinner at home this week using only whole, real foods
I will wait 20 minutes before reaching for a second helping at dinner to make sure I am still hungry before eating more food
I will have breakfast every day this week within 45 minutes of waking
I will choose to drink 1 extra glass of water each day this week
I will gauge my level of hunger this week prior to, during, and after every meal to ensure I eat when I am at 3 or 4/10, and stop eating when I reach 7 or 8/10 on that gauge
This week I will check in to see if my hunger is above or below my neck before reaching for a snack
I will use smaller dinner plates this week
Sample action steps related to activity
I will take the stairs up to my office rather than taking the elevator each morning this week
I will go bike riding this Sunday with my partner
I will take 5 minutes each morning just before I brush my teeth to do 4 resistance training activities at least 3 times this week
I will walk on campus for ten minutes between my classes this week
I will stand on one foot while I brush my teeth this week
I will integrate interval training into my activity routine this week
I will stand up and walk around every time I talk on the phone at home this week
I will do 10 push-ups during one commercial break a day this week
Sample action steps related to lifestyle
I will find an opportunity to volunteer in my community this week
I will perform the 4 – 7 – 8 breaths every time I feel overwhelmed this week
I will only smoke one cigarette each day this week
I will not smoke in my car this week
I will make an appointment this week to visit my doctor for an annual check-up
I will maintain proper posture while sitting at the computer this week
I will go to bed 15 minutes earlier this week

As you move forward, focus on taking one action step at a time. Each new week, select one new action step to embark upon. By focusing on one small action step at a time, it not only makes achievement of your overall goal more manageable, it also creates the opportunity for frequent feel good and confidence building moments along the way with each successful step! You will see that this approach will propel you along the path towards your ultimate goal. Each subsequent accomplishment will motivate you further, building your confidence and capacity for achieving other positive changes in your habits and behaviors. (Remember that slippery slope I described in the Preface?) Before you know it, you will be closer and closer to your overall goal.

Be certain that your accomplishments do not go unnoticed. Each time you achieve one of your short term goals - each action step - celebrate your success! No matter how big or small, each action step is meaningful in supporting and defining your new *manner of living*, so find joy in each successful step and celebrate each one with gusto! Just remember not to celebrate with food or drink; celebrate with a movie, indulge in a great book, a massage, a facial, by dancing around your living room, or by spending a day at the beach or park with the family. Make this journey one that feels great each step of the way.

ACTION STEP#5: Assemble the list of your rewards! List out all the ways you can celebrate accomplishment of each action step. List at least ten rewards that feel good, are fun, and/or meaningful to you. Again, the rewards should not involve food or drink; but they should involve something that brings you joy, including special experiences or little things or moments that make you smile.

If for any reason you do not succeed in achieving your defined action step one week, take a moment to contemplate and explicitly identify the reason why. Then, determine how to overcome that obstacle or modify the action step so that it can become more manageable. If necessary, *ask for help*. Talking with a trusted friend, a doctor, or other expert may help you see things differently and strategize a new way to approach that challenge.

Also, recognize that while you may not have achieved the desired outcome, even little improvements are worth acknowledging. For example, if you had a particularly tough week, acknowledge that even though you may not have completed that week's action step entirely at least you still made some positive steps that week, despite major competing priorities. Perhaps you did not manage to take the stairs every day that week as you had set out to do, but you still managed to take the stairs two times more than you did the week before! That is still a wonderful step in the right direction. Do not focus on and be discouraged by what you did not do; focus on what you *did*. Acknowledge that and then, simply move forward with that same action step the following week. Never get discouraged or give up; this is your life. Trust in your ability and resilience, *you can and will get there.*

Regardless of the goals you have defined for yourself, I encourage you to keep a log of your daily food and drink choices along with your activity for at least one month. While admittedly a little tedious, you will see this will be very helpful particularly during the first few weeks of initiating behavioral change. In fact, studies have consistently show that the mere act of documenting what we eat - self monitoring - is one of our greatest allies in supporting a change in our body composition, and more importantly, in maintaining that change over time.[441,442,443,444]

ACTION STEP#6: Purchase a journal (I encourage you to choose an appealing looking one that you will proudly carry around with you each day) or download one of the free tracking apps listed in the Additional Resources section of this book (such as "LoseIt!" or "MyFitnessPal") to monitor your daily dietary intake and activity.

TIP! Instead of just tracking your activity and what you eat and drink, also make note of how you feel that day. Use the following three expressions to gauge your attitude and feelings each day:

1. Rocked it! I feel great!
2. Challenged me, but I made it through!
3. Tough day, but I can do this!

As you progress, you will see more and more "rocked it! I feel great!" days appear, and there is no better feeling than that!

ACTION STEP#7: Look at today's date on a calendar. Now, jump ahead to exactly one year from today's date and mark that date on your calendar as the one year anniversary of your new *manner of living*! From today on, whether you implement small or major changes to your daily routine, celebrate that anniversary. Your goals may or may not all be achieved by then, but progress certainly will, and that is worth celebrating!

A Final Thought

Make it happen. You *can* do this. And remember: you are never alone. Use this book as a guide along your journey and as a resource that you can turn back to whenever new questions or challenges arise. If you cannot find the answer you are looking for within these pages then the final section of this book that follows, offers a plethora of additional supportive resources with everything from recommended readings, apps, and social networks, to places you can buy products and websites that help you find volunteer opportunities, special blood tests, or healthcare providers.

If that is not enough, then join the *A Manner of Living*® community.

By visiting www.AMannerofLiving.com or the *A Manner of Living*® Facebook page, or by following my blog, you join me and a community of like-minded people sharing ideas, challenges, and solutions. You can also keep in touch with me.

I know it may be unorthodox to do so, but as I end my story and you begin to embark upon yours, I want to thank you for supporting me by reading my words. I hope they have served you well and I look forward to being an ongoing support to you both within the pages of this book and online, as you continue to move forward with your new *manner of living*.

Enjoy the journey ahead. It is an exceptional one.

Additional Resources

Self-Tracking and Motivational Tools

Equipment, wearable sensors, and mobile apps to help monitor your health and to help motivate you to achieve your health goals.

Nike+ FuelBand: tracks each step taken and calories burned.
www.nike.com/us/en_us/lp/nikeplus-fuelband

FitBit: tracks activity, calories burned, calories consumed, and sleep habits.
www.fitbit.com

Jawbone: tracks each step taken and calories burned and measures sleep and eating habits.
www.jawbone.com/up

Ihealth: Wireless blood pressure monitor
www.ihealthlabs.com/wireless-blood-pressure-wrist-monitor-feature_33.htm

Withings: Wireless blood pressure monitor
www.withings.com/en/bloodpressuremonitor

LumoBack: An app and device that you wear around your waist designed to help improve your posture.
www.lumoback.com

Pedometer (step counter)
Pocket Pedometer: HJ-112
www.omronwebstore.com/detail/OMR+HJ-112

Resperate: Biofeedback device to help with blood pressure regulation
www.resperate.com

At Home Body Composition Monitoring
Scales for monitoring weight, lean muscle mass, and body fat percentage at home.

Full Body Sensor Body Composition Monitor & Scale: HBF-514C
www.omronwebstore.com/detail/OMR+HBF-514C

Full Body Sensor Body Composition Monitor & Scale: HBF-510W
www.omronwebstore.com/detail/OMR+HBF-510W

Full Body Sensor Body Composition Monitor & Scale: HBF-516B
www.omronwebstore.com/detail/OMR+HBF-516B

Tobacco Cessation
Helpful resources to support smoking cessation.

Nicotine Anonymous: www.nicotine-anonymous.org

My Last Cigarette: An app that offers help for smokers to quit by mapping out changes in their health as they quit.

Smoke Signals: A device to help you quit smoking that was funded by the National Institutes of Health. It is a smart, interactive case that holds a pack of cigarettes. It monitors your habits, and signals when to smoke, gradually weaning you off the habit. www.smokesignals.net

Helpful Health Apps

Lose It! An app that helps you lose fat by tracking your food consumption, comparing it to previous meals, monitoring your nutrient-intake (protein, carbs, fat, etc.), and even has a barcode scanner that can help you log foods by scanning the package.

MyFitnessPal: An app that includes a food diary with a huge database of food items to track calorie intake.

Glooko: A digital logbook app that helps track and monitor blood sugar levels.

I treadmill: A pedometer app that works in your pocket or purse to counts steps, record distance in miles or kilometers and track calories burned.

Runkeeper: An app that allows you to track your walks, runs, bike rides, hikes, etc. It keeps stats on each activity, compares those stats, sets short-term and long-term goals, offers customizable training plans, and voice coaching.

Lift: An app that helps you break down your challenging personal goals into micro habits in order to make it easier to achieve those goals.

Keas: An app for corporate wellness allowing companies to pick health goals and compete against each other to lose weight and get in shape, incentivized by a reward system which offers both real and virtual prizes.

GymPact and **Stikk:** Apps that use peer pressure and cash as incentives to help you achieve your health goals! If you meet your goal you earn a cash reward and if not, the money goes into a community pot and is given to those who do achieve their milestones.

Zombies, run: If you enjoy video games this one's for you. This app immerses you into a game every time you run on a treadmill or outdoors by having zombies chase you as you run! Talk about motivation!

7 minute workout: A free app based on the "scientific 7-minute workout" routine published in the American College of Sports Medicine's Health and Fitness Journal. A great way to incorporate activity into your daily routine.

Locavore: This app lets you find the fruits and vegetables that are in season based on your location and includes a farmer's market finder.

Find Me Gluten Free: This app helps you find gluten-free restaurants, bars, cafes and grocery stores.

CSPI Chemical Cuisine: A searchable list of food additives, their descriptions, and safety ratings from the Center for Science in the Public Interest (CSPI).

Dirty Dozen: From the Environmental Working Group (EWG), this app helps you chose fruits and veggies with the least amount of pesticide residues. Using the EWG's "Dirty Dozen" and "Clean Fifteen" lists, the app can help you decide when to splurge on organic, and when it is okay to choose conventionally-grown food if organic is not available (or if is cost prohibitive).

HarvestMark Food Traceability: Learn where your food comes from with this app that lets you trace your food back to its source. Want to know which farm those eggs are from? Use this app to learn when, where, and how your food was grown, and whether it is safe.

Get Moving
Helpful resources to support increasing your daily activity.

Need a partner to move with? Find like-minded people in your area looking to get fit together. From jogging to group yoga sessions, the activities span every interest and budget.
www.fitness.meetup.com

Need some guidance on a budget? Download activity videos at:
www.exercisetv.tv/workout-videos/all/?videotype=free-full-length

Every day activity site: Great for those with "no time to work out". Great tips and techniques to add activity throughout the day!
www.squeezeitin.com

Lifestyle Medicine Institute founded by Harvard Medical School. Visit their *tools and resources* page to check out their "Drop Everything and Exercise" video for a quick and easy 10 minute workout.
www.instituteoflifestylemedicine.org

Walk/Run Event Locator
www.active.com

Special Activities and Programs for Older Adults
www.silversneakers.com

Eating Well

Helpful resources to support your new manner of eating.

Zipongo: Think Groupon® for health; this website offers personalized discounts and coupons for healthy foods at local grocery stores. www.zipongo.com/signup-wizard

NatureBox: Distributes its own brand of nutritionist-approved health foods and for every box that the company delivers, it donates a meal to feed the hungry in the U.S. www.naturebox.com

Portion control plates

www.theportionplate.com/abouttheplate.html

www.oodora.com/health-and-food/product-reviews/portion-control-plate.html

Online resource for food safety and freshness

Answers to common questions regarding prep and storage
www.stilltasty.com

Finding healthy, safe and sustainable, local seafood

Seafood Watch
www.seafoodwatch.org

National Geographic: Seafood Decision Guide
www.ocean.nationalgeographic.com/ocean/take-action/seafood-decision-guide

Find your local food bank
www.feedingamerica.org

Gluten free dining and restaurant guide
www.triumphdining.com

Vegan and vegetarian friendly restaurants
http://www.happycow.net

Learn whether chemical food additives are safe or not
The Center for Science in the Public Interest
http://cspinet.org/reports/chemcuisine.htm

Nutritional Supplements
Reputable, quality nutritional supplement manufacturers.
NOTE: these are only available through licensed healthcare professionals. Visit their website to find practitioners in your area.

Metagenics: www.metagenics.com
Pure Encapsulations: www.pureencapsulations.com
Standard Process: www.standardprocess.com (for select organic, whole food supplements)

Dietary Supplement Quality Check
Is your supplement doing more harm than good? Check the quality of your supplements by visiting these websites that offer 3rd party testing for nutritional supplements.

1. **Consumer Labs:** www.consumerlabs.org
2. **NSF:** www.nsf.org/certified/gmp/Listings.asp?Program
3. **Natural Products Association:** www.naturalproductsassoc.org
4. **TGA:** www.tga.gov.au
5. **USP:**www.usp.org/USPVerified/dietarySupplements/companies.html

Volunteering
Excellent site to help you connect and give back to a cause in your area that you value: www.volunteermatch.org

Staying Well

Helpful resources for finding practitioners in your area.

Finding a Certified Nutrition Specialist
The Board for Certification of Nutrition Specialists is the certifying body for the Certified Nutrition Specialist (CNS®) www.cbns.org

Finding a Chiropractor
Resources to help you find licensed chiropractors in your area include:
American Chiropractic Association: www.aca.org
Canadian Chiropractic Association: www.chiropracticcanada.ca
Chiropractic Worldwide: www.wfc.org

Finding an Acupuncturist
The National Certification Commission for Acupuncture and Oriental Medicine (NCCAOM®): www.nccaom.org/find-a-nccaom-certified-practitioner

Finding an Ayurvedic Medicine Practitioner
National Ayurvedic Medical Association: www.ayurvedanama.org

Finding a Naturopathic Doctor
American Association of Naturopathic Physicians
www.naturopathic.org

General Holistic Health Resource
An impartial on-line clearing house for holistic approaches to health. The website includes articles of interests, blogs, and a practitioner database: www.ahha.org

Finding a Guided Imagery Practitioner
Academy for Guided Imagery (AGI): www.acadgi.com

Guided Imagery for Health and Healing
Resource for finding guided imagery products.
www.thehealingmind.org

Specialized Lab Testing
Facilities that offer specialized laboratory testing. Speak with your doctor to determine which tests are right for you.

General Screening and Monitoring
WellnessFx: offers self-directed lab screening of common risk factors. www.wellnessfx.com

Health Diagnostic Laboratory Inc.: offers comprehensive laboratory testing for early detection and monitoring of biomarkers for cardiovascular and related diseases. www.hdlabinc.com

Singulex: offers comprehensive testing for cardiopathology/heart function, vascular inflammation/inflammatory, dyslipidemia/lipids, and cardiometabolic status. www.singulex.com

Genetic Testing
Navigenics: uses a saliva sample to give you a view into your DNA, revealing genetic predisposition for select health conditions. www.navigenics.com

Functional laboratory Testing
Genova Diagnostics: offers functional laboratory testing in a wide range of areas including nutritional, digestive, immunology, metabolic function, and endocrinology. www.genovadiagnostics.com

Food Allergy Testing
The ALCAT Test: identifies cellular reactions to over 350 foods, chemicals, and herbs. www.alcat.com

NMR Testing of Cholesterol Particle Size
It is not only quantity of cholesterol that matter but quality. Even if you have low cholesterol, it is important to learn about the size of those cholesterol particles. This test uses nuclear magnetic resonance (NMR) technology to test for cholesterol particle size. Small, dense particles are more likely to cause the plaque in arteries that leads to heart attacks, than large cholesterol particles. www.liposcience.com and www.labcorp.com

About the Author

Practicing What I Preach

Most books limit the *about the author* section to describing the author's credentials and some impressive highlights of their career. While I am proud of my accomplishments and am happy to share them to enhance the credibility of my work, if you are like me you may be curious about more than just my credentials. Often when I read a book about health, food, activity, or lifestyle I wonder; does the author practice what they preach? What do *they* eat? What sort of activity do they do?

So, for those of you that are curious about me, I have decided to take some creative liberties with the *about the author* section of this book. In addition to sharing my professional credentials with you, I will use this section to give you some insight into how I practice what I preach. I also hope this insight will offer you a practical example of how to put *A Manner of Living*® into practice. I therefore dedicate the next few pages to opening the doors to a day in my life: my food, my activity, my *manner of living*. My professional credentials will follow.

My Daily Routine

My daily alarm is set for 5:04 AM. The number 4 is my signature; being born on the 4th day of the 4th month I was destined to have 4 as my lucky number! No clock of mine has ever been set to a time that did not include a number 4.

I brew organic, free-trade certified coffee and start my day, every day, with a warm cup of strong coffee with a splash of unsweetened, carrageenan-free, organic almond milk. The almond milk lends a subtle sweetness to the coffee, rounding out the edge of the strong espresso blends I tend to prefer. Enjoying that warm cup of coffee is as much ritual as it is about sustenance. It is a pleasurable and relaxing reprise before taking on the day; a transition ritual to take me from sleep to the actions that are about to define my day. I enjoy breakfast with my coffee, always within the first 30 minutes of waking and then as the day unfolds, I will eat something every 3 to 4 hours thereafter.

I snack a little in the evening after I get home from work and enjoy my last meal within 2 hours prior to bedtime. I wrap up each day with a decaffeinated ginger tea about 30 minutes prior to bed. Like my morning coffee this too is a sort of ritual, a calming moment marking the end of my day and my preparation for slumber. I purchase a brand of teas that have inspiring messages written on the paper attached to each tea bag. This is a fun little pleasure to look forward to as I unwrap each tea bag and wrap up my day. My head typically hits my pillow by 10:00 PM and sweet slumber comes soon after. Weekend or weekday, my wake-up time remains essentially the same. The only time I tend to deviate from this routine is while travelling or on holiday.

My Activity

My typical day is quite active. After a long commute, (the one seemingly nonnegotiable aspect of living in Southern California) my day usually involves some sedentary time at my desk, interspersed with opportunities to walk across campus for meetings and walking around in front of a class in a lecture hall for at least 2 hours each day. (I can never stand still as I speak!) Whenever possible, I take the stairs, park a little further, walk a little faster (not an easy feat in 4 inch heels – my guilty pleasure!) and inject activity into my day whenever I can.

As far as formal workouts go, I enjoy group activities and have bounced between different types of fitness classes over the years. I cannot resist trying new things and have therefore dabbled in a diverse array of activities including ballet, Pilates, fitness boot camps, stand-up paddle boarding, spinning, yoga, and even aerial silks, and Pound Rockout Workout™ which is a high energy rock and roll inspired workout using drumsticks! However, the activities for which I have the greatest loyalty are ballet and the ballet inspired barre class. Roughly three times a week for years I have participated in classical ballet and barre classes. I have attended various barre studios in Southern California and each has its own distinct style, but my favorite is Cardio Barre. While ballet allows me to dance gracefully to intoxicatingly beautiful classical music, Cardio Barre offers an intense, whole body engaging barre class that is set to fast-paced, high energy music. The class incorporates graceful, yet challenging ballet inspired moves and even after years of loyal attendance, each time I make even just small refinements to my posture, position, or alignment during a class I can feel the transformative effects of their signature movements. Cardio Barre is truly my addiction! I aim to challenge my muscles and my cardiovascular system at least three times each week so on the rare occasion that I cannot attend a class I will either practice ballet at home using Mary Helen Bowers' *Ballet Beautiful* videos or Elise Gulan's *Ballet Conditioning* video as my guide or I will opt to spend 30 to 45 minutes on a treadmill running intervals (alternating between high and low intensity movements). I follow the running with light weight lifting and gentle stretching and balance activities to maintain flexibility and joint stability. This back-up routine also comes in handy when I am travelling.

What Do I Eat?

I adhere to the precise food plan and manner of eating that I describe in this book. The foods in chapter 6 are the foods that are in my pantry and refrigerator and the recipes in chapter 10 are most of the foods I regularly enjoy. In fact, as I mentioned in chapter 10, it is hard for me to break down my meals in terms of conventional breakfast, lunch, and dinner foods since I tend not to make a major distinction between the foods that make-up each of these meals. This likely stems from that fact that when I was a child, my dad would often prepare our breakfast in the morning. It was simply a matter of convenience. My dad had more flexibility with his work schedule while my mom had to be at work early so often he would prepare breakfast for my brother and me. The only problem with this was that my dad's culinary background was limited to the *fend for yourself* bachelor manner of eating! Ergo, my brother and I grew up with breakfast that included sardines on crackers, Hungarian goulash soup, roasted chicken, grilled salmon... in other words; whatever we had as left-over from dinner, whatever we had in cans, or any innovative combination of the two! Many times this slipped over into lunch as well. Traditional lunch foods were foreign to me. Case in point, I never had a peanut butter sandwich until I was in my twenties! Then, my snack afterschool was not a snack in the conventional sense but rather, it was often whatever food my grandmother was preparing for dinner later that night. Sneaking one of her famous wiener schnitzels fresh and steaming hot just as she was making it used to be one of my favorites! (In hindsight, that deep fried European staple was one snack that would now fall into the 20 category of my 80-20 rule!) Dinner was often a delicious meal from my mom; the most intuitively skilled and talented chef I know. My mom rarely follows a recipe, she has an innate talent for cooking and each meal is different but equally delicious. She too showed me there are no rules for cooking; even the rules imposed by recipes are made to be broken! And every meal is more special and better for it.

While I love eating out and experimenting with new foods, my daily routine tends to be quite consistent. Keep in mind that this consistency might be a strategy you wish to adopt as well. Many nutrition experts agree that adhering to a rather routine albeit healthful manner of eating each day is an effective way to maintain a healthy body composition.

As mentioned, my typical choices for breakfast, lunch, and/or dinner will generally include the recipes I listed in chapter 10. I really do eat that stuff! Other than that, **some quick and easy prep or grab and go options I turn to often include one of the combinations described below:**

- ➤ Oven baked fish with a pinch of sea salt, fresh ground pepper, and a drizzle of extra virgin olive oil with mushrooms and other roasted vegetables.
- ➤ A Greek salad with oregano, extra-virgin olive oil, feta cheese, and large chopped red and green peppers, purple onions, tomatoes over greens. I may have this with grilled fish on the side or just on its own.
- ➤ Ratatouille made with tons of veggies including eggplant, peppers, mushrooms, tomatoes, and extra virgin olive oil.
- ➤ 2 poached or sunny-side up eggs, dill, salt, and pepper to taste.
- ➤ 2 egg omelet with mushrooms, peppers, asparagus or any other vegetables I have. I chop up the veggies, and then add spices to taste.
- ➤ Greek yogurt, blueberries, 1 tsp almond butter.
- ➤ A huge, Nicoise style salad with all the veggies I can find and either fresh or canned salmon or tuna.
- ➤ Grilled salmon burger and mushrooms, over mixed greens including baby kale, with Dijon mustard drizzled with aged balsamic vinegar.

➢ Sardines, canned in spring water or spicy marinara sauce, grilled, or as is over gluten free whole grain crackers, jicama slices, or my almond crackers recipe from chapter 10.

➢ Sardines, canned in spring water, mashed with lemon juice over gluten free whole grain crackers or my almond crackers.

➢ Half an avocado or a hollowed out tomato with salmon or tuna salad inside.

➢ Mackerel, canned in spring water, add fresh ground pepper and dill over gluten free whole grain crackers or my almond crackers or mixed into a chopped vegetable salad.

➢ Oysters, canned in extra virgin olive oil, over chopped veggies or shredded green cabbage with lemon pepper.

➢ Canned salmon or tuna with dill, Greek yogurt, a pinch of cayenne pepper and sea salt with you guessed it, gluten free whole grain crackers or my almond crackers. I also like the salmon or tuna salad wrapped in organic seaweed, mixed into a chopped vegetable salad, or over shredded cabbage. It also tastes great with apple or jicama slices.

Remember: Canned mackerel, sardines, salmon, and oysters are all great and inexpensive sources of protein and omega 3 fatty acids.

Snacks that I always keep on hand at the office and on the go:

➢ Raw, unsalted almonds
➢ Pistachio nuts (low sodium)
➢ Raw mixed nuts (always with walnuts)
➢ Hummus and cut veggies
➢ Avocado cut in half with a pinch of pepper and lemon juice
➢ All natural protein bar (if you enjoy the convenience of bars, look for those with less than 10 grams of sugar, at least 5 grams of fiber and that only contain whole, real ingredients with no added sugar)
➢ Hardboiled or deviled egg
➢ Cherry tomatoes, sugar snap peas, raw broccoli, and/or carrot sticks (I will enjoy these with a source of fat such as nuts, black olives, or a dip like hummus or guacamole to help support absorption of the fat soluble nutrients and to improve satiety)

My favorite type of food when I dine out at a restaurant:

No competition: Japanese food. More specifically, sashimi and sushi wins every time, hands down! When dining out, I tend to gravitate towards ethnic flavors like Indian, Japanese, Vietnamese, or Thai food with complex recipes, creative ingredients that are healthy and taste wonderful but that I do not typically have time to prepare at home. I also enjoy Mediterranean food and creative restaurants with chefs that are not afraid to think outside the culinary box. I often consider dining out as entertainment, so I also gravitate towards raw vegan chefs that can do magic with simple ingredients, molecular gastronomy chefs that combine science with whole fresh foods, and chef that are not afraid to break the culinary rules; the meal becomes like a theater for the palate!

And just for fun... my favorite dining out, decadent dessert culinary indulgence:

It is a tie! My first choice would be real Italian coconut gelato or fresh ice cream (the kind with bits of real coconut in it) and while I have had many great ones the best was possibly from the famous Berthillon on Rue Saint-Louis en l'Ile in Paris, France. My other favorite indulgence would have to be the flourless molten dark chocolate cake from True Food Kitchen in Newport Beach, California. They serve it with cocoa nibs and fresh, real vanilla bean ice cream that gives it the most perfect balance of texture and taste. It is pure delightful, decadence. Both are made with whole, real ingredients and you know what? Both really do taste better when you share them!

To clarify, these indulgences are not part of my daily or even my weekly *manner of living*; these are treats I enjoy on rare, special occasions. That said, it is probably best to describe these delicious indulgences by paraphrasing the famous quote from the movie *Sideways* that anytime one delights in these types of delicious treats, that moment *becomes* a special occasion!

So, now that you have a little insight into me personally, what follows is information about my professional background; how I got here.

Professionally speaking…

I am Dr. Gena E. Kadar. I am a Professor, a Certified Nutrition Specialist, and a licensed Doctor of Chiropractic. While I have been published in scholarly journals, *A Manner of Living*® is my first book.

The Training

My professional path began as I graduated from McGill University in Montreal, Canada after completing studies at University of Salamanca, Spain and the Paris Sorbonne University, France. I received my Doctor of Chiropractic Degree from the Southern California University of Health Sciences and my Certified Nutrition Specialist designation was granted through the Certification Board for Nutrition Specialists.

The Doctor

For nearly a decade I led a successful clinical nutrition and chiropractic practice. I also served as a Corporate Wellness Consultant leading multinational companies in the development and implementation of innovative wellness initiatives and worked as Executive Director of *The Dick Butkus Center for Cardiovascular Wellness*, a nonprofit organization committed to preventing the loss of life from sudden cardiac arrest and cardiovascular disease. I previously served on the board of directors of the *Orange County California Chiropractic Association* and currently serve on the board of directors of the *American Holistic Health Association*. For four consecutive years I had the privilege of serving as Chair of *University of California Irvine, School of Medicine's Susan Samueli Center for Integrative Medicine's* Annual Women's Wellness Conference, and I am truly humbled that among a distinguished group of honorees, this same institution selected me as a recipient of a 2012 Teaching Award.

The Professor

In 2010, I assumed the role of teacher, initially as an Assistant Professor and now as an Associate Professor of Clinical Nutrition at *Southern California University of Health Sciences (SCU)*. This was intended as a temporary move in order to gain experience in research, but little did I know that teaching would become my passion; a calling I never knew I had.

At SCU I had the distinction of serving as President of the Faculty Senate, and Chair of the Department of Healthcare and Community Integration, Chair of the Professional Personnel Committee, Chair of the Academic Programs Task Force, and Chair of the Task force on Interdisciplinary Education. I have also been granted various awards and recognitions for my teaching, service to the institution, and research. Most recently I was appointed Chair of the Division of Integrative Health Sciences.

The Inspiration

My proudest achievement to date is the completion of this, my first book. I began writing *A Manner of Living*® in 2009 as I sat by my father's bedside in a hospital in Canada. My father was a brilliant intellectual, a fearless trailblazer, an eminent aerospace engineer, and an overall exceptional human being. I do not use these descriptions frivolously as he personified each of these qualities more than any person I have ever met. He was truly one of a kind. Too many stories to tell, but in his battle with advanced pancreatic cancer he reinvented the way patients deal with this dreaded disease. Over the course of six years he achieved two previously unheard of remissions and in the process, inspired and supported at least 60 other individuals from across the world that were battling the same disease. My father passed away on November 2nd, 2009 but not before forging a brightly lit path for others to follow. His brilliance and fortitude is ever-present, and inspires me each day. It is my father's drive that infused me with the inspiration to craft this book.

A Manner of Living® evolved organically; the vision and outline of the entire text emerged one night in my mind's eye as I sat by my father's side in that Canadian hospital room. Over the last few months that my dad fought his relentless battle, each night as I sat at my dad's side, the keystrokes on my laptop could barely keep up with the pace of the thoughts emerging from my mind. Soon, the draft for *A Manner of Living*® materialized; its content took well over four years to complete. The completion of *A Manner of Living*® is now just the beginning; the blog by the same name is an extension of my voice from the pages of this book and plans for additional books and exciting collaborations are already in progress. I hope *A Manner of Living*® inspires and supports you to live your healthiest and most *exceptional* life, just as my father has done for me.

348

Keeping in Touch

So dear reader that is *my* story; how I got here and my typical day, my typical food, my typical activity: my *manner of living*. I hope my daily routine serves not as a template for you, but rather as an example of one way to apply the advice outlined in the pages of this book. As you develop your new *manner of living* I hope that through my website, blog, and Facebook page you will share with me and the other members of the *A Manner of Living*® community, an example of a day in *your* life; *your manner of living*. I look forward to hearing from you.

> ## Join the **A Manner of Living**® community at:
>
> www.AMannerofLiving.com
>
> www.AMannerofLiving.wordpress.com
>
> www.facebook.com/AMannerofLiving

References

[1] Fraga M, Ballestar, E, Paz, MF, Ropero, S, Setien, F, Ballestar, ML, et al. Epigenetic differences arise during the lifetime of monozygotic twins, Proc Natl Acad Sci USA. 2005 Jul 26; 102(30):10604-10609.

[2] Dolinoy DC, Huang D, Jirtle RL. Maternal nutrient supplementation counteracts bisphenol A-induced DNA hypomethylation in early development. Proc Natl Acad Sci USA. 2007; 104:13056-13061.

[3] Waterland RA, Jirtle RL. Transposable elements: targets for early nutritional effects on epigenetic gene regulation. Mol Cell Biol. 2003; 23:5293-5300.

[4] Guerrero-Bosagna C, Valladares L. Endocrine disruptors, epigenetically induced changes, and transgenerational transmission of characters and epigenetic states. In: Gore, Andrea C (ed.), Endocrine-disrupting chemicals: from basic research to clinical practice. New York, New York: Humana Press 2007; 175-189.

[5] Anway MD, Skinner MK. Epigenetic programming of the germ line: effects of endocrine disruptors on the development of transgenerational disease. Reprod Biomed Online. 2008; 16:23-25.

[6] Yang BZ, Zhang H, Ge W, Weder N, Douglas-Palumberi H, Perepletchikova F, et al. Child Abuse and Epigenetic Mechanisms of Disease Risk. Am J Prev Med. 2013 Feb; 44(2):101–107.

[7] Fahey J, Zhang Y, Talalay P. Broccoli sprouts: an exceptionally rich source of inducers of enzymes that protect against chemical carcinogens. Proc Natl Acad Sci USA. 1997; 94: 10367–10372.

[8] Ho E, Clarke J, Dashwood R. Dietary sulforaphane, a histone deacetylase inhibitor for cancer prevention. J Nutr. 2009; 139: 2393–2396.

[9] Xiao D, Powolny A, Antosiewicz J, Hahm E, Bommareddy A, et al. Cellular responses to cancer chemopreventive agent D,L-sulforaphane in human prostate cancer cells are initiated by mitochondrial reactive oxygen species. Pharm Res. 2009; 26: 1729–1738.

[10] Myzak M, Tong P, Dashwood W, Dashwood R, Ho E. Sulforaphane retards the growth of human PC-3 xenografts and inhibits HDAC activity in human subjects. Exp Biol Med (Maywood). 2007; 232: 227–234.

[11] Waterland RA, Jirtle RL. Transposable elements: targets for early nutritional effects on epigenetic gene regulation. Mol Cell Biol. 2003 Aug; 23(15):5293-300.

[12] Pembrey ME, Bygren LO, Kaati G, et al. Sex-specific, male-line transgenerational responses in humans. Eur J Hum Genet. 2006; 14:159-166.

[13] Nestler EJ. Epigenetics: Stress makes its molecular mark. Nature. 2012 Oct 11; 490,171–172.

[14] Talens RP, Christensen K, Putter H, Willemsen G, Christiansen L, Kremer D, et al. Epigenetic variation during the adult lifespan: cross-sectional and longitudinal data on monozygotic twin pairs. Aging Cell. 2012; 11:694–703.

[15] Wing RR, Hill JO. Successful weight loss maintenance. Annu Rev Nutr. 2001; 21:323-341.

[16] Beavers KM, Lyles MF, Davis CC, Wang X, Beavers DP, Nicklas BJ. Is lost

lean mass from intentional weight loss recovered during weight regain in postmenopausal women? Am J Clin Nutr. 2011 Sep; 94(3): 767-74.

[17]Anderson JW, Konz EC, Frederich RC, Wood CL. Long-term weight-loss maintenance: a meta-analysis of US studies. Am J Clin Nutr. 2001;74:579-584

[18] Mason C, Foster-Schubert KE, Imayama I, Xiao L, Kong A, Campbell KL, et al. History of weight cycling does not impede future weight loss or metabolic improvements in postmenopausal women. Metabolism. 2013 Jan; 62(1): 127-36.

[19] Metter EJ, Talbot LA, Schrager M, Conwit R. Skeletal muscle strength as a predictor of all-cause mortality in healthy men. J Gerontol A Biol Sci Med Sci. 2002 Oct; 57(10):B359-65.

[20] Source: www.nlm.nih.gov/medlineplus/ency/article/007196.htm

[21] Janssen I. The epidemiology of sarcopenia. Clin Geriatr Med. 2011 Aug; 27(3): 355-63.

[22] Rosenberg IH. Sarcopenia: origins and clinical relevance. J Nutr. 1997 May; 127(5 Suppl):990S-991S.

[23] Stenholm S, Harris TB, Rantanen T, Visser M, Kritchevsky SB, Ferrucci L. Sarcopenic obesity: definition, cause and consequences. Curr Opin Clin Nutr Metab Care. 2008 Nov; 11(6):693-700.

[24] Frontera WR, Hughes VA, Fielding RA, Fiatarone MA, Evans WJ, Roubenoff R. Aging of skeletal muscle: a 12-yr longitudinal study. J Appl Physiol. 2000; 88:1321–1326.

[25] Roubenoff R. Sarcopenic Obesity: The Confluence of Two Epidemics. Obes Res. 2004 Jun; 12(6):887-8.

[26] Beaufrere B, Morio B. Fat and protein redistribution with aging: metabolic considerations. Eur J Clin Nutr. 2000; 54(Suppl 3):S48–53.

[27] Khamseh ME, Malek M, Aghili R, Emami Z. Sarcopenia and diabetes: pathogenesis and consequences, British Journal of Diabetes & Vascular Disease Sept/Oct 2011; 11(5): 230-234.

[28] Karakelides H, Nair KS. Sarcopenia of aging and its metabolic impact. Curr Top Dev Biol. 2005; 68:123-48.

[29] Roubenoff R. Sarcopenic Obesity: The Confluence of Two Epidemics. Obes Res. 2004 Jun; 12(6):887-8.

[30]Sam S, Haffner S, Davidson MH, D'Agostino RB Sr, Feinstein S, et al. Relation of Abdominal Fat Depots to Systemic Markers of Inflammation in Type 2 Diabetes. Diabetes Care. 2009 May; 32(5): 932–937.

[31] Ross R. Atherosclerosis - an inflammatory disease. N Engl J Med 1999; 340:115-126.

[32] Donath MY, Shoelson SEType 2 diabetes as an inflammatory disease.Nat Rev Immunol. 2011 Feb; 11(2):98-107.

[33] Wilcock DM. A Changing Perspective on the Role of Neuroinflammation in Alzheimer's Disease. Int J Alzheimers Dis. 2012; 2012:495243.

[34] Porta C, Larghi P, Rimoldi M, Totaro MG, Allavena P, Mantovani A, Sica A. Cellular and molecular pathways linking inflammation and cancer. Immunobiology. 2009; 214(9-10):761-77.

[35] Bergman, RN, Kim, SP, Catalano, KJ, Hsu, IR, Chiu, JD, Kabir, M, et al. Why

Visceral Fat is Bad: Mechanisms of the Metabolic Syndrome. Obesity. 2006; 14:16S–19S.

[36] Klein S, Allison DB., Heymsfield, SB, Kelley DE, Leibel RL, Nonas C, Kahn R. Waist Circumference and Cardiometabolic Risk: A Consensus Statement from Shaping America's Health: Association for Weight Management and Obesity Prevention; NAASO, The Obesity Society; the American Society for Nutrition; and the American Diabetes Association. Obesity, 2007; 15: 1061–1067.

[37] Source: www.cdc.gov/healthyweight/assessing/index.html

[38] Browning LM, Hsieh SD, Ashwell M. A systematic review of waist-to-height ratio as a screening tool for the prediction of cardiovascular disease and diabetes: 0·5 could be a suitable global boundary value. Nutr Res Rev. 2010; 23: 247–269.

[39] Lee CM, Huxley RR, Wildman RP, Woodward M. Indices of abdominal obesity are better discriminators of cardiovascular risk factors than BMI: a meta-analysis. J Clin Epidemiol. 2008; 61: 646–653

[40] Mombelli G, Zanaboni AM, Gaito S, Sirtori CR. Waist-to-height ratio is a highly sensitive index for the metabolic syndrome in a Mediterranean population. Metab Syndr Relat Disord 2009, 7: 477–484.

[41] Browning LM, Hsieh SD, Ashwell M. A systematic review of waist-to-height ratio as a screening tool for the prediction of cardiovascular disease and diabetes: 0.5 could be a suitable global boundary value. Nutr Res Rev. 2010, 23(2):247–269

[42] Kim HH, Cho S, Lee S, Kim KH, Cho KH, Eun HC, Chung JH. Photoprotective and anti-skin-aging effects of eicosapentaenoic acid in human skin in vivo. J Lipid Res. 2006 May; 47(5):921-30.

[43] Rojas P., Gosch M., Basfi-fer K., Carrasco F., Codoceo J., Inostroza J, et al. Alopecia in women with severe and morbid obesity who undergo bariatric surgery. Nutr. Hosp. 2011 Aug; 26(4): 856-862.

[44] Pollan M. In Defense of Food: An Eater's Manifesto. Penguin; 1 edition, Jan 1, 2008.

[45] Ibid.

[46] Simon, HB. The Harvard Medical School guide to men's health. New York: Free Press. 2002; pp. 31.

[47] Roland PE, Eriksson L, Stone-Elander S, Widen L. Does mental activity change the oxidative metabolism of the brain? J Neuroscience. 1987 Aug 1; 7(8): 2373-2389.

[48] Fairclough SH, Houston K. A metabolic measure of mental effort. Biol Psychol. 2004 Apr;66(2):177-90.

[49] Scholey AB, Harper S, Kennedy DO. Cognitive demand and blood glucose. Physiol Behav. 2001 Jul; 73(4):585-92.

[50] Cahill GF, Herrera MG, Morgan AP, Soeldner JS, Steinke J, Levy PL, Reichard GA, Kipnis DM. Hormone-fuel interrelationships during fasting. J Clin Invest. 1966; 45:1751–1769.

[51] Source: www.circ.ahajournals.org/content/120/11/1011.full.pdf

[52] Source: www.hsph.harvard.edu/nutritionsource/healthy-drinks/how-sweet-is-it/index.html

[53] Source:

www.nhs.uk/chq/Pages/1139.aspx?CategoryID=51&SubCategoryID=167

[54] Krabbe KS, Nielsen AR, Krogh-Madsen R, Plomgaard P, Rasmussen P, Erikstrup C, et al. Brain-derived neurotrophic factor (BDNF) and type 2 diabetes. Diabetologia. 2007 Feb; 50(2):431-8.

[55] Molteni R, Barnard RJ, Ying Z, Roberts CK, Gómez-Pinilla F. A high-fat, refined sugar diet reduces hippocampal brain-derived neurotrophic factor, neuronal plasticity, and learning. Neuroscience. 2002; 112(4):803-14.

[56] Chan YK, Estaki M, Gibson DL. Clinical consequences of diet-induced dysbiosis. Ann Nutr Metab. 2013; 63 Suppl 2:28-40.

[57] Malik VS, Popkin, BM, Bray, GA, Despres, JP, Willett, WC, Hu FB. Sugar-sweetened beverages and risk of metabolic syndrome and type 2 diabetes, Diabetes Care. 2010; 33(11): 2477-2483.

[58] 3. Johnson RK, Appel LJ, Brands M, et al. Dietary sugars intake and cardiovascular health: a scientific statement from the American Heart Association. Circulation. 2009; 120:1011-20.

[59] Mitra A, Gosnell BA, Schiöth HB, Grace MK, Klockars A, Olszewski PK, Levine AS. Chronic sugar intake dampens feeding-related activity of neurons synthesizing a satiety mediator, oxytocin, Peptides. 2010 July; 31(7): 1346–1352.

[60] Yang Q, Zhang Z, Gregg EW, Flanders WD, Merritt R, Hu FB. Added Sugar Intake and Cardiovascular Diseases Mortality among US Adults. JAMA Intern Med. 2014 Apr; 174(4):516-24.

[61] Hallberg L, Brune M, Rossander L. Iron absorption in man: ascorbic acid and dose-dependent inhibition by phytate. Am. J. Clin Nutr.1989; 49:140-144.

[62] Davidsson L, Almgren A, Juillerat MA, Hurrell RF. Manganese absorption in humans: the effect of phytic acid and ascorbic acid in soy formula. Am. J. Clin. Nutr. 1995; 62:984-987.

[63] Weaver CM, Heaney RP, Martin BR, Fitzsimmons ML. Human calcium absorption from whole wheat products. J. Nutr. 1991; 121:1769-1775.

[64] Nävert B, Sandström B, Cederblad A, Reduction of the phytate content of bran by leavening in bread and its effect on zinc absorption in man. Br. J. Nutr. 1985; 53:47-53.

[65] Weaver CM, Kannan S. Phytate and mineral bioavailability. In: Reddy NR, Sathe SK (eds). Food Phytates. CRC Press: Boca Raton, FL, 2002; pp 211–223.

[66] Hurrell RF, Influence of Vegetable Protein Sources on Trace Element and Mineral Bioavailability· J. Nutr. Sep 1, 2003; 133, 92973S-2977S.

[67] Tannenbaum SR, Young VR, Archer MC. Vitamins and minerals. In Fennema OR, ed. Food Chemistry. New York: Marcel Dekker, Inc., 1985; p 445.

[68] Shamsuddin AM, Anti-cancer function of phytic acid. International Journal of Food Science & Technology, 2002; 37: 769–782.

[69] Walker ARP, Fox FW, Irving JT. The Effect of Bread Rich in Phytate Phosphorus on the metabolism of Certain Mineral Salts with Special Reference to Calcium. The Biochemical Journal 1948; 42(1):452-461.

[70] Marero LM, Payumo EM, Aguinaldo AR., Matsumoto I, Homma S. The antinutritional factors in weaning foods prepared from germinated legumes and cereals. Lebensmittelwissenschaft Technol. 1991; 24:177-181.

[71] Sathe SK, Venkatachalam M. Influence of Processing Technologies on Phytate and Its Removal. In: Reddy NR, Sathe SK (eds). Food Phytates, CRC Press, 2001; p 170.

[72] Hallberg L, Brune M, Rossander L. Iron absorption in man: ascorbic acid and dose-dependent inhibition by phytate. Amer J Clin Nutr. Jan 1989. 49(1):140-144.

[73] Tuntawiroon M, Sritongkul N, Rossander-Hultén L, Pleehachinda R, Suwanik R, Brune M, Hallberg L. Rice and Iron absorption in man. Eur J Clin Nutr. 1990 Jul; 44(7):489-97.

[74] Layrisse M, García-Casal MN, Solano L, Barón MA, Arguello F, Llovera D, et al. New property of vitamin A and B carotene on human iron absorption: effect on phytate and polyphenols as inhibitors of iron absorption. Arch Latinoam Nutr. 2000 Sep; 50(3):243-8.

[75] Famularo G, De Simone C, Pandey V, Sahu AR, Minisola G. Probiotic lactobacilli: an innovative tool to correct the malabsorption syndrome of vegetarians? Medical Hypotheses. 2005; 65(6):1132–5.

[76] Bulhões AC, Goldani HAS, Oliveira FS, Matte US, Mazzuca RB, Silveira TR. Correlation between lactose absorption and the C/T-13910 and G/A-22018 mutations of the lactase-phlorizin hydrolase (LCT) gene in adult-type hypolactasia. Brazilian Journal of Medical and Biological Research 2007; 40 (11): 1441–6.

[77] Hawrelak JA, Myers SP. The causes of intestinal dysbiosis: a review. Altern Med Rev. 2004 Jun; 9(2):180-97.

[78] Sekirov I, Russell S, Caetano L, Antunes M, Finlay BB. Gut microbiota in health and disease. Am. Physiol. Soc. 2010; 90:859–904.

[79] Montemurno E, Cosola C, Dalfino G, Daidone G, De Angelis M, Gobbetti M, Gesualdo L., What Would You Like to Eat, Mr CKD Microbiota? A Mediterranean Diet, please! Kidney Blood Press Res. 2014 Jul 29; 39(2-3):114-123.

[80] Chan YK, Estaki M, Gibson DL. Clinical consequences of diet-induced dysbiosis. Ann Nutr Metab. 2013; 63 Suppl 2:28-40.

[81] Power SE, O'Toole PW, Stanton C, Ross RP, Fitzgerald GF, Intestinal microbiota, diet and health. Br J Nutr. 2014 Feb; 111(3):387-402.

[82] Rescigno M. Intestinal microbiota and its effects on the immune system. Cell Microbiol. 2014 Jul; 16(7):1004-13.

[83] Petrof EO, Claud EC, Gloor GB, Allen-Vercoe E., Microbial ecosystems therapeutics: a new paradigm in medicine? Benef Microbes. 2013 Mar 1; 4(1):53-65.

[84] Bested AC, Logan AC, Selhub EM. Intestinal microbiota, probiotics and mental health: from Metchnikoff to modern advances: Part II - contemporary contextual research. Gut Pathog. 2013 Mar 14; 5(1):3.

[85] Montemurno E, Cosola C, Dalfino G, Daidone G, De Angelis M, Gobbetti M, Gesualdo L. What Would You Like to Eat, Mr CKD Microbiota? A Mediterranean Diet, please! Kidney Blood Press Res. 2014 Jul 29; 39(2-3):114-123.

[86] Brown K, DeCoffe D, Molcan E, Gibson DL. Diet-induced dysbiosis of the

intestinal microbiota and the effects on immunity and disease. Nutrients. 2012 Aug;4(8):1095-119.

[87] Lawrence GD. Dietary fats and health: dietary recommendations in the context of scientific evidence. Adv Nutr. 2013 May 1; 4(3):294-302.

[88] Raz O, Steinvil A, Berliner S, Tovit R, Justo D, Shapira I. The effect of two iso-caloric meals containing equal amounts of fats with a different fat composition on the inflammatory and metabolic markers in apparently healthy volunteers. J Inflamm (Lond). 2013 Jan 31; 10(1):3.

[89] Yamagishi K, Iso H, Kokubo Y, Saito I, Yatsuya H, Ishihara J, et al. Dietary intake of saturated fatty acids and incident stroke and coronary heart disease in Japanese communities: the JPHC Study. Eur Heart J. 2013 Apr; 34(16):1225-32.

[90] Thiébaut AC, Jiao L, Silverman DT, Cross AJ, Thompson FE, Subar AF, et al. Dietary fatty acids and pancreatic cancer in the NIH-AARP diet and health study. J Natl Cancer Inst. 2009 Jul 15; 101(14):1001-11.

[91] Chowdhury R, Warnakula S, Kunutsor S, et al. Association of Dietary, Circulating, and Supplement Fatty Acids With Coronary Risk: A Systematic Review and Meta-analysis. Intern Med. 2014; 160(6):398-406.

[92] Paddon-Jones D, Westman E, Mattes RD, Wolfe RR, et al. Protein, weight management, and satiety Am J Clin Nutr May 2008 87: 5 1558S-1561S

[93] Westerterp-Plantenga MS, Lejeune MP. Protein intake and body-weight regulation. Appetite 2005; 45:187–90.

[94] Layman DK. Protein quantity and quality at levels above the RDA improves adult weight loss. J Am Coll Nutr 2004; 23:631S–6S.

[95] Westerterp-Plantenga MS, Lejeune MP, Nijs I, van Ooijen M, Kovacs EM. High protein intake sustains weight maintenance after body weight loss in humans. Int J Obes Relat Metab Disord 2004; 28:57–64.

[96] Larsen TM. Diets with high or low protein content and glycemic index for weight-loss maintenance. N Engl J Med. 2010 Nov 25; 363(22):2102-13.

[97] Pan A, Sun Q, Bernstein AM, Schulze, MB, Manson, JE, Stampfer MJ, Willett WC, Hu FB. Red Meat Consumption and Mortality Results From 2 Prospective Cohort Studies. Arch Intern Med. 2012; 172(7):555-563.

[98] Feskens EJ, Sluik D, van Woudenbergh GJ. Meat Consumption, Diabetes, and Its Complications. Curr Diab Rep. 2013 Apr; 13(2):298-306.

[99] Wollstonecroft MM, Ellis PR, Hillman GC, Fuller DQ, Butterworth PJ. A calorie is not necessarily a calorie: Technical choice, nutrient bioaccessibility, and interspecies differences of edible plants. Proc Natl Acad Sci U S A. 2012 Apr 24; 109(17):E991.

[100] Novotny J, Gebauer S, Baer D. Discrepancy between the Atwater factor predicted and empirically measured energy values of almonds in human diets. Am J Clin Nutr. August 2012; 96(2):296-301.

[101] Barr SB, Wright JC. Postprandial energy expenditure in whole-food and processed-food meals: implications for daily energy expenditure. Food Nutr Res. 2010 Jul 2; 54.

[102] Carmody R, Weintraub G, Wrangham R. Energetic consequences of thermal and nonthermal food processing. Proc Natl Acad Sci U S A. 2011 Nov 29;

108(48):19199-19203.

[103] Aravanis C, Corcondilas A, Dontas AS, Lekos D, Keys A. Coronary heart disease in seven countries, Circulation 1970 Apr; 41 (4 Suppl): I1–211.

[104] Keys A, Aravanis C, Blackburn HW, Van Buchem FS, Buzina R, Djordjević BD, et al. Epidemiological studies related to coronary heart disease: characteristics of men aged 40-59 in seven countries. Acta Med Scand Suppl. 1966; 460:1-392.

[105] Knoops KT, de Groot LC, Kromhout D, Perrin AE, Moreiras-Varela O, Menotti A, van Staveren WA. Mediterranean diet, lifestyle factors, and 10-year mortality in elderly European men and women: the HALE project. JAMA. 2004 Sep 22; 292(12):1433-9.

[106] Sanchez-Villegas A, Delgado-Rodriguez M, Alonso A, Schlatter J, Lahortiga F, Serra Majem L, Martinez-Gonzalez MA. Association of the Mediterranean Dietary Pattern with the Incidence of Depression: The Seguimiento Universidad de Navarra/University of Navarra Follow-up (SUN) Cohort. Arch Gen Psychiatry. 2009; 66(10):1090–1098.

[107] Nuñez-Cordoba JM, Alonso A, Beunza JJ, Palma S, Gomez-Gracia E, Martinez-Gonzalez MA. Role of vegetables and fruits in Mediterranean diets to prevent hypertension. Eur J Clin Nutr. 2009 May; 63(5):605-12.

[108] Psaltopoulou T, Naska A, Orfanos P, Trichopoulos D, Mountokalakis T, Trichopoulou A. Olive oil, the Mediterranean diet, and arterial blood pressure: the Greek European Prospective Investigation into Cancer and Nutrition (EPIC) study, Amer J Clin Nutr. 2004 Oct 80(4): 1012-1018, Errata Col. 81, 1181.

[109] Scarmeas N, Luchsinger JA, Mayeux R, Stern Y. Mediterranean diet and Alzheimer disease mortality. Neurology. 2007 Sep 11; 69(11):1084-93.

[110] Esposito K, Marfella R, Ciotola M, et al. Effect of a Mediterranean style diet on endothelial dysfunction and markers of vascular inflammation in the metabolic syndrome: a randomized trial. JAMA. 2004; 292:1440-1446.

[111] Shai I, Schwarzfuchs D, Henkin Y, Shahar DR, Witkow S, Greenberg I, et al. Weight loss with a low-carbohydrate, Mediterranean, or low-fat diet. N Engl J Med. 2008 Jul 17; 359 (3): 229–241.

[112] Kastorini C-M, Milionis H, Esposito K, Giugliano D, Goudevenos J, Panagiotakos D. The Effect of Mediterranean Diet on Metabolic Syndrome and its Components. J Am Coll Cardiol. 2011; 57 (11): 1299–1313.

[113] Estruch R, Ros E, Salas-Salvado J, Covas MI, Corella D, Arós F, et al. Primary prevention of cardiovascular disease with a Mediterranean diet. N Engl J Med. 2013; 368:1279-1290.

[114] Estruch R, Ros E, Salas-Salvado J, Covas MI, Corella D, Arós F, et al. Primary prevention of cardiovascular disease with a Mediterranean diet. N Engl J Med. 2013; 368:1279-1290.

[115] Ramjee V, Jacobson T. Intensifying Statin Therapy to Maximize Cardiovascular Risk Reduction. Clin Lipidology. 2011;6(2):131-136.

[116] Knoops KT, de Groot LC, Kromhout D, Perrin AE, Moreiras-Varela O, Menotti A, van Staveren WA. Mediterranean diet, lifestyle factors, and 10-year mortality in elderly European men and women: the HALE project. JAMA. 2004 Sep 22; 292(12):1433-9.

[117] Jenkins DJ, Wolever TM, Taylor RH, et al. Glycemic index of foods: a physiological basis for carbohydrate exchange. Am J Clin Nutr. 1981 Mar; 34(3): 362–6.

[118] Jenkins DJ, Kendall CW, McKeown-Eyssen G, Josse RG, Silverberg J, Booth GL, et al. Effect of a low-glycemic index or a high-cereal fiber diet on type 2 diabetes: a randomized trial. JAMA. 2008 Dec; 300(23):2742–53.

[119] Lennerz BS, Alsop DC, Holsen LM, Stern E, Rojas R, Ebbeling CB, Goldstein JM, Ludwig DS. Effects of dietary glycemic index on brain regions related to reward and craving in men. Am J Clin Nutr. 2013 Sep;98(3):641-7.

[120] Thomas DE, Elliott EJ, Baur L. Low glycaemic index or low glycaemic load diets for overweight and obesity. Cochrane Database Syst Rev. 2007 Jul 18; (3):CD005105.

[121] Pereira MA, Swain J, Goldfine AB, Rifai N, Ludwig DS. Effects of a low-glycemic load diet on resting energy expenditure and heart disease risk factors during weight loss. JAMA. 2004:292(20)2482-24900.

[122] ADA Position Paper, July 2009 Journal of the American Dietetic Association

[123] Orlich MJ, Singh PN, Sabaté J, Jaceldo-Siegl K, Fan J, Knutsen S, Beeson WL, Fraser GE. Vegetarian dietary patterns and mortality in Adventist Health Study 2. JAMA Intern Med. 2013 Jul 8; 173(13):1230-8.

[124] Lopez-Garcia E, Schulze MB, Fung TT, Meigs JB, Rifai N, Manson JE, Hu FB. Major dietary patterns are related to plasma concentrations of markers of inflammation and endothelial dysfunction. Am J Clin Nutr. 2004 Oct; 80(4): 1029-35.

[125] Dandona P, Aljada A, Chaudhuri A, Mohanty P, Garg R. Metabolic syndrome: a comprehensive perspective based on interactions between obesity, diabetes, and inflammation. Circulation. 2005; 111:1448–1454.

[126] Donath MY, Shoelson SE. Type 2 diabetes as an inflammatory disease. Nat Rev Immunol. 2011 Feb; 11(2):98-107.

[127] Wilcock DM. A Changing Perspective on the Role of Neuroinflammation in Alzheimer's Disease. Int J Alzheimers Dis. 2012;2012:495243.

[128] Porta C, Larghi P, Rimoldi M, Totaro MG, Allavena P, Mantovani A, Sica A. Cellular and molecular pathways linking inflammation and cancer. Immunobiology. 2009; 214(9-10):761-77.

[129] Ridker PM. C-reactive protein and the prediction of cardiovascular events among those at intermediate risk: moving an inflammatory hypothesis toward consensus. J Am Coll Cardiol. 2007 May 29;49(21):2129-38.

[130] Richard C, Couture P, Desroches S, Lamarche B. Effect of the Mediterranean diet with and without weight loss on markers of inflammation in men with metabolic syndrome. Obesity (Silver Spring). 2013 Jan; 21(1):51-7.

[131] Panagiotakos DB, Dimakopoulou K, Katsouyanni K, Bellander T, Grau M, Koenig W, Lanki T, et al. Mediterranean diet and inflammatory response in myocardial infarction survivors. Int J Epidem. 2009; 38(3):856-866.

[132] Richard C, Couture P, Desroches S, Lamarche B. Effect of the Mediterranean diet with and without weight loss on markers of inflammation in men with metabolic syndrome. Obesity (Silver Spring). 2013 Jan; 21(1):51-7.

[133] O'Keefe JH, Bybee KA, Lavie CJ. Alcohol and cardiovascular health: the razor-sharp double-edged sword. J Am Coll Cardiol. 2007 Sep 11; 50(11):1009-14.

[134] Mifflin MD, St Jeor ST, Hill LA, Scott BJ, Daugherty SA, Koh YO. A new predictive equation for resting energy expenditure in healthy individuals. Am J Clin Nutr. 1990 51 (2): 241–7.

[135] Frankenfield D, Roth-Yousey L, Compher C., Comparison of predictive equations for resting metabolic rate in healthy nonobese and obese adults: a systematic review. J Am Diet Assoc. 2005 May; 105(5):775-89.

[136] Frankenfield DC, Bias and accuracy of resting metabolic rate equations in non-obese and obese adults, Clinical Nutrition 2013 Dec 32(6): 976-982.

[137] Zello GA. Dietary Reference Intakes for the macronutrients and energy: considerations for physical activity. Appl Physiol Nutr Metab. 2006 Feb; 31(1):74-9.

[138] Almoosawi S, Prynne CJ, Hardy R, Stephen AM. Time-of-day of energy intake: association with hypertension and blood pressure 10 years later in the 1946 British Birth Cohort. J Hypertens. 2013 May; 31(5):882-92.

[139] Obesity 2010: The Obesity Society 28th Annual Scientific Meeting. Poster 202-P. Presented October 12, 2010.

[140] Baron KG, Reid KJ, Kern AS, Zee PC. Role of sleep timing in caloric intake and BMI. Obesity (Silver Spring). 2011 Jul; 19(7):1374-81.

[141] Garaulet M, Gómez-Abellán P, Alburquerque-Béjar JJ, Lee YC, Ordovás JM, Scheer FA. Timing of food intake predicts weight loss effectiveness. Int J Obes (Lond). 2013 Apr; 37(4):604-11.

[142] Adapted from: www.webmd.com/diet/healthtool-food-calorie-counter, the Institute of Functional Medicine, www.choosemyplate.gov/food-groups/vegetables.html and www.calorieking.com/foods/

[143] Dr. Seuss, Green Eggs and Ham, Random House, August 12, 1960.

[144] Source:www.fda.gov/food/guidancecomplianceregulatoryinformation/guidance documents/foodlabelingnutrition/ucm053455.htm

[145] Source: www.cancer.gov/cancertopics/factsheet/Risk/artificial-sweeteners

[146] Soffritti M, Belpoggi F, Esposti DD, Lambertini L. Aspartame induces lymphomas and leukaemias in rats. Eur J Oncology. 2005; 10, 107-116.

[147] Swithers, SE. Artificial sweeteners produce the counterintuitive effect of inducing metabolic derangements. Trends Endocrinol Metab. 2013; 24(9): 431-441.

[148] Suez J, Korem T, Zeevi D, Zilberman-Schapira G, Thaiss CA, Maza O, Israeli D, et al. Artificial sweeteners induce glucose intolerance by altering the gut microbiota. Nature. 2014 Oct 9; 514(7521):181-6.

[149] Bray GA, Nielsen SJ, Popkin BM. Consumption of high-fructose corn syrup in beverages may play a role in the epidemic of obesity. Am J Clin Nutr. 2004 Apr; 79(4):537-43. Review. Erratum in: Am J Clin Nutr. 2004 Oct;80(4):1090.

[150] van Buul VJ, Tappy L, Brouns FJ. Misconceptions about fructose-containing sugars and their role in the obesity epidemic. Nutr Res Rev. 2014 Jun; 27(1):119-30.

[151] Bray GA, Nielsen SJ, Popkin BM. Consumption of high-fructose corn syrup in beverages may play a role in the epidemic of obesity. Am J Clin Nutr. 2004; 79(4):537-43. Review.

[152] Pollock NK, Bundy V, Kanto W, Davis CL, Bernard PJ, Zhu H, Gutin B, Dong Y. Greater fructose consumption is associated with cardiometabolic risk markers and visceral adiposity in adolescents. J Nutr. 2012 Feb; 142(2):251-7.

[153] Mozaffarian D, Katan MB, Ascherio A, Stampfer MJ, Willett WC. Trans Fatty Acids and Cardiovascular Disease, N Engl J Med 2006 Apy 13; 354:1601-1613.

[154] Teegala SM, Willett WC, Mozaffarian D. Consumption and health effects of trans fatty acids: A review. J AOAC Int. 2009 Sept-Oct; 92(5):1250-7.

[155] Dietary Reference Intakes for Energy, Carbohydrate, Fiber, Fat, Fatty Acids, Cholesterol, Protein, and Amino Acids. Macronutrients, Food and Nutrition Board, 2005.

[156] McCann D, Barrett A, Cooper A, Crumpler D, Dalen L, Grimshaw K, Kitchin E, Stevenson J. Food additives and hyperactive behaviour in 3-year-old and 8/9-year-old children in the community: a randomised, double-blinded, placebo-controlled trial. Lancet. 2007; 370 (9598): 1560-1567.

[157] Pelsser LM, Frankena K, Toorman J, Savelkoul HF, Dubois AE, Pereira RR, Haagen TA, Buitelaar JK. Effects of a restricted elimination diet on the behaviour of children with attention-deficit hyperactivity disorder (INCA study): A randomised controlled trial. Lancet. 2011; 377(9764): 494-503.

[158] CSPI. Food Dyes: A Rainbow of Risks. Washington, DC: Center for Science in the Public Interest; 2010.

[159] Food Standards Agency. Compulsory Warnings on Colours in Food and Drink [press release] London: Food Standards Agency; Jul 22, 2010.

[160] Beverage ingredients can form carcinogen. Consum Rep. 2006 Oct; 71(10):7.

[161] McCann D, Barrett A, Cooper A, Crumpler D, Dalen L, Grimshaw K, Kitchin E, Stevenson J. Food additives and hyperactive behaviour in 3-year-old and 8/9-year-old children in the community: a randomised, double-blinded, placebo-controlled trial. Lancet. 2007; 370 (9598): 1560-1567.

[162] Source: www.inchem.org/documents/iarc/vol73/73-17.html

[163] Source: www.ntp.niehs.nih.gov/ntp/roc/twelfth/profiles/ButylatedHydroxyanisole.pdf

[164] EFSA Panel on Food Additives and Nutrient Sources added to Food (ANS); Scientific Opinion on the re-evaluation of Butylated hydroxytoluene BHT (E 321) as a food additive. EFSA Journal 2012; 10(3):2588. [43 pp.]

[165] UNEP and OECD, 2,6-di-tert-butyl-p-cresol (BHT) Screening Information Data Set: Initial Assessment Report (Paris: OECD, 2002), Available online: www.inchem.org/documents/sids/sids/128370.pdf.

[166] Source: www.ntp.niehs.nih.gov/?objectid=07066859-E45C-2537-6C80D75BAE99B78D

[167] He K, Du S, Xun P, Sharma S, Wang H, Zhai F, Popkin B. Consumption of monosodium glutamate in relation to incidence of overweight in Chinese adults: China Health and Nutrition Survey (CHNS) Am J Clin Nutr. 2011 June; 93(6): 1328–1336.

[168] Magnuson BA, Burdock GA, Doull J, Kroes RM, Marsh GM, Pariza MW, et al. Aspartame: a safety evaluation based on current use levels, regulations, and toxicological and epidemiological studies". Crit. Rev. Toxicol. 2007; 37 (8): 629-727.

[169] Soffritti M, Belpoggi F, Esposti DD, Lambertini L. Aspartame induces lymphomas and leukaemias in rats. European Journal of Oncology. 2005; 10(2):107–116.

[170] Whitehouse CR, Boullata J, McCauley LA. The potential toxicity of artificial sweeteners. AAOHN J. 2008 Jun; 56(6):251-9; quiz 260-1.

[171] Yang Q. Gain weight by "going diet?" Artificial sweeteners and the neurobiology of sugar cravings Yale J Biol Med. 2010 June; 83(2): 101–108.

[172] Susan S. Schiffman Rationale for Further Medical and Health Research on High-Potency Sweeteners Chem Senses. 2012 October; 37(8): 671–679.

[173] Borthakur A, Bhattacharyya S, Anbazhagan AN, Kumar A, Dudeja PK, Tobacman JK. Prolongation of carrageenan-induced inflammation in human colonic epithelial cells by activation of an NFκB-BCL10 loop. Biochim Biophys Acta. 2012 Aug; 1822(8):1300-7.

[174] Borthakur A, Bhattacharyya S, Dudeja PK, Tobacman JK. Carrageenan induces interleukin-8 production through distinct Bcl10 pathway in normal human colonic epithelial cells. Am J Physiol Gastrointest Liver Physiol. 2007 Mar; 292(3):G829-38.

[175] Bhattacharyya S, O-Sullivan I, Katyal S, Unterman T, Tobacman JK. Exposure to the common food additive carrageenan leads to glucose intolerance, insulin resistance and inhibition of insulin signalling in HepG2 cells and C57BL/6J mice. Diabetologia. 2012 Jan; 55(1):194-203.

[176] Mensinga TT, Speijers GJ, Meulenbelt J. Health implications of exposure to environmental nitrogenous compounds. Toxicol Rev. 2003; 22:41–51.

[177] Powlson DS, Addiscott TM, Benjamin N, et al. When does nitrate become a risk for humans? J Environ Qual. 2008; 37:291–5.

[178] Norat T, Bingham S, Ferrari P, et al. Meat, fish, and colorectal cancer risk: the European Prospective Investigation into cancer and nutrition. J Natl Cancer Inst. 2005; 97:906–16.

[179] Mensinga TT, Speijers GJ, Meulenbelt J. Health implications of exposure to environmental nitrogenous compounds. Toxicol Rev. 2003; 22:41–51.

[180] World Cancer Research Fund. Food, nutrition, physical activity, and the prevention of cancer: a global perspective. Second Expert Report, 2007. Available from: www.dietandcancerreport.org.

[181] Hord NG, Tang Y, Bryan NS. Food sources of nitrates and nitrites: the physiologic context for potential health benefits. Am J Clin Nutr. 2009 Jul; 90(1):1-10.

[182] Ludwig DS, Ebbeling CB. Overweight children and adolescents. N Engl J Med. 2005 Sep 8; 353(10):1070-1.

[183] Lebenthal Y, Horvath A, Dziechciarz P, Szajewska H, Shamir R. Are treatment targets for hypercholesterolemia evidence based? Systematic review and meta-analysis of randomized controlled trials. Arch Dis Child. 2010; 95 (9): 673–80.

[184] Wansink B, Just DR, Payne CR, Klinger MR. Attractive Names Sustain Increased Vegetable Intake in Schools. Prev Med. 2012; 55:4, 330-332.

[185] Agarwal S, Rao AV. Tomato lycopene and its role in human health and chronic diseases. CMAJ. 2000 Sep 19; 163(6):739-44.

[186] Unlu NZ, Bohn T, Francis DM, Nagaraja HN, Clinton SK, Schwartz SJ. Lycopene from heat-induced cis-isomer-rich tomato sauce is more bioavailable than from all-trans-rich tomato sauce in human subjects. Br J Nutr. 2007 Jul; 98(1):140-6.

[187] Conaway CC, Getahun SM, Liebes LL, Pusateri DJ, Topham DK, Botero-Omary M, Chung FL. Disposition of glucosinolates and sulforaphane in humans after ingestion of steamed and fresh broccoli., Nutr Cancer. 2000; 38(2):168-78. Erratum in: Nutr Cancer 2001; 41(1-2):196.

[188] Moreno DA, López-Berenguer C, García-Viguera C. Effects of stir-fry cooking with different edible oils on the phytochemical composition of broccoli. J Food Sci. 2007 Jan; 72(1):S064-8.

[189] Yuan G, Sun B, Yuan J, Wang Q. Effects of different cooking methods on health-promoting compounds of broccoli J Zhejiang Univ Sci B. 2009 Aug; 10(8): 580–588.

[190] Brown MJ, Ferruzzi MG, Nguyen ML, Cooper DA, Eldridge AL, Schwartz SJ, White WS. Carotenoid bioavailability is higher from salads ingested with full-fat than with fat-reduced salad dressings as measured with electrochemical detection, Am J Clin Nutr August 2004 vol. 80 no. 2 396-403.

[191] Katragadda HR, Fullana A, Sidhu S, Carbonell-Barrachina AA. Emissions of volatile aldehydes from heated cooking oils, Food Chemistry 120 (2010) 59–65.

[192] Fullana A, Carbonell-Barrachina AA, Sidhu S. Volatile aldehyde emissions from heated cooking oils. J Sc Food Agri. 2004; 84: 2015–2021.

[193] Katragadda HR, Fullana A, Sidhu S, Carbonell-Barrachina AA, Emissions of volatile aldehydes from heated cooking oils, Food Chemistry, 2010; 120: 59–65.

[194] Baiano A, Gambacorta G, Terracone C, Previtali MA, Lamacchia C, La Notte E, Changes in Phenolic Content and Antioxidant Activity of Italian Extra-Virgin Olive Oils during Storage, J Food Sci. Mar 2009; 74(2) C177 - C183.

[195] Valavanidis A, Nisiotou C, Papageorgiou Y, Kremli I, Satravelas N, Zinieris N, et al., Comparison of the radical scavenging potential of polar and lipidic fractions of olive oil and other vegetable oils under normal conditions and after thermal treatment. Agric Food Chem. 2004 Apr 21; 52(8):2358-65.

[196] Payne GW. Effect of inflammation on the aging microcirculation: impact on skeletal muscle blood flow control. Microcirculation. 2006 Jun; 13(4):343-52.

[197] Carlson MC, Erickson KI, Kramer AF, Voss MW, Bolea N, Mielke M, et al. Evidence for Neurocognitive Plasticity in At-Risk Older Adults: The Experience Corps Program J Gerontol A Biol Sci Med Sci. 2009 January; 64A(1): 132–137.

[198] O'Brien J, Morrissey PA. Nutritional and toxicological aspects of the Maillard browning reaction in foods. Crit Rev Food Sci Nutr. 1989; 28:211–248.

[199] Uribarri J, Woodruff S, Goodman S, Cai W, Chen X, Pyzik R, Yong A, Striker GE, Vlassara H. Advanced glycation end products in foods and a practical guide to their reduction in the diet. J Am Diet Assoc. 2010 Jun; 110(6):911-16.e12.

362

[200] Snow LM, Fugere NA, Thompson LV. Advanced glycation end-product accumulation and associated protein modification in type II skeletal muscle with aging. J Gerontol A Biol Sci Med Sci. 2007 Nov; 62(11):1204-10.

[201] Uribarri J, Woodruff S, Goodman S, Cai W, Chen X, Pyzik R, Yong A, Striker GE, Vlassara H. Advanced glycation end products in foods and a practical guide to their reduction in the diet. J Am Diet Assoc. 2010 Jun; 110(6):911-16.e12.

[202] Vlassara H, Cai W, Crandall J, Goldberg T, Oberstein R, Dardaine V, et al. Inflammatory mediators are induced by dietary glycotoxins, a major risk factor for diabetic angiopathy. Proc Natl Acad Sci U S A 2002 Nov 26; 99(24):15596-601.

[203] Sugimura T, Wakabayashi K, Nakagama H, Nagao M. Heterocyclic amines: Mutagens/carcinogens produced during cooking of meat and fish. Cancer Science. 2004; 95(4):290–299.

[204] Ollberding NJ, Wilkens LR, Henderson BE, Kolonel LN, Le Marchand L. Meat consumption, heterocyclic amines and colorectal cancer risk: the Multiethnic Cohort Study. Int J Cancer. 2012 Oct 1; 131(7):E1125-33.

[205] Cross AJ, Ferrucci LM, Risch A, et al. A large prospective study of meat consumption and colorectal cancer risk: An investigation of potential mechanisms underlying this association. Cancer Research. 2010; 70(6):2406–2414.

[206] Stolzenberg-Solomon RZ, Cross AJ, Silverman DT, et al. Meat and meat-mutagen intake and pancreatic cancer risk in the NIH-AARP cohort. Cancer Epidemiology, Biomarkers, and Prevention. 2007; 16(12):2664–2675

[207] Anderson KE, Sinha R, Kulldorff M, et al. Meat intake and cooking techniques: Associations with pancreatic cancer. Mutation Research. 2002; 506–507:225–231.

[208] Cross AJ, Peters U, Kirsh VA, Andriole GL, Reding D, Hayes RB, et al. A prospective study of meat and meat mutagens and prostate cancer risk. Cancer Research. 2005; 65(24):11779–11784.

[209] Mottram DS, Wedzicha BL, Dodson AT. Acrylamide is formed in the Maillard reaction. Nature. 2002 Oct 3; 419(6906):448-9.

[210] Friedman M. Chemistry, biochemistry, and safety of acrylamide. A review. J Agric Food Chem. 2003 Jul 30; 51(16):4504-26. Review.

[211] Lipworth L, Sonderman JS, Tarone RE, McLaughlin JK. Review of epidemiologic studies of dietary acrylamide intake and the risk of cancer. Eur J Cancer Prev. 2012 Jul; 21(4):375-86.

[212] Lau C, Anitole K, Hodes C, Lai D, Pfahles-Hutchens A, Seed J. Perfluoroalkyl acids: a review of monitoring and toxicological findings. Toxicol. Sci. 2007 Oct; 99 (2): 366–94.

[213] Halldorsson I, Rytter D, Haug LS, Bech BH, Danielsen I, Becher G, et al. Prenatal Exposure to Perfluorooctanoate and Risk of Overweight at 20 Years of Age: A Prospective Cohort Study. Environ Health Perspect. 2012 May; 120(5):668-73.

[214] Quintaes KD, Farfan JA, Tomazini FM, Morgano MA. Mineral migration from stainless steel, cast iron and soapstone (steatite) Brazilian pans to food preparations. Arch Latinoam Nutr. 2006 Sep; 56(3):275-81.

[215] Wansink B, Cheney M, Super Bowls: Serving Bowl Size and Food Consumption. JAMA. 2005 Apr 13; 293(14):1727–1728.

[216] Wansink B, Van Ittersum K. Shape of Glass and Amount of Alcohol Poured: Comparative Study of Effect of Practice and Concentration. BMJ. 2005 Dec 24; 331(7531):1512–1514.

[217] Source: adapted from a recipe by Lisa Cain, Ph.D. writer on healthy snacks

[218] Adapted from recipe in July 2011 issue of Women's Health magazine

[219] Source: adapted from a recipe at www.Skinnytaste.com

[220] Recipe adapted from Palmer, S, (2012) The Plant-Powered Diet: The Lifelong Eating Plan for Achieving Optimal Health Beginning Today. The Experiment; 1 edition.

[221] Source: adapted from a recipe at www.Self.com/fooddiet

[222] Source: adapted from a recipe at www.dailygarnish.com/2011/01/four-ingredient-healthy-peanut-sauce-tofu-marinade.html

[223] Source: adapted from a recipe at www.neverhomemaker.com/2010/01/detox-day-5-back-to-square-one.html

[224] Source: adapted from a recipe at www.menshealth.com/nutrition/meatball-matrix

[225] Source: adapted from a recipe at www.mylifetime.com/shows/cook-yourself-thin/recipes/chocolate-and-cranberry-biscotti

[226] Source: adapted from a recipe at www.theburlapbag.com/2012/07/2-ingredient-cookies-plus-the-mix-ins-of-your-choice/

[227] Source: adapted from a recipe at http://www.mynewroots.org/site/2011/04/the-raw-brownie-2/

[228] Source: adapted from recipe at: http://www.mindbodygreen.com/0-7154/easy-raw-apple-pie.html

[229] Source: adapted from recipe at: http://www.mindbodygreen.com/0-7154/easy-raw-apple-pie.html

[230] Source: adapted from a recipe at www.mylifetime.com/shows/cook-yourself-thin/recipes/vanilla-cupcakes

[231] Source: adapted from a recipe by chef Amanda Freitag and nutritionist Julie Barto

[232] Source: adapted from a recipe at: www.onehungrymess.com/2011/03/03/vegan-avocado-frozen-yogurt/

[233] American Association for the Advancement of Science. "Diet And Disease In Cattle: High-Grain Feed May Promote Illness And Harmful Bacteria." ScienceDaily, 11 May 2001. Web. 11 Nov. 2012.

[234] Source: www.ucsusa.org/assets/documents/food_and_environment/greener-pastures.pdf, p. 58.

[235] Source: www.cancer.org/cancer/cancercauses/othercarcinogens/athome/recombinant-bovine-growth-hormone

[236] Mayer, AM. Historical changes in the mineral content of fruits and vegetables. British Food Journal. 1997; 99(6): 207- 211.

[237] Davis DR, Epp MD, Riordan HD. Changes in USDA Food Composition Data for 43 Garden Crops, 1950 to 1999, J Am Coll Nutr. Dec 2004 23(6): 669-682.

[238] Ruzzin J, Petersen R, Meugnier E, Madsen L, Lock EJ, Lillefosse H, et al.

Persistent organic pollutant exposure leads to insulin resistance syndrome. Environ Health Perspect. 2010 Apr; 118(4):465-71.

[239] Ibrahim MM, Fjære E, Lock EJ, Naville D, Amlund H, Meugnier E, et al. Chronic consumption of farmed salmon containing persistent organic pollutants causes insulin resistance and obesity in mice. PLoS One. 2011; 6(9):e25170.

[240] Ukropec J, Radikova Z, Huckova M, Koska J, Kocan A, et al. High prevalence of prediabetes and diabetes in a population exposed to high levels of an organochlorine cocktail. Diabetologia. 2010; 53: 899–906.

[241] Ruzzin J, Petersen R, Meugnier E, Madsen L, Lock EJ, et al. Persistent Organic Pollutant Exposure Leads to Insulin Resistance Syndrome. Environ Health Perspect. 2010; 118: 465–471.

[242] World Health Organization (2010) Source: http://www.who.int/mediacentre/factsheets/fs225/en/

[243] Midtbo LK, Ibrahim MM, Myrmel LS, Aune UL, Alvheim AR, Liland NS, et al. Intake of farmed Atlantic salmon fed soybean oil increases insulin resistance and hepatic lipid accumulation in mice. PLoS One. 2013; 8(1):e53094.

[244] Monterey Bay Aquarium. Source: www.montereybayaquarium.org/cr/seafoodwatch.aspx

[245] National Geographic. Source: www.ocean.nationalgeographic.com/ocean/take-action/seafood-decision-guide/

[246] Yorifuji T, Tsuda T, Harada M. Minamata Disease: Catastrophic food poisoning by methylmercury and a challenge for democracy and justice. Pages 63-99 in TKTK (Eds.), Late Lessons From Early Warnings-2012: Science, Precaution, Innovation. Volume II. European Environment Agency.

[247] Source: www.water.epa.gov/scitech/swguidance/fishshellfish/outreach/advice_index.cfm

[248] Mozaffarian D, Rimm EB. Fish intake, contaminants, and human health: evaluating the risks and the benefits. JAMA. 2006 Oct 18; 296(15):1885-99.

[249] United States Department of Agriculture. Source: www.ams.usda.gov

[250] Smith-Spangler C, Brandeau ML, Hunter GE, Bavinger JC, Pearson M, Eschbach PJ, et al. Are Organic Foods Safer or Healthier Than Conventional Alternatives? A Systematic Review. Ann Intern Med. 2012 Sep; 157(5):348-366.

[251] Environmental Protection Agency. Source: www.epa.gov/pesticides/factsheets/riskassess.htm

[252] Bouchard MF, Bellinger DC, Wright RO, Weisskopf MG. Attention-Deficit/Hyperactivity Disorder and Urinary Metabolites of Organophosphate Pesticides. Pediatrics. 2010 Jun 1; 125(6):e1270-e1277.

[253] Grandjean P, Harari R, Barr DB, Debes F. Pesticide exposure and stunting as independent predictors of neurobehavioral deficits in Ecuadorian school children. Pediatrics. 2006; 117(3).

[254] Furlong CE, PON1 status of farmworker mothers and children as a predictor of organophosphate sensitivity. Pharmacogenet Genomics. 2006;16(3):183–190

[255] Weiss B. Vulnerability of children and the developing brain to neurotoxic hazards. Environ Health Perspect. 2000; 108(suppl 3):375–381.

[256] Source:

www.progressreport.cancer.gov/doc_detail.asp?pid=1&did=2007&chid=71&coid
=713&mid#pesticides

[257] Source: www.ornl.gov/sci/techresources/Human_Genome/elsi/gmfood.shtml

[258] Séralini GE, Clair E, Mesnage R, Gress S, Defarge N, Malatesta M, et al. Long term toxicity of a Roundup herbicide and a Roundup-tolerant genetically modified maize. Food Chem Toxicol. 2012 Nov; 50(11):4221-31.

[259] Glassner B, The Gospel of Food: Everything You Think You Know About Food Is Wrong, Ecco. Jan 2, 2007.

[260] Wansink B, Mindless Eating, Bantam Books. 2006.

[261] Kapleau, P, The Three pillars of Zen: teaching, practice, and enlightenment. New York: Anchor Books. 1989; pp. 43–44.

[262] Kokkinos A, le Roux CW, Alexiadou K, Tentolouris N, Vincent RP. Kyriaki D, et al. Eating slowly increases the postprandial response of the anorexigenic gut hormones, peptide YY and glucagon-like peptide-1. J Clin Endocrinol Metab. 2010 Jan; 95(1):333-7.

[263] Grotto D, Zied E. The Standard American Diet and its relationship to the health status of Americans. Nutr Clin Pract. 2010 Dec; 25(6):603-12.

[264] Surén P, Roth C, Bresnahan M, Haugen M, Hornig M, Hirtz D, et al. Association between maternal use of folic acid supplements and risk of autism spectrum disorders in children. JAMA. 2013 Feb 13; 309(6):570-7.

[265] Forrest KY, Stuhldreher WL. Prevalence and correlates of vitamin D deficiency in US adults. Nutr Res. 2011 Jan; 31(1):48-54.

[266] U.S. Department of Agriculture, Agricultural Research Service. 2011. USDA National Nutrient Database for Standard Reference, Release 24. Nutrient Data Laboratory Home Page, available at: www.ars.usda.gov/ba/bhnrc/ndl

[267] Institute of Medicine, Food and Nutrition Board. Dietary Reference Intakes for Calcium and Vitamin D. Washington, DC: National Academy Press, 2010.

[268] Norman AW, Henry HH. Vitamin D. In: Bowman BA, Russell RM, eds. Present Knowledge in Nutrition, 9th ed. Washington DC: ILSI Press, 2006.

[269] Krause R, Bühring M, Hopfenmüller W, Holick MF, Sharma AM. Ultraviolet B and blood pressure. Lancet 1998; 352:709-10.

[270] Munger KL, Levin LI, Hollis BW, Howard NS, Ascherio A. Serum 25-hydroxyvitamin D levels and risk of multiple sclerosis. JAMA. 2006; 296:2832-8.

[271] Hyppönen E, Läärä E, Reunanen A, Järvelin MR, Virtanen SM. Intake of vitamin D and risk of type 1 diabetes: a birth-cohort study. Lancet. 2001; 358:1500-3.

[272] Pittas AG, Dawson-Hughes B, Li T, Van Dam RM, Willett WC, Manson JE, et al. Vitamin D and calcium intake in relation to type 2 diabetes in women. Diabetes Care. 2006; 29:650-6.

[273] Schleithoff SS, Zittermann A, Tenderich G, Berthold HK, Stehle P, Koerfer R. Vitamin D supplementation improves cytokine profiles in patients with congestive heart failure: a double-blind, randomized, placebo-controlled trial. Am J Clin Nutr. 2006; 83:754-9.

[274] Salehi-Tabar R, Nguyen-Yamamoto L, Tavera-Mendoza LE, Quail T, Dimitrov V, An BS, et al. Vitamin D receptor as a master regulator of the c-

MYC/MXD1 network. Proc Natl Acad Sci U S A. 2012 Nov 13; 109(46):18827-32.

[275] Institute of Medicine, Food and Nutrition Board. Dietary Reference Intakes for Calcium and Vitamin D. Washington, DC: National Academy Press, 2010.

[276] Garland CF, Gorham ED, Mohr SB, Garland FC. Vitamin D for cancer prevention: global perspective. Ann Epidemiol. 2009 Jul; 19(7):468-83.

[277] Deng X, Song Y, Manson JE, Signorello LB, Zhang SM, Shrubsole MJ, et al. Magnesium, vitamin D status and mortality: results from US National Health and Nutrition Examination Survey (NHANES) 2001 to 2006 and NHANES III. BMC Med. 2013 Aug 27; 11:187.

[278] Clayton JA, Rodgers S, Blakey J. Thiazide diuretic prescription and electrolyte abnormalities in primary care. Br J Clin Pharmacol. 2006 Jan; 61:87-95.

[279] Khedun SM, Naicker T, Maharaj B. Zinc, hydrochlorothiazide and sexual dysfunction. Cent Afr J Med. 1995; 41:312-315.

[280] Langsjoen PH, Langsjoen AM. The clinical use of HMG CoA-reductase inhibitors and the associated depletion of coenzyme Q10: A review of animal and human publications. Biofactors 2003; 18(1-4):101-111.

[281] Akhtar N, Haqqi TM. Current nutraceuticals in the management of osteoarthritis: a review. Ther Adv Musculoskelet Dis. 2012 Jun; 4(3):181-207.

[282] Aslam T, Delcourt C, Silva R, Holz FG, Leys A, Garcià Layana A, Souied E. Micronutrients in Age-Related Macular Degeneration. Ophthalmologica. 2013; 229(2):75-9.

[283] Hegarty B, Parker G. Fish oil as a management component for mood disorders - an evolving signal. Curr Opin Psychiatry. 2013 Jan; 26(1):33-40.

[284] Rosenbaum CC, O'Mathúna DP, Chavez M, Shields K. Antioxidants and antiinflammatory dietary supplements for osteoarthritis and rheumatoid arthritis. Altern Ther Health Med. 2010 Mar-Apr; 16(2):32-40.

[285] Xu Q, Parks CG, DeRoo LA, Cawthon RM, Sandler DP, Chen H. Multivitamin use and telomere length in women. Am J Clin Nutr. 2009 Jun;89(6):1857-63.

[286] Cawthon RM, Smith KR, O'Brien E, Sivatchenko A, Kerber RA. Association between telomere length in blood and mortality in people aged 60 years or older. Lancet. 2003 Feb 1; 361(9355):393-5.

[287] Martin-Ruiz C, Dickinson HO, Keys B, Rowan E, Kenny RA, Von Zglinicki T. Telomere length predicts poststroke mortality, dementia, and cognitive decline. Ann Neurol. 2006; 60:174–80.

[288] Fitzpatrick AL, Kronmal RA, Gardner JP, Psaty BM, Jenny NS, Tracy RP, et al. Leukocyte telomere length and cardiovascular disease in the Cardiovascular Health Study. Am J Epidemiol. 2007; 165:14–21.

[289] Wu X, Amos CI, Zhu Y, Zhao H, Grossman BH, Shay JW, et al. Telomere dysfunction: a potential cancer predisposition factor. J Natl Cancer Inst. 2003; 95:1211–8.

[290] McGrath M, Wong JY, Michaud D, Hunter DJ, De Vivo I. Telomere length, cigarette smoking, and bladder cancer risk in men and women. Cancer Epidemiol Biomarkers Prev. 2007; 16:815–9.

[291] Gaziano JM, Sesso HD, Christen WG, Bubes V, Smith JP, MacFadyen J, et al.

Multivitamins in the prevention of cancer in men: the Physicians' Health Study II randomized controlled trial. JAMA. 2012 Nov 14; 308(18):1871-80.

[292] Sesso HD, Christen WG, Bubes V, Smith JP, MacFadyen J, Schvartz M, et al. Multivitamins in the prevention of cardiovascular disease in men: the Physicians' Health Study II randomized controlled trial. JAMA. 2012 Nov 7; 308(17):1751-60.

[293] Meulepas JM, Newcomb PA, Burnett-Hartman AN, Hampton JM, Trentham-Dietz A. Multivitamin supplement use and risk of invasive breast cancer Public Health Nutr. 2010 October; 13(10): 1540–1545.

[294] Mursu J, Robien K, Harnack LJ, Park K, Jacobs DR Jr. Dietary supplements and mortality rate in older women: the Iowa Women's Health Study. Arch Intern Med. 2011 Oct 10; 171(18):1625-33.

[295] Lonn E, Bosch J, Yusuf S, Sheridan P, Pogue J, Arnold JM. Effects of Long-term Vitamin E Supplementation on Cardiovascular Events and Cancer: A Randomized Controlled Trial. JAMA. 2005; 293(11):1338-1347.

[296] Li K, Kaaks R, Linseisen J, Rohrmann S. Associations of dietary calcium intake and calcium supplementation with myocardial infarction and stroke risk and overall cardiovascular mortality in the Heidelberg cohort of the European Prospective Investigation into Cancer and Nutrition study (EPIC-Heidelberg) Heart. 2012; 98:920-925.

[297] Rizos EC, Ntzani EE, Bika E, Kostapanos MS, Elisaf MS. Association Between Omega-3 Fatty Acid Supplementation and Risk of Major Cardiovascular Disease Events: A Systematic Review and Meta-analysis. JAMA. 2012; 308(10): 1024-1033.

[298] Albanes D, Heinonen OP, Taylor PR, Virtamo J, Edwards BK, Rautalahti M, et al. α-Tocopherol and β-carotene supplements and lung cancer incidence in the Alpha-Tocopherol, Beta-Carotene Cancer Prevention Study: effects of base-line characteristics and study compliance. J Natl Cancer Inst. 1996; 88(21): 1560-1570.

[299] Omenn GS, Goodman GE, Thornquist MD, Balmes J, Cullen MR, Glass A, et al., Risk Factors for Lung Cancer and for Intervention Effects in CARET, the Beta-Carotene and Retinol Efficacy Trial. J Natl Cancer Inst. 1996; 88 (21): 1550-1559.

[300] Banim PJ, Luben R, McTaggart A, Welch A, Wareham N, Khaw KT, Hart AR. Dietary antioxidants and the aetiology of pancreatic cancer: a cohort study using data from food diaries and biomarkers. Gut. 2013 Oct; 62(10):1489-96.

[301] Brasky TM, Darke AK, Song X, Tangen CM, Goodman PJ, Thompson IM, et al. Plasma Phospholipid Fatty Acids and Prostate Cancer Risk in the SELECT Trial. J Natl Cancer Inst. 2013 Aug 7; 105(15): 1132-1141.

[302] Source: www.nsf.org/certified/gmp/Listings.asp?Program

[303] Source: www.naturalproductsassoc.org.

[304] Source: www.tga.gov.au/

[305] Source: www.consumerlab.com

[306] Source: www.usp.org/USPVerified/dietarySupplements/companies.html

[307] Swinburn B, Eggar G, Raza F. Dissecting obesogenic environments; the development and application of a framework for identifying and prioritizing

environmental interventions for obesity. Prev Med. 1999; 29(6), 563-570.
[308] Source:
www.blogs.hbr.org/cs/2013/01/sitting_is_the_smoking_of_our_generation.html
[309] Dunstan DW, Barr EL, Healy GN, Salmon J, Shaw JE, Balkau B, et al.
Television viewing time and mortality: the Australian Diabetes, Obesity and
Lifestyle Study (AusDiab). Circulation. 2010 Jan 26; 121(3):384-91.
[310] Pavey TG, Peeters GG, Brown WJ. Sitting-time and 9-year all-cause mortality
in older women. Br J Sports Med. 2012 Dec 15.
[311] Patel AV, Bernstein L. Deka A, Feigelson HS, Campbell PT, Gapstur SM, et al.
Leisure Time Spent Sitting in Relation to Total Mortality in a Prospective Cohort
of US Adults. Am. J. Epidemiol. 2010; 172 (4):419-429.
[312] Katzmarzyk PT, Church TS, Craig CL, Bouchard C. Sitting time and mortality
from all causes, cardiovascular disease, and cancer. Med Sci Sports Exerc. 2009
May; 41(5):998-1005.
[313] Zderic TW, Hamilton MT. Identification of hemostatic genes expressed in
human and rat leg muscles and a novel gene (LPP1/PAP2A) suppressed during
prolonged physical inactivity (sitting) Lipids in Health and Disease 2012; 11:137.
[314] Buettner D. The Blue Zones: Lessons for Living Longer From the People
Who've Lived the Longest [Deluxe Edition] [Mass Market Paperback] National
Geographic; Reprint edition, Oct 19, 2010.
[315] Loprinzi PD, Cardinal BJ. Association between Biologic Outcomes and
Objectively Measured Physical Activity Accumulated in ≥10-Minute Bouts and
<10-Minute Bouts. Am J Health Promotion: 2013 Jan/Feb; 27(3):143-151.
[316] Source: www.acefitness.org/getfit/studies/bestworstabexercises.pdf
[317] Shiraev T, Barclay G. Evidence based exercise - clinical benefits of
high intensity interval training. Aust Fam Physician. 2012 Dec; 41(12):960-2.
[318] De Bock K, Richter EA, Russell AP, Eijnde BO, Derave W, Ramaekers M, et
al. Exercise in the fasted state facilitates fibre type-specific intramyocellular lipid
breakdown and stimulates glycogen resynthesis in humans. J Physiol. 20005; 564:
649–660.
[319] De Glisezinski I, Harant I, Crampes F, Trudeau F, Felez A, Cottet-Emard JM,
et al. Effect of carbohydrate ingestion on adipose tissue lipolysis during long-
lasting exercise in trained men. J Appl Physiol. 1998; 84: 1627–1632.
[320] De Bock K, Derave W, Eijnde BO, Hesselink MK, Koninckx E, Rose AJ, et al.
Effect of training in the fasted state on metabolic responses during exercise with
carbohydrate intake. J Appl Physiol. 2008 Apr; 104(4):1045-55.
[321] Van Proeyen K, Szlufcik K, Nielens H, Ramaekers M, Hespel P. Beneficial
metabolic adaptations due to endurance exercise training in the fasted state. J Appl
Physiol. 2011 Jan; 110(1):236-45.
[322] Beelen M, Burke LM, Gibala MJ, van Loon L JC. Nutritional strategies to
promote postexercise recovery. Int J Sport Nutr Exerc Metab. 2010 Dec; 20(6):
515-32.
[323] Ivy JL, Goforth HW Jr, Damon BM, McCauley TR, Parsons EC, Price TB.
Early postexercise muscle glycogen recovery is enhanced with a carbohydrate-
protein supplement. J Appl Physiol (1985). 2002 Oct; 93(4):1337-44.

[324] Baer DJ, Stote KS, Paul DR, Harris GK, Rumpler WV, Clevidence BA. Whey protein but not soy protein supplementation alters body weight and composition in free-living overweight and obese adults. J Nutr. 2011 Aug; 141(8):1489-94.

[325] Liu ZM, Ho SC, Chen YM, Ho YP. A mild favorable effect of soy protein with isoflavones on body composition--a 6-month double-blind randomized placebo-controlled trial among Chinese postmenopausal women. Int J Obes (Lond). 2010 Feb; 34(2):309-18.

[326] Messina M. A brief historical overview of the past two decades of soy and isoflavone research. J Nutr. 2010 Jul; 140(7):1350S-4S.

[327] Lidder S, Webb AJ. Vascular effects of dietary nitrate (as found in green leafy vegetables & beetroot) via the Nitrate-Nitrite-Nitric Oxide pathway. Br J Clin Pharmacol. 2012 Aug 13.

[328] Hernández A, Schiffer TA, Ivarsson N, Cheng AJ, Bruton JD, Lundberg JO, et al. Dietary nitrate increases tetanic [Ca2+]i and contractile force in mouse fast-twitch muscle. J Physiol. 2012 Aug 1; 590 (Pt 15):3575-83.

[329] Milkowski A, Garg HK, Coughlin JR, Bryan NS. Nutritional epidemiology in the context of nitric oxide biology: a risk-benefit evaluation for dietary nitrite and nitrate. Nitric Oxide. 2010 Feb 15; 22(2):110-9.

[330] Murphy M, Eliot K, Heuertz RM, Weiss E. Whole beetroot consumption acutely improves running performance. J Acad Nutr Diet. 2012 Apr; 112(4):548-52.

[331] Cooke JP, Ghebremariam YT. Dietary nitrate, nitric oxide, and restenosis. J Clin Invest. 2011 April 1; 121(4): 1258–1260.

[332] Kuo LE. Neuropeptide Y acts directly in the periphery on fat tissue and mediates stress-induced obesity and metabolic syndrome. Nat Med. 2007 Jul; 13(7):803-11.

[333] Melhorn SJ, Krause EG, Scott KA, Mooney MR, Johnson JD, Woods SC, et al., Meal Patterns and Hypothalamic NPY Expression During Chronic Social Stress and Recovery. Am J Physiol Regul Integr Comp Physiol. 2010 Sept; 299(3): R813–R822.

[334] Vance DE, Roberson AJ, McGuinness TM, Fazeli PL. How neuroplasticity and cognitive reserve protect cognitive functioning.J Psychosoc Nurs Ment Health Serv. 2010 Apr; 48(4):23-30.

[335] Piazza JR, Charles ST, Sliwinski MJ, Mogle J, Almeida DM. Affective Reactivity to Daily Stressors and Long-Term Risk of Reporting a Chronic Physical Health Condition. Ann Behav Med. 2012 Oct 19. [Epub ahead of print]

[336] Dusek JA, Otu HH, Wohlhueter AL, Bhasin M, Zerbini LF, Joseph MG, Benson H, Libermann TA. Genomic counter-stress changes induced by the relaxation response. PLoS One. 2008 Jul 2; 3(7):e2576.

[337] Walach H, Jonas WB. Review Placebo research: the evidence base for harnessing self-healing capacities. J Altern Complement Med. 2004; 10 Suppl 1:S103-12.

[338] Eccles R. The power of the placebo. Curr Allergy Asthma Rep. 2007 May; 7(2):100-4.

[339] Lang E, Benotsch E, Fick I, Lutgendorf S, Berbaum ML, Berbaum KS, et al.

Adjunctive non-pharmacological analgesia for invasive medical procedures: A randomized trial. Lancet 2000, 355: 1486-90.

[340] Posadzki P, Ernst E. Guided imagery for musculoskeletal pain: a systematic review. Clin J Pain 2011; 27:648–53.

[341] Tusek DL. Guided imagery; a significant advance in the care of patients undergoing elective colorectal surgery. Dis Colon Rectum. 1997; 40(2):172-178.

[342] Brouziyne M, Molinaro C. Mental imagery combined with physical practice of approach shots for golf beginners. Perceptual and Motor Skills. 2005 Aug; 101(1): 203-11.

[343] Hudetz JA, Hudetz AG, Klayman J. Relationship between relaxation by guided imagery and performance of working memory. Psychol Rep. 2000 Feb; 86(1):15-20.

[344] Trakhenberg EC. The effects of guided imagery on the immune system: A critical review. Int J Neurosci. 2008 June: 118(6)839-55.

[345] Panagioti M, Gooding PA, Tarrier N. An empirical investigation of the effectiveness of the broad-minded affective coping procedure (BMAC) to boost mood among individuals with posttraumatic stress disorder (PTSD). Behav Res Ther. 2012 Oct; 50(10):589-95.

[346] Luckhaupt SE. National Institute for Occupational Safety and Health, CDC. Short Sleep Duration Among Workers, United States, 2010, April 27, 2012 /Morbidity and Mortality Weekly Report (MMWR) 61(16);281-285.

[347] Ruiter, M, et al. June 11, 2012, SLEEP 2012 conference, Boston.

[348] Haus EL, Smolensky MH. Shift work and cancer risk: potential mechanistic roles of circadian disruption, light at night, and sleep deprivation. Sleep Med Rev. 2013 Aug; 17(4):273-84.

[349] Spiegel K, Tasali E, Penev P, Van Cauter E. Brief communication: Sleep curtailment in healthy young men is associated with decreased leptin levels, elevated ghrelin levels, and increased hunger and appetite. Ann Intern Med. 2004; 141(11):846–850.

[350] Nogueiras R, Tschop MH, Zigman JM. Central nervous system regulation of energy metabolism: ghrelin versus leptin. Ann N Y Acad Sci. 2008;1126:14–19

[351] Markwald RR, Melanson EL, Smith MR, Higgins J, Perreault L, Eckel RH, Wright KP. Impact of insufficient sleep on total daily energy expenditure, food intake, and weight gain. Proc Natl Acad Sci U S A. 2013 Apr 2; 110(14):5695-700.

[352] Nedeltcheva AV, Kilkus JM, Imperial J, Schoeller DA, Penev PD. Insufficient sleep undermines dietary efforts to reduce adiposity. Ann Intern Med. 2010 Oct 5; 153(7):435-41.

[353] Watson NF, Harden KP, Buchwald D, Vitiello MV, Pack AI, Weigle DS, Goldberg J. Sleep duration and body mass index in twins: a gene-environment interaction. SLEEP 2012; 35(5):597-603.

[354] Mollicone, DJ, Van Dongen, HPA, Rogers NL, Dinges DF. Optimizing sleep/wake schedules in space: Sleep during chronic nocturnal sleep restriction with and without diurnal naps. Acta Astronautica 2007; 60 (4–7): 354.

[355] Lahl O, Wispel C, Willigens B, Pietrowsky R. An ultra-short episode of sleep is

sufficient to promote declarative memory performance. Journal of Sleep Research 2008; 17 (1): 3–10.

[356] Brooks A, Lack L. A brief afternoon nap following nocturnal sleep restriction: Which nap duration is most recuperative? Sleep 2006; 29:831-840.

[357] Ibid.

[358] Mednick S, Nakayama K, Stickgold R.Sleep-dependent learning: a nap is as good as a night. Nat Neurosci. 2003 Jul; 6(7):697-8.

[359] Boden-Albala B, Roberts ET, Bazil C, Moon Y, Elkind MS, Rundek T, et al. Daytime sleepiness and risk of stroke and vascular disease: findings from the Northern Manhattan Study (NOMAS). Circ Cardiovasc Qual Outcomes. 2012 Jul 1; 5(4):500-7.

[360] Haus EL, Smolensky MH. Shift work and cancer risk: potential mechanistic roles of circadian disruption, light at night, and sleep deprivation. Sleep Med Rev. 2013 Aug; 17(4):273-84.

[361] Source: www.nccam.nih.gov/health/stress/relaxation.htm#status

[362] De Oliveira C, Watt R, Hamer M. Toothbrushing, inflammation, and risk of cardiovascular disease: Results from Scottish Health Survey. BMJ. 2010; 340:c2451.

[363] Mustapha IZ, Debrey S, Oladubu M, Ugarte R. Cardiovascular disease markers of systemic bacterial exposure in periodontal disease and risk: a systematic review and meta-analysis. J Periodontol. 2007; 78:2289-302.

[364] Chen ZY, Chiang CH, Huang CC, Chung CM, Chan WL, Huang PH, et al. The Association of Tooth Scaling and Decreased Cardiovascular Disease: A Nationwide Population-based Study. Am J Med. 2012 Jun; 125(6): 568-575.

[365] Bock SA, Sampson HA, Sampson HA, Atkins FM, Zeiger RS, Lehrer S, Sachs M, et al. Double-blind, placebo-controlled food challenge (DBPCFC) as an office procedure: a manual, J Allergy Clin Immunol. 1988 Dec; 82(6):986-97.

[366] Sinclair S. Migraine Headaches: nutritional, botanical and other alternative approaches. Alt Med Rev. 1999; 4(2):86-95.

[367] Pelsser L, Frankena K, Toorman J, Savelkoul HF, Dubois AE, Pereira RR, et al. Effects of a restricted elimination diet on the behaviour of children with attention-deficit hyperactivity disorder (INCA study): a randomised controlled trial. Lancet. 2011 Feb 5; 377(9764): 494-503.

[368] Darlington LG, Ramsey NW, Mansfield JR. Placebo controlled blind study of dietary manipulation therapy in rheumatoid arthritis. Lancet. 1986; 1(8475), 236–38.

[369] Gibson PR, Shepherd SJ. Evidence Based Dietary Management of Functional Gastrointestinal Symptoms: The FODMAP Approach, J Gastroenterol Hepatol. 2010 Feb; 25(2):252-8.

[370] Catassi C, Fasano A. Celiac disease. Curr Opin Gastroenterol. 2008; 24:687–691.

[371] Sapone A, Bai JC, Ciacci C, Dolinsek J, Green PHR, Hadjivassiliou M, et al. Spectrum of gluten related disorders: consensus on new nomenclature and classification, BMC Med. 2012 Feb 7;10:13.

[372] Ferguson A, Gillett H, Humphreys K, Kingstone K. Heterogeneity of celiac

disease: clinical, pathological, immunological, and genetic. Ann N Y Acad Sci. 1998; 859:112–120.

[373] Anderson LA, McMillan SA, Watson RG, Monaghan P, Gavin AT, Fox C, Murray LJ. Malignancy and mortality in a population-based cohort of patients with coeliac disease or "gluten sensitivity". World J Gastroenterol. 2007; 13:146–151.

[374] Fasano A. Physiological, pathological, and therapeutic implications of zonulin-mediated intestinal barrier modulation: living life on the edge of the wall. Am J Pathol. 2008 Nov; 173(5):1243-52.

[375] Drago S, El Asmar R, Di Piero M, Clemente MG, Tripathi A, Sapone A, et al. Gliadin, zonulin and gut permeability: effects on celiac and non-celiac intestinal mucosa and intestinal cell lines. Scand J Gastroenterol. 2006; 41:408–419.

[376] Sapone A, Lammers K, Casolaro V, Cammarota M et al., Divergence of gut permeability and mucosal immune gene expression in two gluten-associated conditions: celiac disease and gluten sensitivity BMC Med. 2011; 9: 23.

[377] Ludvigsson JF, Montgomery SM, Ekbom A, Brandt L, Granath F. Small-intestinal histopathology and mortality risk in celiac disease. JAMA. 2009 Sep 16; 302(11):1171-8.

[378] Sapone A, Lammers K, Casolaro V, Cammarota M, et al. Divergence of gut permeability and mucosal immune gene expression in two gluten-associated conditions: celiac disease and gluten sensitivity BMC Med. 2011; 9: 23.

[379] Vilppula A, Collin P, Mäki M, et al. Undetected coeliac disease in the elderly: a biopsy-proven population-based study. Dig. Liver Dis. 2008, 40(10), 809–813.

[380] Van den Broeck HC, De Jong HC, Salentijn EM, et al. Presence of celiac disease epitopes in modern and old hexaploid wheat varieties: wheat breeding may have contributed to increased prevalence of celiac disease. Theor. Appl. Genet. 2010, 121(8), 1527–1539.

[381] Lebenthal-Bendor Y, Theuer RC, Lebenthal A, Tabi I, Lebenthal E. Malabsorption of modified food starch (acetylated distarch phosphate) in normal infants and in 8–24-month-old toddlers with non-specific diarrhea, as influenced by sorbitol and fructose. Acta Paediatr. 2001, 90(12), 1368–1372.

[382] Brown AC. Problems of an Emerging Condition Separate From Celiac Disease, Expert Rev Gastroenterol Hepatol. 2012; 6(1):43-55.

[383] Brown AC. Problems of an Emerging Condition Separate From Celiac Disease, Expert Rev Gastroenterol Hepatol. 2012; 6(1):43-55.

[384] Catassi C, Fabiani E, Iacono G, D'Agate C, Francavilla R, Biagi F, et al. A prospective, double-blind, placebo-controlled trial to establish a safe gluten threshold for patients with celiac disease. Am J Clin Nutr. 2007; 85:160–166.

[385] Gibert A, Espadaler M, Angel Canela M, Sanchez A, Vaque C, Rafecas M. Consumption of gluten-free products: should the threshold value for trace amounts of gluten be at 20, 100 or 200 ppm? Eur J Gastroenterol Hepatol. 2006; 18:1187–1195.

[386] Norris JM, Barriga K, Hoffenberg EJ, Taki I, Miao D, Haas JE, et al. Risk of celiac disease autoimmunity and timing of gluten introduction in the diet of infants at increased risk of disease. JAMA. 2005; 293(19), 2343–2351.

[387] Brown AC. Problems of an Emerging Condition Separate From Celiac Disease, Expert Rev Gastroenterol Hepatol. 2012; 6(1):43-55.

[388] Marietta EV, Gomez AM, Yeoman C, Tilahun AY, Clark CR, et al. (2013) Low Incidence of Spontaneous Type 1 Diabetes in Non-Obese Diabetic Mice Raised on Gluten-Free Diets Is Associated with Changes in the Intestinal Microbiome. PLoS ONE 8(11): e78687.

[389] Krismer M, van Tulder M. Strategies for prevention and management of musculoskeletal conditions. Low back pain (non-specific). Best Pract Res Clin Rheumatol. 2007 Feb; 21(1):77-91.

[390] Buckwalter JA. Activity vs. rest in the treatment of bone, soft tissue and joint injuries. Iowa Orthop J. 1995; 15: 29–42.

[391] Malmivaara A, Hakkinen V, Aro T, et al. Treatment of acute low back pain: bed rest, exercises, or ordinary activity? N Engl J Med. 1995; 332:351.

[392] Saltzman CL, Hillis SL, Stolley MP, Anderson DD, Amendola A. Motion versus fixed distraction of the joint in the treatment of ankle osteoarthritis: a prospective randomized controlled trial. J Bone Joint Surg Am. 2012 Jun 6; 94(11):961-70.

[393] Waddell G. Simple low back pain: rest or active exercise? Ann Rheum Dis. 1993; 52:317.

[394] Dettori JR, Bullock SH, Sutlive TG, Franklin RJ, Patience T. The effects of spinal flexion and extension exercises and their associated postures in patients with acute low back pain. Spine. 1995; 20:2303.

[395] Engel KG, Buckley BA, Forth VE, McCarthy DM, Ellison EP, Schmidt MJ, Adams JG. Patient understanding of emergency department discharge instructions: Where are knowledge deficits greatest? Acad Emerg Med. 2012 Sep; 19(9):1035-1044.

[396] Ibid.

[397] Chou R, Huffman LH. Medications for acute and chronic low back pain: a review of the evidence for an American Pain Society/American College of Physicians clinical practice guideline. Ann Intern Med. 2007; 147(7):505-14.

[398] Dagenais S, Haldeman S. Evidence-Based Management of Low Back Pain, Mosby; 1 edition, February 25, 2011, p.2.

[399] Ibid., p.3.

[400] Wiesel SW, Tsourmas N, Feffer HL, Citrin CM, Patronas N. A study of computer-assisted tomography. I. The incidence of positive CAT scans in an asymptomatic group of patients. Spine (Phila Pa 1976). 1984 Sep; 9(6):549-51.

[401] Wheeler AH, Hanley EN Jr. Nonoperative treatment for low back pain. Rest to restoration. Spine (Phila Pa 1976). 1995 Feb 1; 20(3):375-8.

[402] Jensen MC, Brant-Zawadzki MN, Obuchowski N, Modic MT, Malkasian D, Ross JS. Magnetic Resonance Imaging of the Lumbar Spine in People without Back Pain. N Engl J Med. 1994 Jul 14; 331:69-7.

[403] Source: www.uptodate.com/contents/nonsteroidal-antiinflammatory-drugs-nsaids-beyond-the-basics

[404] Tarone RE, Blot WJ, McLaughlin JK. Nonselective nonaspirin nonsteroidal anti-inflammatory drugs and gastrointestinal bleeding: Relative and absolute risk

estimates from recent epidemiologic studies. Am J Ther. 2004; 11(1):17–25.

[405] Singh G, Triadafilopoulos G. Epidemiology of NSAID induced gastrointestinal complications. J Rheumatol. 1999; 26(suppl):18–24.

[406] Trelle S, Reichenbach S, Wandel S, Hildebrand P. Tschannen B, Villiger PM, et al. Cardiovascular safety of non-steroidal anti-inflammatory drugs: Network meta-analysis. BMJ. 2011 Jan 11;342:c7086.

[407] Yu Y, Ricciotti E, Scalia R, Tang SY, Grant G, Yu Z, et al. Vascular COX-2 Modulates Blood Pressure and Thrombosis in Mice. Sci Transl Med. 2012 May 2; 4:132ra54.

[408] McGettigan P, Henry D. Cardiovascular Risk with Non-Steroidal Anti-Inflammatory Drugs: Systematic Review of Population-Based Controlled Observational Studies. PLoS Med 2011; 8(9): e1001098.

[409] Greene J. Cost-conscious prescribing of nonsteroidal anti-inflammatory drugs for adults with arthritis. Archives of Internal Medicine. 1992; 152:1995-2002.

[410] Almekinders, L. An in vitro investigation into the effects of repetitive motion and nonsteroidal anti-inflammatory medication on human tendon fibroblasts. Am J Sp Med. 1995; 23:119-123.

[411] Roelofs PDDM, Deyo RA, Koes BW, Scholten RJPM, van Tulder MW. Non-steroidal anti-inflammatory drugs for low back pain. Cochrane Database of Syst Rev. 2008, Issue 1. Art. No.: CD000396.

[412] Choi BKL, Verbeek JH, Tam WWS, Jiang JY. Exercises for prevention of recurrences of low-back pain. Cochrane Database of Syst Rev. 2010, Issue 1. Art. No.: CD006555.

[413] Furlan A, Yazdi F, Tsertsvadze A, et al. Complementary and Alternative Therapies for Back Pain II. Evidence Report/Technology Assessment No. 194. Prepared by the University of Ottawa Evidence-based Practice Center under Contract No. 290-2007-10059-I (EPCIII). AHRQ Publication No. 10(11)E007. Rockville, MD: Agency for Healthcare Research and Quality 2010.

[414] Goertz CM, Long CR, Hondras MA, Petri R, Delgado R, Lawrence DJ, Owens EF, Meeker WC. Adding chiropractic manipulative therapy to standard medical care for patients with acute low back pain: results of a pragmatic randomized comparative effectiveness study. Spine. 2013 Apr 15; 38(8):627-34.

[415] Kizhakkeveettil A, Rose K, Kadar GE. Integrative Complementary and Alternative Medical Care for Low Back Pain: A Systematic Review, Global Adv Health Med. 2014; 3(5):49-64.

[416] Bronfort G, Evans R, Anderson AV, Svendsen KH, Bracha Y, Grimm RH. Spinal Manipulation, Medication, or Home Exercise with Advice for Acute and Subacute Neck Pain. Ann Intern Med. 2012 Jan 3; 156(1 Pt 1):1-10.

[417] Liliedahl RL, Finch MD, Axene DV, Goertz CM. Cost of care for common back pain conditions initiated with chiropractic doctor vs medical doctor/doctor of osteopathy as first physician: experience of one Tennessee-based general health insurer. J Manipulative Physiol Ther. 2010 Nov-Dec; 33(9):640-3.

[418] Hertzman-Miller RP, Morgenstern H, Hurwitz EL, et al. Comparing the satisfaction of low back pain patients randomized to receive medical or chiropractic care: results from the UCLA low back pain study. Am J Public

Health. 2002; 92(10):1628-1633.

[419] Meeker WC, Haldeman S. Chiropractic: a profession at the crossroads of mainstream and alternative medicine. Ann Intern Med. 2002; 136(3):216-227.

[420] Bronfort G, Evans R, Anderson AV, Svendsen KH, Bracha Y, Grimm RH. Spinal Manipulation, Medication, or Home Exercise with Advice for Acute and Subacute Neck Pain. Ann Intern Med. 2012 Jan 3; 156(1 Pt 1):1-10.

[421] Hsu C, Bluespruce J, Sherman K, Cherkin D. Unanticipated benefits of CAM therapies for back pain: an exploration of patient experiences. J Altern Complement Med. 2010 Feb; 16(2):157-63.

[422] Tseng CY, Lee JP, Tsai YS, Lee SD, Kao CL, Liu TC, Lai C, Harris MB, Kuo CH. Topical cooling (icing) delays recovery from eccentric exercise-induced muscle damage. J Strength Cond Res. 2013 May; 27(5):1354-61.

[423] Source: www.medicine.ox.ac.uk/bandolier/booth/painpag/Chronrev/Analges/CP063.html

[424] Smith J. No-Drug, Anti-Inflammatory Diet Yields Positive Clinical-Trial Results, Including Marked Improvement Of Metabolic Abnormalities And Rapid Weight Loss. Medical News Today. MediLexicon, Intl., 20 Jun. 2006. Web. 20 Dec. 2012.

[425] Raz O, Steinvil A, Berliner S, Rosenzweig T, Justo D, Shapira I. The effect of two iso-caloric meals containing equal amounts of fats with a different fat composition on the inflammatory and metabolic markers in apparently healthy volunteers. J Inflamm (Lond). 2013 Jan 31; 10(1):3.

[426] Watkins B, Li Y, Lippman HE, Feng S. Modulatory effects of omega-3 polyunsaturated fatty acids on osteoblast function and bone metabolism. Prostaglandins, Leukotrienes and Essential Fatty Acids, 2003 Jun; 68: 387-98.

[427] Kiecolt-Glaser, J. Psychosomatic Medicine. 2007 Apr; 69: 217-224.

[428] Barrett J, Curran V, Glynn L, Godwin M. Canadian Health Services Research Foundation synthesis: interprofessional collaboration and quality primary health care. Ottawa: Health Canada. Canadian Health Services Research Foundation, 2007.

[429] Boyce RA, Moran MC, Nissen LM, Chenery HJ, Brooks PM. Interprofessional education in health sciences: the University of Queensland Health Care Team Challenge. Med J Aust. 2009; 190(8):433-6.

[430] Farley TA, Dalal MA, Mostashari F, Frieden TR. Deaths preventable in the U.S. by improvements in use of clinical preventive services. Am J Prev Med. 2010, 38:600-9.

[431] Fielding JE, Teutsch SM. Integrating clinical care and community health. JAMA. 2009; 302:317-9.

[432] Kaplan RS, Porter ME. How to solve the cost crisis in health care. Harv Bus Rev. 2011; 89(9):46-52, 54, 56-61.

[433] Wilt TJ, Brawer MK, Jones KM, Barry MJ, Aronson WJ, Fox S, et al. Prostate Cancer Intervention versus Observation Trial (PIVOT) Study Group, Radical prostatectomy versus observation for localized prostate cancer. N Engl J Med. 2012 Jul 19; 367(3):203-13.

[434] Kechagias S, Ernersson A, Dahlqvist O, Lundberg P, Lindström T, Nystrom

FH, et al. Fast-food-based hyper-alimentation can induce rapid and profound elevation of serum alanine aminotransferase in healthy subjects Gut. 2008; 57:649-654.

[435] Ekstedt M, Franzen LE, Mathiesen UL, Thorelius L, Holmqvist M, Bodemar G, et al. Long-term follow-up of patients with NAFLD and elevated liver enzymes. Hepatology. 2006; 44:865–73.

[436] Bennet AM, Di Angelantonio E, Ye Z, Wensley F, Dahlin A, Ahlbom A, et al. Association of apolipoprotein E genotypes with lipid levels and coronary risk. JAMA. 2007 Sep 19; 298(11):1300-11.

[437] Stojakovic T, Scharnagl H, März W. ApoE: crossroads between Alzheimer's disease and atherosclerosis. Semin Vasc Med. 2004 Aug; 4(3):279-85.

[438] Slomski A. Mammography No Benefit in Reducing Deaths From Breast Cancer. JAMA. 2014; 311(12):1191.

[439] Hayes JH, Barry MJ. Screening for Prostate Cancer with the Prostate-Specific Antigen Test: A Review of Current Evidence. JAMA. 2014; 311(11): 1143-1149.

[440] Prochaska JO, DiClemente CC. Stages and processes of self-change of smoking: toward an integrative model of change. J Consult Clin Psychol. 1983 Jun; 51(3):390–5.

[441] Hollis JF, Gullion CM, Stevens VJ, Brantley PJ, Appel LJ, Ard JD, et al. Weight loss during the intensive intervention phase of the weight-loss maintenance trial. Am J Prev Med. 2008 Aug; 35(2):118-26.

[442] Kong A, Beresford SA, Imayama I, Duggan C, Alfano CM, Foster-Schubert KE, et al. Adoption of diet-related self-monitoring behaviors varies by race/ethnicity, education, and baseline binge eating score among overweight-to-obese postmenopausal women in a 12-month dietary weight loss intervention. Nutr Res. 2012 Apr; 32(4):260-5.

[443] Burke LE, Wang J, Sevick MA. Self-monitoring in weight loss: a systematic review of the literature. J Am Diet Assoc. 2011 Jan; 111(1):92-102.

[444] Kong A, Beresford SA, Alfano CM, Foster-Schubert KE, Neuhouser ML, Johnson DB, et al. Self-monitoring and eating-related behaviors are associated with 12-month weight loss in postmenopausal overweight-to-obese women. J Acad Nutr Diet. 2012 Sep; 112(9):1428-35.

36715795R00236

Made in the USA
Middletown, DE
17 February 2019